Perioperative Anesthetic Care of the Obese Patient

Perioperative Anesthetic Care of the Obese Patient

Edited by

Vilma E. Ortiz
Massachusetts General Hospital
Boston, Massachusetts, USA

Jeanine Wiener-Kronish
Massachusetts General Hospital
Boston, Massachusetts, USA

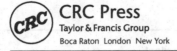

CRC Press
Taylor & Francis Group
Boca Raton London New York

CRC Press is an imprint of the
Taylor & Francis Group, an **informa** business

Cover illustration source: Nguyen, NT and Wolfe, BM. The Physiologic effects of Pneumoperitoneum in the morbidly obese. Annals of Surgery. Feb 2005; 241 (2): 219-226. Used with permission from Wolters Kluwer Health.

CRC Press
Taylor & Francis Group
6000 Broken Sound Parkway NW, Suite 300
Boca Raton, FL 33487-2742

First issued in paperback 2019

© 2010 by Taylor & Francis Group, LLC
CRC Press is an imprint of Taylor & Francis Group, an Informa business

No claim to original U.S. Government works

ISBN-13: 978-1-4200-9530-2 (hbk)
ISBN-13: 978-0-367-38510-1 (pbk)

Library of Congress Cataloging-in-Publication Data

Perioperative anesthetic care of the obese patient / edited by
Vilma E. Ortiz, Jeanine Wiener-Kronish.
    p. ; cm.
    Includes bibliographical references and index.
    ISBN-13: 978-1-4200-9530-2 (hardcover : alk. paper)
    ISBN-10: 1-4200-9530-7 (hardcover : alk. paper) 1. Anesthesia. 2. Obesity—
Complications. 3. Overweight persons—Surgery. I. Ortiz, Vilma E. (Vilma Enid),
II. Wiener-Kronish, Jeanine P., 1951-.
    [DNLM: 1. Anesthesia. 2. Surgical Procedures, Operative. 3. Obesity. 4.
Perioperative Care. WO 200 P445 2009]
    RD87.3.O23P47 2009
    617.9′6743—dc22

                                                                    2009025805

Visit the Taylor & Francis Web site at
http://www.taylorandfrancis.com

and the CRC Press Web site at
http://www.crcpress.com

Preface

The prevalence of obesity in the United States and worldwide is increasing at a worrisome rate. The World Health Organization (WHO) projects that by 2015 approximately 2.3 billion adults will be overweight [body mass index (BMI) ≥ 25] and more than 700 million will be obese (BMI ≥ 30). Some chronic conditions associated with obesity include peripheral vascular disease, liver disease, polycythemia, cardiorespiratory derangements, and diabetes. More and more frequently, obese and severely obese patients are seen in the operating room for procedures ranging from elective to emergency surgery. Perioperative healthcare providers are faced with the challenge of caring for this complex patient population while ensuring their safety. The issues facing the anesthesiologist are myriad: increase in co-morbidities, potential for airway complications, and postoperative adverse events. An understanding of the associated co-morbidities will impact the perioperative anesthetic approach as well as the postoperative management of these patients.

This handbook is divided into four sections: preoperative assessment, intraoperative management, postoperative care, and special situations. The discussion within the preoperative assessment section is divided into the main areas of concern, including cardiac, pulmonary, renal, gastrointestinal, and endocrine systems. Additionally, preoperative and psychological evaluations are discussed. The following section on intraoperative management will continue the in-depth discussion to the next stage of care with thorough coverage of drug administration, airway management, monitoring issues, intraoperative challenges, and bariatric surgery. Postoperative care provides the clinician with the information needed for optimal patient recovery, and as the increase in obesity affects all age groups, the last heading covers the perioperative concerns in the obese parturient, the obese trauma patient as well as in the obese child/adolescent. The information contained herein is meant to complement knowledge gained from the study of textbook and journal articles on the subject.

With the goal of optimizing medical care and improving patient safety, the handbook of *Perioperative Anesthetic Care of the Obese Patient* provides an efficient way for the healthcare provider to obtain clear, updated information in a format that is concise and easy to access. It is designed to be a valuable tool for practicing anesthesiologists and will also be of great use to anesthesia residents, medical and surgical residents, medical students, nurse anesthetists, and nurses caring for this patient population in the United States and abroad. As an easy to carry resource, it will make the information available where the clinician needs it most: the preoperative evaluation area, the clinic, the operating room, and the recovery room.

Vilma E. Ortiz
Jeanine Wiener-Kronish

Contents

Contributors

Aalok V. Agarwala MD MBA   Instructor in Anesthesia, Harvard Medical School, Assistant in Anesthesia, Department of Anesthesia and Critical Care, Massachusetts General Hospital, Boston, Massachusetts, U.S.A.

Meredith A. Albrecht MD PhD   Instructor in Anesthesia, Harvard Medical School, Assistant in Anesthesia, Department of Anesthesia and Critical Care, Massachusetts General Hospital, Boston, Massachusetts, U.S.A.

Ronald F. Albrecht II MD   Associate Professor of Anesthesia, University of Illinois at Chicago College of Medicine, Chief of Anesthesia, Jesse Brown Veteran's Administration Medical Center, Chicago, Illinois, U.S.A.

William J. Benedetto MD   Instructor in Anesthesia, Harvard Medical School, Assistant in Anesthesia, Department of Anesthesia and Critical Care, Massachusetts General Hospital, Boston, Massachusetts, U.S.A.

Lorenzo Berra MD   Clinical Fellow in Anesthesia, Harvard Medical School, Resident, Department of Anesthesia and Critical Care, Massachusetts General Hospital, Boston, Massachusetts, U.S.A.

Edward A. Bittner MD PhD   Instructor in Anesthesia, Harvard Medical School, Assistant in Anesthesia and Intensivist, Department of Anesthesia and Critical Care, Massachusetts General Hospital, Boston, Massachusetts, U.S.A.

Roland Brusseau MD   Instructor, Harvard Medical School, Assistant in Anesthesia, Department of Anesthesiology, Perioperative and Pain Medicine, Children's Hospital Boston, Boston, Massachusetts, U.S.A.

Tim Canty MD   Instructor in Anesthesia, Harvard Medical School, Assistant in Anesthesia, Department of Anesthesia and Critical Care, Massachusetts General Hospital, Boston, Massachusetts, U.S.A.

Jonathan E. Charnin MD   Instructor in Anesthesia, Harvard Medical School, Assistant in Anesthesia, Department of Anesthesia and Critical Care, Massachusetts General Hospital, Boston, Massachusetts, U.S.A.

Hovig V. Chitilian MD   Instructor in Anesthesia, Harvard Medical School, Assistant in Anesthesia, Department of Anesthesia and Critical Care, Massachusetts General Hospital, Boston, Massachusetts, U.S.A.

Marc de Moya MD   Assistant Professor of Surgery, Division of Trauma, Emergency Surgery, and Surgical Critical Care, Massachusetts General Hospital, Boston, Massachusetts, U.S.A.

Matthias Eikermann MD PhD   Assistant Professor of Anesthesia, University Duisburg-Essen, Essen, Germany, Assistant in Anesthesia, Department of Anesthesia and Critical Care, Massachusetts General Hospital, Boston, Massachusetts, U.S.A.

Gregory Ginsburg MD   Instructor in Anesthesia, Harvard Medical School, Assistant in Anesthesia, Department of Anesthesia and Critical Care, Massachusetts General Hospital, Boston, Massachusetts, U.S.A.

Mark A. Hoeft MD   Clinical Fellow in Anesthesia, Harvard Medical School, Resident, Department of Anesthesia and Critical Care, Massachusetts General Hospital, Boston, Massachusetts, U.S.A.

Fawsi S. Khayat MD   Minimally Invasive Surgery Fellow, Harvard Medical School, Department of Surgery, Massachusetts General Hospital, Boston, Massachusetts, U.S.A.

William R. Kimball MD PhD   Assistant Professor of Anesthesia and Critical Care, Harvard Medical School, Associate Anesthetist, Department of Anesthesia and Critical Care, Massachusetts General Hospital, Boston, Massachusetts, U.S.A.

Jean Kwo MD   Assistant Professor of Anesthesia, Harvard Medical School, Assistant Anesthetist, Department of Anesthesia and Critical Care, Massachusetts General Hospital, Boston, Massachusetts, U.S.A.

Vilma E. Ortiz MD   Assistant Professor in Anesthesia, Harvard Medical School, Department of Anesthesia and Critical Care, Associate Anesthetist, Massachusetts General Hospital, Boston, Massachusetts, U.S.A.

Heather A. Panaro MD   Clinical Fellow in Anesthesia, Harvard Medical School, Resident, Department of Anesthesia and Critical Care, Massachusetts General Hospital, Boston, Massachusetts, U.S.A.

Janey S. A. Pratt MD FACS   Instructor in Surgery, Harvard Medical School, Assistant Surgeon, Department of Surgery, Massachusetts General Hospital, Boston, Massachusetts, U.S.A.

Shubha V. Y. Raju MBBS MHS   Clinical Fellow in Anesthesia, Harvard Medical School, Resident, Department of Anesthesia and Critical Care, Massachusetts General Hospital, Boston, Massachusetts, U.S.A.

Heena P. Santry MD   Fellow and Assistant in Surgery, Division of Trauma, Emergency Surgery, and Surgical Critical Care, Massachusetts General Hospital, Boston, Massachusetts, U.S.A.

Torin D. Shear MD   Instructor in Anesthesia, Harvard Medical School, Assistant in Anesthesia, Department of Anesthesia and Critical Care, Massachusetts General Hospital, Boston, Massachusetts, U.S.A.

Stephanie Sogg PhD   Staff Psychologist, MGH Weight Center, Boston, Massachusetts, U.S.A.

John L. Walsh MD   Assistant Professor of Anesthesia, Harvard Medical School, Assistant Anesthetist, Department of Anesthesia and Critical Care, Massachusetts General Hospital, Boston, Massachusetts, U.S.A.

Nicholas C. Watson MD   Fellow in Critical Care Anesthesiology, Harvard Medical School, Department of Anesthesia and Critical Care, Massachusetts General Hospital, Boston, Massachusetts, U.S.A.

1 | Cardiovascular Effects of Obesity

Meredith A. Albrecht[1] and Ronald F. Albrecht[2] II

[1]Instructor in Anesthesia, Harvard Medical School, Assistant in Anesthesia, Department of Anesthesia and Critical Care, Massachusetts General Hospital, Boston, Massachusetts, U.S.A.

[2]Associate Professor of Anesthesia, University of Illinois at Chicago College of Medicine, Chief of Anesthesia, Jesse Brown Veteran's Administration Medical Center, Chicago, Illinois, U.S.A.

INTRODUCTION

Obesity dramatically alters the cardiovascular system in several ways that can lead to persistent and escalating dysfunction. Obesity can cause both specific hemodynamic changes that are deleterious to myocardial function as well as demonstrable structural alterations in the heart. It is also associated with several pathologic disease states. Significant increases in morbidity are directly related to a patient's overweight body habitus and can have a profound impact on both quality of life as well as life expectancy. Weight loss can reduce many of these changes.

PATHOPHYSIOLOGICAL EFFECTS OF OBESITY ON THE CARDIOVASCULAR SYSTEM

Hemodynamic Changes

Obesity leads to a constant state of cardiovascular stress, much akin to persistent exercise. Excessive fat accumulation results in a relatively hyperdynamic circulation due to an increase in blood volume, arteriovenous oxygen difference, and oxygen consumption. Cardiac output is elevated due to an increase in oxygen demand. This increase in cardiac output is accomplished mainly through a larger stroke volume which, in time, leads to left ventricular hypertrophy (LVH) and left ventricular (LV) dilatation. One may also see an increase in both pulmonary arterial pressure and as well as pulmonary vascular resistance (1–3). Conversely, obesity results in lower total peripheral and renal vascular resistances (4). Even though obesity increases sympathetic outflow, renin, and aldosterone levels and enhances sodium retention, the obese patient's total peripheral resistance is demonstrably decreased. Messerli has shown that in normotensive, obese patients there is a reduction in systemic vascular resistance (SVR), especially in the splanchnic vascular bed (4–6), supporting this counter-intuitive finding.

Structural Changes

Post mortem Studies

Post-mortem studies of obese subjects by Carpenter et al. demonstrate the frequent presence of excess epicardial fat. While some post-mortem studies of the obese also demonstrate fatty infiltration of the myocardium, similar infiltration can be seen in autopsy studies of lean individuals. This is an incidental finding and consists of epicardial fat cords infiltrating atrophic muscle. More ominously, however, in patients with coronary artery disease, islands of fat are surrounded by fibrosis in the myocardium (2,7). Other autopsy findings commonly seen in obese subjects are LVH and LV dilatation. Right ventricular hypertrophy (RVH) and left atrial hypertrophy are less common findings (8,9).

Echocardiographic Studies
Echocardiographic studies in severely obese patients by Alpert et al., demonstrate LV dilation, increased LV wall thickness, increased LV mass or LVH, left atrial enlargement, and right ventricular (RV) enlargement. LVH is almost always present in symptomatic obese patients (10). The Lauer group studied a large cohort of patients enrolled in the Framingham Study and determined how these changes occurred with increasing body mass index (BMI). A significant positive correlation was observed between LV mass and increasing BMI (11,12). It has also been shown by Nakajima et al. that those who were obese for greater than 15 years were more likely to have LV dilation (13).

Functional Changes
Left Ventricular Diastolic Function
The presence of LVH is associated with reduced LV compliance. The stiffened LV, in association with obesity-induced increases in blood volume and high cardiac output state, results in a high LV filling pressure (2,14). LV filling pressure is known to correlate with BMI, especially in severe obesity (15). Non-invasive measures of LV diastolic filling (or relaxation) are significantly more impaired in obese than in lean patients (16–18). Diastolic relaxation is impaired whether or not there is concomitant hypertension (HTN). Furthermore, the degree of diastolic dysfunction is increased if congestive heart failure (CHF) is present. A transient increase in the cardiac output due to the increased demand dictated by exercise or stress causes an increase in the LV filling pressure that can lead to pulmonary edema or CHF (2). Diastolic dysfunction and increased LV filling pressures result in a decreased ability to perfuse an increased myocardial muscle mass in the patient with LVH, potentially leading to increases in ischemia.

Ventricular Systolic Function
Stoddard et al. compared LV systolic function (i.e., ejection fraction, fractional shortening, etc.) in obese and lean patients and demonstrated no changes in LV systolic function while Scaglione et al. showed decreased function in obese patients (2,17,19). Interpreted as a group, the overall trend from these studies is increasing LV loading conditions and worsening LV function as BMI increases. The longer the duration of obesity, the more pronounced the effect on LV function. However, while LV function is decreased in obesity, it is still in the normal range for the majority of patients (2). Unfortunately, very little information is currently available regarding RV function and obesity, but it is most likely normal unless the right ventricle is dilated (2).

Effects of HTN on Cardiovascular Function
LV dilation and secondary eccentric hypertrophy are sequelae of disease states characterized by volume overload (e.g., obesity). Conversely, isolated HTN is a pressure overload state which promotes concentric LVH. When both conditions are present there is a melding of the two remodeling strategies resulting in less dilation and less LVH than would occur with just one of these conditions at the same level of severity.

The obese hypertensive patient is at significant risk for cardiac dysfunction, including CHF. Despite having less LVH than a strict hypertensive patient, there is more total LV mass due to LV dilation, resulting in severe diastolic relaxation dysfunction (2,6).

Metabolic and Endocrine Effects of Obesity on the Cardiovascular System

Visceral obesity promotes a pro-inflammatory environment causing increased levels of resistin, free fatty acids, and interleukins. These mediators cause increased dyslipidemia and increased insulin resistance leading to a higher incidence of the metabolic syndrome and diabetes mellitus (DM) (20). Visceral adipose cells are not inert as previously believed. These cells release cytokines and adhesion molecules (such as tumor necrosis factor) which stimulate the production of interleukin-6, C-reactive protein, and other mediators resulting in increased atherogenic plaque formation and insulin resistance. A pro-inflammatory state is created with dyslipidemia as well as elevated glucose and insulin levels. This condition increases oxidative stress, endothelial dysfunction, and further plaque formation. A pro-thrombotic milieu is also correlated with increasing BMI (20–22).

Anesthetic Implications

Obese patients have an increased incidence of LVH and derangement of diastolic relaxation. Some also have impaired systolic function. These patients are particularly sensitive to changes in preload and afterload. Patients should be carefully evaluated for the presence of CHF preoperatively as changes in intravascular fluid status during the surgical procedure could easily impair heart function (2). In addition, alterations in patient position can affect shifts in intravascular volume. Both Tsueda and Paul demonstrated that suddenly placing severely obese individuals supine can lead to cardiac collapse. This presumably results from acute right heart failure precipitated by abrupt volume overloading, increased myocardial oxygen demand, and resultant ischemia (23,24).

COMMON COMORBIDITIES OF OBESITY AND THEIR EFFECTS ON THE CARDIOVASCULAR SYSTEM

Mortality and Obesity

Cardiovascular disease is still the leading cause of morbidity and mortality in the world. Obesity is associated with an increased risk of all cause and cardiovascular mortality, that is, a 2 to 3× greater risk for a BMI > 35 kg/m² compared with normal BMI (18.5–24.9 kg/m²) (25). It is not completely clear if obesity is an independent predictor of cardiovascular risk or if the comorbid conditions associated with obesity are confounding variables. However, Calle et al. used the participants in the Framingham Heart Study to identify obesity as an independent risk factor for death from cardiovascular causes (26). In addition, a recent analysis of the CRUSADE registry by Madala et al. demonstrated that a BMI > 40 kg/m² was associated with a patient's first non-ST-segment elevation myocardial infarction occurring 12 years prematurely compared to normal controls after adjustment for other risk factors (27).

While calculating the BMI is generally relatively easy, it is a poor predictor of mortality risk. This is because it does not take into account the relative components of an individual's weight (muscle vs. adipose, etc.) An assessment of adiposity such as waist circumference (measured halfway between the last rib and the iliac crest) or waist-hip ratio is generally a better predictor of mortality (28). It was recently shown in a meta-analysis by de Koning et al. that a 1 cm increase in waist circumference was associated with a 2% increase in the relative risk of a cardiovascular event (29).

Obesity Paradox

Being overweight or obese increases the risk of acquiring HTN, DM, and coronary artery disease (CAD). Interestingly, however, the overweight/obese patient who suffers from a chronic disease has a lower mortality than a patient with the same disease who is not overweight/obese. For example, Curtis et al. demonstrated that mortality in heart failure patients decreases with an increasing BMI (30). McAuley et al. studied obese veterans without heart failure. These patients had a 22% decrease in all cause mortality versus the non-obese. If the data were adjusted for cardiopulmonary fitness level, the obese patients had a 35% lower mortality (31). Uretsky et al. recently examined all causes of mortality in the INVEST cohort of patients with HTN and CAD, most of whom were studied over an average of 2.7 years. Obese patients (BMI 30–35 kg/m²) had the most reduced risk of death, myocardial infarction or stroke with a hazard ratio of 0.68 (32). Researchers frequently describe a U-shaped curve where overweight (BMI 25–29.9 kg/m²) or obese (BMI 30–35 kg/m²) patients have the lowest risk of mortality and the underweight (BMI < 18.5 kg/m²) and severely obese (BMI > 35 kg/m²) have an increased risk. The mechanism for increased survival in obese patients is unclear. Importantly, these data focus on mortality and it may well be that obese patients live longer but are less free from disability.

Coronary Artery Disease

Obesity is an independent risk factor for the development of CAD, especially if insulin resistance, dyslipidemia, and HTN are present. Peiris et al. have found that abdominal and visceral fat are particularly correlated with an increased incidence of CAD (33). This risk of CAD is proportional to the duration of obesity. However, not all obese patients have significant CAD. In fact >40% of obese patients with angina do not have significant CAD. The angina is caused by an oxygen supply/demand imbalance from cardiac hypertrophy (LVH) (34,35).

Hypertension

Obesity is strongly related to hypertensive disease. With the Framingham Heart Study, Garrison et al. demonstrated that the vast majority of HTN was due to excess weight in young adults (aged 20–49 years) (36). El-Atat el al. showed a linear relationship between BMI and both systolic and diastolic blood pressure (37). Engeli's group found that obesity causes sympathetic stimulation and activates the renin–angiotensin–aldosterone system (38,39). The upregulated renin–angiotensin–aldosterone axis causes sodium retention and increased extracellular volume, leading to HTN (40). Fortunately, weight loss is very successful in reducing the obese patient's systemic blood pressure. A meta-analysis by He and Whelton demonstrated that decreasing systolic blood pressure by more than 10 mm Hg reduced the risk of cardiovascular mortality by 25% (41). Obese, hypertensive patients incur an increase in both sympathetic outflow as well as in the renin–angiotensin system due to increased levels of leptin, a modulatory molecule secreted by adipose cells (42). Recent changes in national guidelines suggest a much lower target acceptable blood pressure (<120/80 mm Hg) for the general population. To date, there have been no randomized control trials to help select the best medications for treatment of HTN in the obese. Beta blockers are commonly used to decrease cardiovascular morbidity and mortality in patients with a history of ischemic heart disease and heart failure. They also can decrease the high sympathetic tone often present in obesity. The long term effects of treatment with beta blockers have not been specifically studied in the obese. Beta-blockers do promote weight gain (range, 0.4–3.5 kg), most likely due to a resultant decrease in metabolic rate. They also have adverse effects on lipid metabolism and often increase insulin resistance which predisposes patients to the development of DM. Accordingly, Pischon and Sharma do not recommend beta blockers as first line agents in the treatment of the uncomplicated HTN of obesity (43). In contrast, angiotensin-converting enzyme inhibitors or angiotensin-receptor blockers lower blood pressure and also delay the onset of diabetes and heart failure. They have also been shown to reduce insulin resistance (43–46).

Dyslipidemia

An increase in cholesterol levels is one of the most predictive indicators of coronary risk in obesity. Increasing BMI is correlated with an increase in triglycerides (TG) and low density lipoprotein (LDL), small, dense particles which are associated with increased production of plaques. Levels of high density lipoprotein (HDL) are lower in the obese. This lipid pattern is worsened if DM, the metabolic syndrome, or poor nutritional status is present (20,47,48). Treatment of these lipid derangements is associated with reduction in both cardiovascular events and mortality. Successful therapy may lead to a decrease in systemic inflammation, improvement of endothelial function, and stabilization (as well as possible reduction) of atherosclerotic plaques, ameliorating the risk of adverse cardiac events and death (49). For example, statin use is very effective in the reduction of LDL and TG and increasing HDL. Fibrates are effective in reducing TG levels and increasing HDL levels. Fibrates are particularly effective in patients with insulin resistance, such as patients with metabolic syndrome or DM (20,50).

Diastolic Dysfunction or Obesity-Related Cardiomyopathy

After adjusting for cardiovascular disease, HTN, and LVH, obesity is an independent risk factor for developing heart failure. After adjusting for other risk factors in the Framingham study, Kenchaiah et al. demonstrated a doubling of the risk of developing heart failure in obese (BMI > 30 kg/m^2) versus lean patients (51). In this study, obesity increased the risk of developing both systolic and diastolic heart failure (51). Cardiomyopathy (CM) is seen primarily in the morbidly obese. The mechanism for developing heart failure is unclear but is likely due to the physiological stress of the increased body mass, hyperdynamic circulation, and comorbid conditions, especially obstructive sleep apnea. To compensate for these changes and an increased cardiac output, the heart develops LVH and LV dilation. The resulting impaired relaxation can lead to diastolic dysfunction. The combination of LVH, impaired diastolic filling, and a high cardiac output state causes increased LV filling pressures and can result in diastolic LV failure. If the LV wall stress continues to increase, LV systolic failure can also occur (14).

A direct effect of obesity on the myocardium has also been implicated in the development of CHF, specifically the direct infiltration of lipids in the muscle and vasculature which escalates with increasing body mass (52). One theory suggests that excessive body fat predisposes an individual to elevated levels of free fatty acids and triglycerides in the circulation and the myocardium. These new fat deposits release hormones and inflammatory mediators that aggravate CAD. Byproducts also lead to cellular death causing left ventricular remodeling and diastolic dysfunction resulting in an obesity-specific dilated non-ischemic CM. The presence of LV failure by either of these mechanisms leads to a further increase in pulmonary arterial pressure which, if high enough, can lead to RVH and/or failure. Obesity CM is always associated with LV failure. If isolated RV failure is present it is generally due to pulmonary pathology. Obesity CM, a dilated CM, can also be arrhythmogenic (20). CHF from obesity CM is treated similarly to CHF from any other etiology.

Atrial Fibrillation

Obesity has been associated with a two to five times increase in the risk of stroke compared to non-obese individuals as shown by Go et al. (53). Perhaps related, Wang et al. demonstrated an increased incidence of atrial fibrillation in the obese using the Framingham study (adjusted hazard ratios of 1.52 for men and 1.46 for women) (54). Larger cohort studies by Frost et al. have also shown an increased risk of atrial fibrillation in obesity (55). Not surprisingly, Pritchett et al. found that increasing BMI is associated with increasing left atrial diameter, a known predictor of atrial fibrillation (56). Left atrial enlargement in obesity could be explained by elevated plasma volume, HTN, LVH, diastolic dysfunction, increased sympathetic tone, and/or obstructive sleep apnea (20).

EFFECTS OF WEIGHT LOSS ON THE CARDIOVASCULAR SYSTEM
Mortality

Weight loss offers the best long-term solution for improvement/resolution of the various coexisting diseases of obesity. It also offers substantial mortality reduction (2,20).

Effects on Hemodynamics, Morphology, and Function

Many of the hemodynamics changes induced by obesity can be reversed by weight loss. Weight loss causes a decrease in circulating blood volume, oxygen consumption, arteriovenous oxygen difference, cardiac output, and stroke volume. SVR often returns to normal. RV and LV filling pressures do not normalize due to the extensive remodeling of the heart. However, Alexander's group found a more robust increase in cardiac output with exercise after weight loss (2,57). As shown by Alpert et al., when obese patients with LVH lose a substantial amount of weight following bariatric surgery, the LV chamber size and wall thickness decrease. Most likely the improvement in cardiovascular loading conditions, i.e., decreased LV filling pressures, results in the regression of LVH over time (58). In addition, Alpert et al. found that LV systolic function can improve in the severely obese with substantial weight loss, probably secondary to reduction in body mass (2,59).

Effects on Patients with Obesity CM
Alpert et al. also showed that weight loss is followed by a decrease in the severity of a patient's CHF symptoms as demonstrated by an improvement in the New York Heart Association functional class. A reduction in BMI can not only reverse the deleterious hemodynamic changes incurred with obesity but may also result in a regression of the myocardial remodeling that has occurred (2,60).

Effects of Weight Loss Drugs
1. *Orlistat (Alli™, Xenical™)* is an inhibitor of gastric and pancreatic lipases that reduces the absorption of dietary fats by up to 30%. It is associated with no significant cardiac effects (61).
2. *Sibutramine (Meridia™)* works by blocking the neuronal uptake of norepinephrine, serotonin, and (to a lesser extent) dopamine. It can be associated with tachycardia, vasodilation, and HTN. It has also been associated with primary pulmonary HTN if the patient is on another agent with serotonergic activity (62).
3. *Rimonabant* is not approved in the United States but is used internationally for weight loss. It is an endocannabinoid receptor antagonist (63).
4. *Diethylpropion* is a sympathomimetic amine with properties similar to amphetamines. It reduces appetite by stimulation of the hypothalamus to release norepinephrine. It has been associated with arrhythmias, HTN, pulmonary HTN, tachycardia, and regurgitant cardiac valvular disease (64).
5. *Phentermine (Adipex-P™, Fastin™, Ionamin™)* is a sympathomimetic amine which has similar properties to amphetamines, reducing appetite by stimulation of the hypothalamus to release norepinephrine. It has been associated with HTN, primary pulmonary HTN (especially if also given with fenfluramine or dexfenfluramine), regurgitant cardiac valvular disease, and tachycardia (65).
6. *Fenfluramine (Pondimin™)* a sympathomimetic amine that promotes the release of serotonin and blocks its neuronal uptake. This increase in serotonin decreases appetite. It is no longer clinically used in the United States (66).
7. *Dexfenfluramine (Redux™)* is a dextroisomer of fenfluramine and its activity is due to serotonergic pathways in the brain. It is no longer clinically available in the United States (66).
8. *Combination therapy of fenfluramine (or dexfenfluramine) and phentermine (fen-phen)* is highly associated with regurgitant valvular disease (67,68). The mechanism is believed to be due to increased amounts of serotonin which stimulate fibroblast growth and fibrogenesis, possibly causing plaque formation on the valves and thickening of valve leaflets. The resultant aortic and mitral regurgitation are similar to the cardiac lesions of carcinoid heart disease (69). These valvular derangements may also be due to drug-mediated effects of the serotonin-2B receptor present on heart valves (70). All bariatric patients should be asked if they have ever received combination therapy.
9. *Ephedra/ephedrine supplements* have been associated with significant cardiovascular risks and adverse events documented in several case reports, including cerebral vascular accident (CVA). This subset of weight reduction drugs has been shown by Shekelle et al. to increase heart rate, blood pressure, and incidence of palpitations (71). However, Hallas et al. in a recent case-control study in Denmark found that there was no significant increase in death, myocardial infarction, or CVA in chronic users of caffeine/ephedrine supplements compared to new users (72).

REFERENCES

1. Alexander JK. Obesity and cardiac performance. Am J Cardiol 1964; 14: 860–5.
2. Alpert MA. Cardiac morphology and ventricular function. In: Alvarez AO, Brodsky JB, Alpert MA, Cowan GSM, eds. Morbid Obesity: Peri-operative Management. Cambridge: Cambridge University Press, 2004: 59–68.
3. Messerli FH, Sundgaard-Riise K, Reisin ED, et al. Dimorphic cardiac adaptation to obesity and arterial hypertension. Ann Intern Med 1983; 99: 757–61.
4. Messerli FH. Cardiovascular effects of obesity and hypertension. Lancet 1982; 1: 1165–8.
5. Rocchini AP. Hemodynamic and cardiac consequences of childhood obesity. Ann N Y Acad Sci 1993; 699: 46–56.
6. Messerli FH, Sundgaard-Riise K, Reisin E, et al. Disparate cardiovascular effects of obesity and arterial hypertension. Am J Med 1983; 74: 808–12.
7. Carpenter HM. Myocardial fat infiltration. Am Heart J 1962; 63: 491–6.
8. Amad KH, Brennan JC, Alexander JK. The cardiac pathology of chronic exogenous obesity. Circulation 1965; 32: 740–5.
9. Warnes CA, Roberts WC. The heart in massive (more than 300 pounds or 136 kilograms) obesity: analysis of 12 patients studied at necropsy. Am J Cardiol 1984; 54: 1087–91.
10. Alpert MA, Terry BE, Kelly DL. Effect of weight loss on cardiac chamber size, wall thickness and left ventricular function in morbid obesity. Am J Cardiol 1985; 55: 783–6.
11. Lauer MS, Anderson KM, Kannel WB, et al. The impact of obesity on left ventricular mass and geometry. The Framingham Heart Study. JAMA 1991; 266: 231–6.
12. Lauer MS, Anderson KM, Levy D. Separate and joint influences of obesity and mild hypertension on left ventricular mass and geometry: the Framingham Heart Study. J Am Coll Cardiol 1992; 19: 130–4.
13. Nakajima T, Fujioka S, Tokunaga K, et al. Noninvasive study of left ventricular performance in obese patients: influence of duration of obesity. Circulation 1985; 71: 481–6.
14. Alpert MA. Obesity cardiomyopathy: pathophysiology and evolution of the clinical syndrome. Am J Med Sci 2001; 321: 225–36.
15. de Divitiis O, Fazio S, Petitto M, et al. Obesity and cardiac function. Circulation 1981; 64: 477–82.
16. Chakko S, Mayor M, Allison MD, et al. Abnormal left ventricular diastolic filling in eccentric left ventricular hypertrophy of obesity. Am J Cardiol 1991; 68: 95–8.
17. Stoddard MF, Tseuda K, Thomas M, et al. The influence of obesity on left ventricular filling and systolic function. Am Heart J 1992; 124: 694–9.
18. Mureddu GF, de Simone G, Greco R, et al. Left ventricular filling pattern in uncomplicated obesity. Am J Cardiol 1996; 77: 509–14.
19. Scaglione R, Dichiara MA, Indovina A, et al. Left ventricular diastolic and systolic function in normotensive obese subjects: influence of degree and duration of obesity. Eur Heart J 1992; 13: 738–42.
20. Zalesin KC, Franklin BA, Miller WM, et al. Impact of obesity on cardiovascular disease. Endocrinol Metab Clin North Am 2008; 37: 663–84, ix.
21. Lefebvre AM, Laville M, Vega N, et al. Depot-specific differences in adipose tissue gene expression in lean and obese subjects. Diabetes 1998; 47: 98–103.
22. Rosito GA, D'Agostino RB, Massaro J, et al. Association between obesity and a prothrombotic state: the Framingham Offspring Study. Thromb Haemost 2004; 91: 683–9.
23. Paul DR, Hoyt JL, Boutros AR. Cardiovascular and respiratory changes in response to change of posture in the very obese. Anesthesiology 1976; 45: 73–8.
24. Tsueda K, Debrand M, Zeok SS, et al. Obesity supine death syndrome: reports of two morbidly obese patients. Anesth Analg 1979; 58: 345–7.

25. Calle EE, Thun MJ, Petrelli JM, et al. Body-mass index and mortality in a prospective cohort of U.S. adults. N Engl J Med 1999; 341: 1097–105.
26. Hubert HB, Feinleib M, McNamara PM, et al. Obesity as an independent risk factor for cardiovascular disease: a 26-year follow-up of participants in the Framingham Heart Study. Circulation 1983; 67: 968–77.
27. Madala MC, Franklin BA, Chen AY, et al. Obesity and age of first non-ST-segment elevation myocardial infarction. J Am Coll Cardiol 2008; 52: 979–85.
28. Visscher TL, Seidell JC, Molarius A, et al. A comparison of body mass index, waist-hip ratio and waist circumference as predictors of all-cause mortality among the elderly: the Rotterdam study. Int J Obes Relat Metab Disord 2001; 25: 1730–5.
29. de Koning L, Merchant AT, Pogue J, et al. Waist circumference and waist-to-hip ratio as predictors of cardiovascular events: meta-regression analysis of prospective studies. Eur Heart J 2007; 28: 850–6.
30. Curtis JP, Selter JG, Wang Y, et al. The obesity paradox: body mass index and outcomes in patients with heart failure. Arch Intern Med 2005; 165: 55–61.
31. McAuley P, Myers J, Abella J, et al. Body mass, fitness and survival in veteran patients: another obesity paradox? Am J Med 2007; 120: 518–24.
32. Uretsky S, Messerli FH, Bangalore S, et al. Obesity paradox in patients with hypertension and coronary artery disease. Am J Med 2007; 120: 863–70.
33. Peiris AN, Sothmann MS, Hoffmann RG, et al. Adiposity, fat distribution, and cardiovascular risk. Ann Intern Med 1989; 110: 867–72.
34. Adams JP, Murphy PG. Obesity in anaesthesia and intensive care. Br J Anaesth 2000; 85: 91–108.
35. McNulty PH, Ettinger SM, Field JM, et al. Cardiac catheterization in morbidly obese patients. Catheter Cardiovasc Interv 2002; 56: 174–7.
36. Garrison RJ, Kannel WB, Stokes J 3rd, et al. Incidence and precursors of hypertension in young adults: the Framingham Offspring Study. Prev Med 1987; 16: 235–51.
37. El-Atat F, Aneja A, McFarlane S, et al. Obesity and hypertension. Endocrinol Metab Clin North Am 2003; 32: 823–54.
38. Engeli S, Sharma AM. Emerging concepts in the pathophysiology and treatment of obesity-associated hypertension. Curr Opin Cardiol 2002; 17: 355–9.
39. Engeli S, Sharma AM. The renin-angiotensin system and natriuretic peptides in obesity-associated hypertension. J Mol Med 2001; 79: 21–9.
40. Hall JE, Hildebrandt DA, Kuo J. Obesity hypertension: role of leptin and sympathetic nervous system. Am J Hypertens 2001; 14: 103S–115S.
41. He J, Whelton PK. Elevated systolic blood pressure and risk of cardiovascular and renal disease: overview of evidence from observational epidemiologic studies and randomized controlled trials. Am Heart J 1999; 138: 211–19.
42. Vasan RS, Larson MG, Leip EP, et al. Assessment of frequency of progression to hypertension in non-hypertensive participants in the Framingham Heart Study: a cohort study. Lancet 2001; 358: 1682–6.
43. Pischon T, Sharma AM. Use of beta-blockers in obesity hypertension: potential role of weight gain. Obes Rev 2001; 2: 275–80.
44. Sharma AM, Pischon T, Engeli S, et al. Choice of drug treatment for obesity-related hypertension: where is the evidence? J Hypertens 2001; 19: 667–74.
45. Effects of ramipril on cardiovascular and microvascular outcomes in people with diabetes mellitus: results of the HOPE study and MICRO-HOPE substudy. Heart Outcomes Prevention Evaluation Study Investigators. Lancet 2000; 355: 253–9.
46. Yusuf S, Sleight P, Pogue J, et al. Effects of an angiotensin-converting-enzyme inhibitor, ramipril, on cardiovascular events in high-risk patients. The Heart Outcomes Prevention Evaluation Study Investigators. N Engl J Med 2000; 342: 145–53.
47. Garber AM, Avins AL. Triglyceride concentration and coronary heart disease. BMJ 1994; 309: 1440–1.

48.   Austin MA, King MC, Vranizan KM, et al. Atherogenic lipoprotein phenotype. A proposed genetic marker for coronary heart disease risk. Circulation 1990; 82: 495–506.
49.   Grundy SM, Cleeman JI, Merz CN, et al. Implications of recent clinical trials for the National Cholesterol Education Program Adult Treatment Panel III guidelines. Circulation 2004; 110: 227–39.
50.   Keech A, Simes RJ, Barter P, et al. Effects of long-term fenofibrate therapy on cardiovascular events in 9795 people with type 2 diabetes mellitus (the FIELD study): randomised controlled trial. Lancet 2005; 366: 1849–61.
51.   Kenchaiah S, Evans JC, Levy D, et al. Obesity and the risk of heart failure. N Engl J Med 2002; 347: 305–13.
52.   Malavazos AE, Ermetici F, Coman C, et al. Influence of epicardial adipose tissue and adipocytokine levels on cardiac abnormalities in visceral obesity. Int J Cardiol 2007; 121: 132–4.
53.   Go AS, Hylek EM, Phillips KA, et al. Prevalence of diagnosed atrial fibrillation in adults: national implications for rhythm management and stroke prevention: the AnTicoagulation and Risk Factors in Atrial Fibrillation (ATRIA) Study. JAMA 2001; 285: 2370–5.
54.   Wang TJ, Parise H, Levy D, et al. Obesity and the risk of new-onset atrial fibrillation. JAMA 2004; 292: 2471–7.
55.   Frost L, Hune LJ, Vestergaard P. Overweight and obesity as risk factors for atrial fibrillation or flutter: the Danish Diet, Cancer, and Health Study. Am J Med 2005; 118: 489–95.
56.   Pritchett AM, Jacobsen SJ, Mahoney DW, et al. Left atrial volume as an index of left atrial size: a population-based study. J Am Coll Cardiol 2003; 41: 1036–43.
57.   Alexander JK, Peterson KL. Cardiovascular effects of weight reduction. Circulation 1972; 45: 310–18.
58.   Alpert MA, Lambert CR, Terry BE, et al. Effect of weight loss on left ventricular mass in nonhypertensive morbidly obese patients. Am J Cardiol 1994; 73: 918–21.
59.   Alpert MA, Terry BE, Lambert CR, et al. Factors influencing left ventricular systolic function in nonhypertensive morbidly obese patients, and effect of weight loss induced by gastroplasty. Am J Cardiol 1993; 71: 733–7.
60.   Alpert MA, Terry BE, Mulekar M, et al. Cardiac morphology and left ventricular function in normotensive morbidly obese patients with and without congestive heart failure, and effect of weight loss. Am J Cardiol 1997; 80: 736–40.
61.   Orlistat: drug information. [Accessed January 2009, from: http://www.utdol.com/online/content/topic.do?topicKey=drug_l_z/58480&selectedTitle=1~37&source=search_result]
62.   Sibutramine: drug information. [Accessed January 2009, from: http://www.utdol.com/online/content/topic.do?topicKey=drug_l_z/16297&selectedTitle=1~99&source=search_result]
63.   Rimonabant: International drug information. [Accessed January 2009, from: http://www.utdol.com/online/content/topic.do?topicKey=int_drug/62385&selectedTitle=1~9&source=search_result]
64.   Diethylpropion: drug information. [Accessed January 2009, from: http://www.utdol.com/online/content/topic.do?topicKey=drug_a_k/79496&selectedTitle=1~5&source=search_result]
65.   Phentermine: drug information. [Accessed January 2009, from: http://www.utdol.com/online/content/topic.do?topicKey=drug_l_z/198514&selectedTitle=1~10&source=search_result]
66.   Valvular heart disease induced by drugs. *UpToDate*, 2008. [Accessed January 2009, from: http://www.utdol.com/online/content/topic.do?topicKey=valve_hd/14218&selectedTitle=1~18&source=search_result]
67.   Connolly HM, Crary JL, McGoon MD, et al. Valvular heart disease associated with fenfluramine-phentermine. N Engl J Med 1997; 337: 581–8.
68.   Graham DJ, Green L. Further cases of valvular heart disease associated with fenfluramine-phentermine. N Engl J Med 1997; 337: 635.

69. Pellikka PA, Tajik AJ, Khandheria BK, et al. Carcinoid heart disease. Clinical and echocardiographic spectrum in 74 patients. Circulation 1993; 87: 1188–96.
70. Rothman RB, Baumann MH, Savage JE, et al. Evidence for possible involvement of 5-HT(2B) receptors in the cardiac valvulopathy associated with fenfluramine and other serotonergic medications. Circulation 2000; 102: 2836–41.
71. Shekelle PG, Hardy ML, Morton SC, et al. Efficacy and safety of ephedra and ephedrine for weight loss and athletic performance: a meta-analysis. JAMA 2003; 289: 1537–45.
72. Hallas J, Bjerrum L, Stovring H, et al. Use of a prescribed ephedrine/caffeine combination and the risk of serious cardiovascular events: a registry-based case-crossover study. Am J Epidemiol 2008; 168: 966–73.

2 | Respiratory Concerns in the Obese Patient

Matthias Eikermann

Assistant Professor of Anesthesia, University Duisburg-Essen, Essen, Germany, Assistant in Anesthesia, Department of Anesthesia and Critical Care, Massachusetts General Hospital, Boston, Massachusetts, U.S.A.

INTRODUCTION

There is substantial evidence to suggest that obesity is associated with an increased incidence of perioperative complications (1–6) such as wound infections and break-down (3), venous thromboembolism (4), adverse cardiac events (5), and respiratory complications (7,6). The mechanisms by which obesity may increase the incidence of perioperative respiratory complications have not yet been completely elucidated. Obese patients breathe rapidly and shallowly, and 80% of morbidly obese middle-aged subjects report shortness of breath while climbing two flights of stairs (8). Obese patients also have a higher incidence of difficult mask ventilation, airway obstruction, major oxygen desaturation, and overall critical respiratory adverse events (2,9). This chapter aims to provide some insight into the mechanisms by which obesity may affect the upper airway and pulmonary function. Obesity can alter respiratory physiology by two main mechanisms: effects of excessive tissue on upper airway and pulmonary function, and effects of obesity on neurologic control of upper airway dilator and respiratory muscles.

Even a modest increase in body weight substantially worsens exercise performance against gravity, such as climbing stairs (10). Weight loss in morbidly obese patients often results in a marked improvement in their clinical state and in their arterial blood gas tensions (11,12). In addition, excess tissue in the oropharyngeal airway is a main mechanism of obstructive sleep apnea (OSA) (13,14). Surgical removal may lead to an improvement of sleep apnea symptoms in some patients (15).

The direct effects of excess tissue do not explain the entire respiratory pathology observed in the obese. Alveolar hypoventilation develops in some obese individuals and the correlation between the degree of obesity and the extent of hypoventilation is poor (16). Control of breathing is influenced by a variety of factors that might be more important than body weight: age, sex, body size, changes in physical characteristics, metabolic rate, acid-base status, high altitude residence, and smoking habits (17,18). Most patients with obesity hypoventilation syndrome can hyperventilate when requested and normalize then their arterial carbon dioxide tension (19). Thus, the mechanical disadvantage of obesity alone does not provide an adequate explanation for hypoventilation in these patients. It has, therefore, been hypothesized that alveolar hypoventilation is a consequence of an obesity induced impairment of ventilatory drive (16). Several studies have shown that patients with obesity hypopnea syndrome have significantly reduced hypoxic and hypercapnic ventilatory drives compared with normal subjects (20,21).

EFFECTS OF OBESITY ON PULMONARY FUNCTION

Pulmonary function is determined by the interaction of the lungs, chest wall, and respiratory muscles. Obesity influences lung function through its effect on the chest wall and the respiratory muscles. In general, the mechanical properties of the lungs are normal but the compliance of the chest wall is reduced (22). The most persistent abnormality is a restrictive respiratory impairment (17,23). Although the volume restriction is mild, vital capacity (VC) in obese patients is inversely related to body mass index (BMI) (24). However, in non-obese individuals VC increases with BMI. Consequently, in large populations the relation of VC and BMI shows an initial increase. Morbidly obese patients typically have a reduced tidal volume, which seems to be primarily the result of a reduction in inspiratory time rather than a reduction in respiratory drive (25).

• Respiratory Muscles and Pulmonary Workload

Cherniack and colleagues (22) have shown inefficient respiratory muscle contractions in obese individuals. Other data show that maximal inspiratory (PI_{max}) and expiratory (PE_{max}) pressures are lower than that predicted in obese individuals (26). These findings may result from either reduced chest wall compliance or lower lung volume at which ventilation takes place. It is also possible that obesity impairs respiratory muscle function. Respiratory muscles become fatigued when an imbalance occurs between energy supply and energy demand. The percentage of cardiac output and total body oxygen consumption dedicated to respiratory muscle work during quiet breathing (VO_2Resp) is very small (<3%) in non-obese subjects (27,28). Some data suggest that morbidly obese patients dedicate a disproportionately high percentage of total VO_2 to conduct respiratory work, even during quiet breathing (29). Severe obesity in humans constitutes a load on the respiratory muscles that changes their force–length characteristics (30). The diaphragm's volume-generating function is reduced as well (31). After weight loss surgery, respiratory muscle endurance and, to a lesser degree, muscle strength increases (32).

Functional Residual Capacity

Obesity results in decreased functional residual capacity (FRC) due to diminution of expiratory reserve volume (ERV) (17). The decrease in ERV is often so marked that FRC approaches residual volume. In consequence, ventilation in the lung bases is reduced, especially in those with the smallest ERV, leading to arterial hypoxemia (33).

Recent studies evaluated the effects of weight-loss surgery on ERV and FRC. Weiner and coworkers showed that a decrease in BMI of 10 kg/m^2 was paralleled by an increase of FRC and ERV of approximately 10%, suggesting a cause-effect relationship between obesity and impairment of lung volumes. The effects of obesity on FRC are particularly important in the perioperative period. Neuromuscular blockade and anesthesia decrease FRC in obese and non-obese patients, but the magnitude of the decrease seems to be greater in obese patients than in patients of normal weight (34).

Asthma

It is unclear if obesity is an independent risk factor for asthma (35). A meta-analysis of seven prospective epidemiological studies in which BMI was self-reported showed that the incidence of asthma increased by 50% in overweight/obese individuals. There was a dose-response relationship between body weight and asthma, with no significant gender disparity (36). However, it has also been suggested that this may be because obesity decreases lung volumes and increases airway resistance, leading to symptoms that could mimic asthma (37). It is less controversial that obesity increases the prevalence, incidence, and severity of asthma, whereas

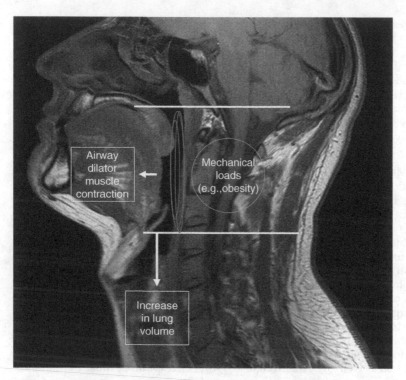

Figure 1 Upper airway patency depends on the balance between collapsing forces (circles) that put a mechanical load to the upper airway (e.g., obesity), and the dilating forces (arrows), i.e., neuromuscular responses that activate the upper airway dilator muscles, and increases in lung volume. Increasing upper airway collapsibility induces nocturnal symptoms of increasing severity ranging from mild snoring to complete apnea.

weight loss in obese individuals improves asthma outcomes (38). Long-term steroids increase appetite and may lead to weight gain which may worsen already established asthma (39).

UPPER AIRWAY FUNCTION
Upper Airway Anatomy in the Obese
The tendency for the upper airway to collapse during sleep is related to the balance between dilating forces and collapsing forces (Fig. 1). Airway anatomy influences pharyngeal patency. In obese patients, an increased amount of pharyngeal soft tissue renders the upper airway prone to collapse (13,40). In non-obese individuals, when muscle activity is completely inhibited (e.g., during complete neuromuscular blockade), the airway generally remains patent and requires about –5 cm H_2O to collapse (41). In obese patients airway patency is challenged by increased pharyngeal soft tissue (42), such that positive pressure [e.g., continuous positive airway pressure (CPAP)] may be required to keep the upper airway open (43).

Sleep Apnea
OSA is a common disorder with a prevalence linked to the obesity epidemic in Western society (44). In patients with OSA, the upper airway collapses at higher

pharyngeal pressures, usually expressed as a less negative critical upper airway closing pressure (P_{crit}). The mechanism for this increased upper airway collapsibility has both an anatomic and a physiologic basis (Fig. 1).

Clinical Presentation

OSA is characterized by repetitive collapse of the upper airway during sleep. Episodic hypoxaemia, hypercapnia, large negative intrathoracic pressure swings (to −120 mm Hg), surges in systemic blood pressure associated with arousals from sleep, and sleep fragmentation characterize the condition. Loud snoring is a typical feature of OSA and in most cases the culmination of a respiratory event is associated with a brief awakening from sleep (arousal). During apneic or hypopneic episodes, the reduction of airflow often leads to acute impairments in gas exchange and recurrent arousals from sleep. The health consequences of sleep apnea are numerous. If left untreated, it leads to excessive daytime sleepiness, cognitive dysfunction, impaired work performance, and decrements in health-related quality of life (45).

Epidemiology

OSA is a common chronic disease in Western society with a prevalence estimated at 2% of women and 4% of men in the general population (46). Several risk factors, including obesity, male sex, age (47), and heritable factors, have been associated with this increased prevalence (46). Among these, obesity is the strongest (48,49). Mild-to-moderate obesity has been associated with markedly increased risk of sleep apnea (46). In severe obesity (BMI > 40 kg/m²), the prevalence of sleep apnea was estimated to vary between 40% and 90% (50), and the severity of sleep apnea was generally greater than that found in leaner clinical populations (50,51).

Genetic factors seemingly play a role in the pathogenesis of OSA. After accounting for socioeconomic status, age, geographic region, and period of diagnosis, men with at least one sibling with OSA have a markedly higher incidence of OSA (52).

Pathophysiology

The pathophysiological causes of OSA vary considerably between individuals. Important components include upper airway anatomy, the ability of the upper airway dilator muscles to respond to respiratory challenge during sleep, the propensity to wake from increased respiratory drive during sleep (arousal threshold), the stability of the respiratory control system (loop gain), and the potential for state-related changes in lung volume to influence these factors. Of these, obesity explains 30% to 50% of the variance in apnea–hypopnea (AHI) and is the only variable that can be modified (53).

Upper airway muscle function. Pharyngeal muscles may be activated during inspiration (phasic pattern) with less activity during expiration (54) or have a similar level of activity across the respiratory cycle (tonic pattern). The genioglossus, an inspiratory phasic muscle, is the best studied such muscle. There are three primary neural inputs controlling the genioglossus muscle:

1. Mechanoreceptors located mainly in the larynx, leading to increased hypoglossal output to the genioglossal muscle in response to negative pressure (55,56)
2. The respiratory pattern generating neurons in the medulla that activate the genioglossus muscle about 50 to 100 msec before diaphragmatic activation (57)
3. Brainstem arousal promoting neurons mediating the "wakefulness stimulus" (58)

With these three inputs, pharyngeal muscle activity is linked to respiration, local conditions in the airway (negative pressure), and arousal state (wake vs. sleep). In patients with OSA, the genioglossus muscle has significantly more activity in both inspiration and expiration compared to control subjects (59). With the onset of sleep, the control of these muscles changes. The negative-pressure reflex is substantially reduced during non-REM sleep and is further decreased during rapid eye movement (REM) sleep (60,61). The "wakeful" input to these muscles is diminished during sleep as well (62), rendering the airway vulnerable during sleep.

Role of ventilatory instability in OSA.   While a small (narrow lumen) upper airway increases the risk of collapse, other mechanisms, such as ventilatory control instability, might further increase the risk. This is because the upper airway muscles, like the diaphragm, are linked to ventilatory control. An increase in ventilatory drive activates the upper airway muscles and promotes patency (63), whereas a decrease in ventilatory drive relaxes the upper airway muscles and facilitates closure (64). Consequently, fluctuations in ventilatory drive (due to ventilatory control instability) can lead to upper airway instability and potentially collapse at the nadir of ventilatory drive (65). It has recently been shown in patients with OSA that the ventilatory variability index and AHI are strongly correlated (66).

Changes in lung volume.   Changes in lung volume can also influence pharyngeal patency. Lung inflation applies caudal traction on the trachea and larynx, thereby inducing a longitudinal tension on the pharyngeal airway (67). Because of the redistribution of tissue at higher lung volumes, tissue pressure may change as well. This caudal force tends to stiffen the airway and reduces collapsibility. This has been convincingly demonstrated in animals and in humans (67,68). Thus, decrements in lung volume, which occur as a consequence of obesity, changes in posture (upright to supine) and transitions from wakefulness to sleep result in less tension on the airway walls (69), a condition that promotes airway collapse.

Diagnosis

A detailed clinical assessment forms an important part of the evaluation of patients suspected of having OSA. When interviewing a patient with suspected OSA, it is highly desirable to interview the partner, who can usually provide important additional information based on direct observation of the patient's sleeping habits (70). The partner's input is valuable in the identification of apnea episodes, and may also provide a different perspective on the patient's daytime symptoms such as sleepiness and cognitive function. It is common for the patient to report a lesser degree of functional impairment than that observed by the partner.

Nocturnal symptoms.   Snoring is the main symptom of sleep apnea as it reflects the basic pathophysiology underlying the disorder, namely a critical narrowing of the upper airway (71). In population surveys, 25% of men and 15% of women are habitual snorers. The prevalence of snoring increases progressively with age; reports indicate that 60% of men and 40% of women between the ages of 41 and 65 years habitually snore (46). Snoring is the most frequent symptom of OSAS, occurring in up to 95% of patients, but has poor predictive value because of the high prevalence in the general population (72). Witnessed apneas are a good diagnostic predictor of OSAS but do not predict severity of the disorder (73).

Daytime symptoms.   Although sleep apnea is the most common cause of excessive daytime sleepiness, it has not been found useful as a clinical feature to discriminate between patients with and without the disorder. Between 30% and 50% of the general population reports significant sleepiness (46,49), but the severity of daytime sleepiness and sleep apnea do not correlate very well (74). This may reflect the fact that many other sleep disorders also cause daytime sleepiness. A patient's report of a brief episode of sleeping while driving might be more specific for the diagnosis OSA.

Anatomic factors that predispose to upper airway narrowing should be sought in the physical examination of a patient suspected of having OSA. These include: retrognathia, micrognathia, tonsillar hypertrophy, macroglossia, and inferior displacement of the hyoid. However, the most common physical finding in patients with OSA is a nonspecific narrowing of the oropharyngeal airway, with or without an increase in soft tissue deposition (73). Accordingly, it is not a surprise that the Mallampati score has been reported to be a good predictor of OSA (75). Obesity is common in OSA, particularly upper body obesity. Neck circumference is a strong predictor of OSA (76), and values <37 cm and >48 cm are associated with a low and high risk, respectively. Recently, the STOP questionnaire, consisting of four yes/no questions related to snoring, tiredness during daytime, observed apnea, and high blood pressure, has been validated against the AHI obtained from monitored polysomnography (77). Combined with BMI, age, neck size, and gender, it had a high sensitivity, especially for patients with moderate to severe OSA (77).

Treatment

Since the original description of CPAP treatment by Sullivan and coworkers (78) in 1983, positive airway pressure (PAP) remains the mainstay of treatment for moderate-to-severe OSA in adults (79). Positive airway pressure treatment is considered the treatment of choice in patients with moderate-to-severe OSA usually defined as AHI ≥ 15/hr. Since the introduction of CPAP as a treatment of OSA, additional modes of pressure delivery have been developed (bilevel PAP, autoadjusting PAP, flexible PAP). The downside of positive airway pressure therapy is the insufficient compliance with its use, amounting to approximately 50% of ideal use (6). Therefore, surgical treatment is considered a second line treatment for this condition. Current definition of surgical success is a greater than 50% reduction of the AHI and/or an AHI of <20 events per hour (80).

The goal of nasal reconstructive surgery is to improve nasal airway blockage caused by bony, cartilaginous, or hypertrophied tissues in order to restore normal breathing and optimize nasal CPAP use. Uvulopalatopharyngoplasty aims to enlarge the retropalatal airway by trimming and reorienting the posterior and anterior lateral pharyngeal pillars, and by excising the uvula and posterior portion of the palate. Mandibular osteotomy with genioglossus advancement addresses upper airway obstruction at the base of the tongue. The genioglossus muscle is attached to the lingual surface of the mandible at the geniotubercle and also to the hyoid complex just above the larynx. Movement forward of either or both of these anatomic structures will stabilize the tongue base along with the associated pharyngeal dilatators.

Paradoxically, recent data suggest that treatment with certain hypnotics may improve this condition (81–83). Arousal from sleep is traditionally believed to be an important mechanism for re-establishing airway patency in OSA. However, an excessively low arousal threshold may predispose an individual to recurrent arousals, and the hyperventilation that occurs during these episodes may produce hypocapnia during subsequent sleep (84). In such cases, CO_2 values below the apnea threshold will lead to either central or obstructive apnea, depending on the prevailing upper airway mechanics. Thus, a low arousal threshold may contribute to sleep apnea, at least in some individuals (84,85). In theory, hypnotics could improve breathing stability by raising the arousal threshold (82) and allowing respiratory stimuli to accumulate. This accumulation, in turn, may activate pharyngeal dilator muscles and improve airway mechanics. Sedatives have been shown to increase the arousal threshold in response to airway occlusion in normal subjects (86), and some clinicians have already used sedatives to treat unselected sleep apnea patients (81,82). Prospective controlled studies are required to evaluate if treatment with sleep promoting agents might be a viable treatment approach for patients with OSA.

Perioperative Concerns

Risk of perioperative complications. OSA may increase a patient's risk of developing perioperative complications. An association of sleep-disordered breathing with postoperative complications has recently been demonstrated in a prospective controlled study (87). The mechanisms by which OSA increases the patients' risk of perioperative complications have not yet been completely elucidated. During the first 24 hours after laparoscopic bariatric surgery in morbidly obese subjects, OSA does not seem to increase the risk of postoperative hypoxemia (88,89). Therefore, it might be possible that the increased risk of perioperative complications is due to a high vulnerability of their upper airway on the second or third postoperative day. These mechanisms include, but are not limited to, residual drug effects, positional changes required as a consequence of surgery, and perioperative changes in sleep architecture (Fig. 2).

General anesthetic agents (90–92), including propofol (93,94), isoflurane (92), and thiopentone (91) can predispose the upper airway to collapse, at least in part by decreasing upper airway muscle activity and impairing hypoxic and hypercapnic drive (90,91,93). Other data show that partial neuromuscular transmission failure, even to a degree that does not evoke dyspnea or oxygen desaturation, markedly decreases inspiratory upper airway volume and can evoke partial inspiratory airway collapse (95). Enhanced monitoring may be useful when patients with OSA are exposed to additional risk factors for development of neuromuscular transmission failure, for example, following anesthesia, or when given drugs known to enhance neuromuscular blockade (magnesium, certain antibiotics).

It has been shown that the lateral position structurally improves maintenance of the passive pharyngeal airway in patients with OSA. In the postoperative period, however, patients are frequently positioned supine which increases airway collapsibility (96). Severe changes in sleep architecture, such as reduced or lack of REM sleep and slow wave sleep (SWS), occur during the first three nights after major general surgery. A subsequent rebound of REM sleep and gradual increase in SWS occur on the third and fourth nights (97). The latter might put patients with OSA at risk for perioperative complications. Frequency and intensity of apneic episodes are markedly higher during REM compared with non-REM sleep.

Preoperative testing. Polysomnography remains the "gold standard" for diagnosing and treating OSA. However, restricted access, practical application, and cost may limit its utility in the preoperative setting. Anesthesiologists should work with surgeons to develop a protocol whereby patients in whom OSA is suspected on clinical grounds are evaluated long enough before the day of surgery to allow preparation of a perioperative management plan. This evaluation should be initiated in a pre-anesthesia clinic whenever possible. It may be useful to routinely include the use of a validated questionnaire [e.g., the STOP questionnaire (98)] in the preoperative workup algorithm. Polysomnography and a subsequent CPAP titration study should be considered in patients at high risk of OSA scheduled for major surgery. This strategy allows patients to receive CPAP treatment in the perioperative period, an approach which has been suggested to reduce perioperative complications (99).

Perioperative management. Preoperative evaluation of a patient for potential identification of OSA includes (i) medical record review, (ii) patient or family interview,

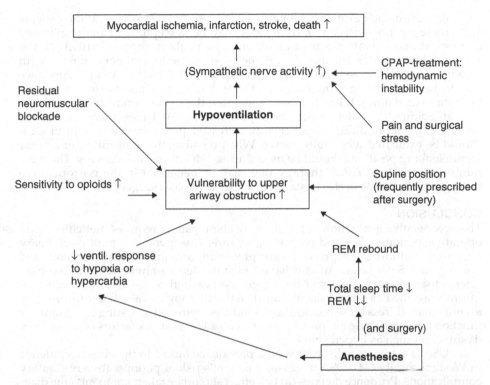

Figure 2 Possible mechanisms by which obstructive sleep apnea may induce an increased risk of develop perioperative respiratory complications. Drug effects (anesthetics, sedatives, opioids, and/or neuromuscular blocking agents), increased REM sleep (a "REM-rebound" occurs typically during the second or third postoperative night), as well as positional changes can increase the vulnerability of the upper airway to collapse, leading to hypoventilation and sympathetic nerve system activation during sleep. The sympathetic nervous system activation might be aggravated by inadequately treated pain and/or positive airway pressure treatment during hypovolemia. *Abbreviations*: CPAP, continuous positive airway pressure; REM, rapid eye movement.

(iii) physical examination, (iv) sleep studies, and (v) preoperative X-rays for cephalometric measurement in selected cases.

Optimally, the patient *and* family interview should include focused questions related to snoring, apneic episodes, frequent arousals during sleep (vocalization, shifting position, extremity movements), morning headaches, and daytime somnolence. A physical examination should include an evaluation of the airway, nasopharyngeal characteristics, neck circumference, tonsil, and tongue size. If any of these characteristics suggest that the patient has OSA, the anesthesiologist and surgeon should jointly decide whether to (i) manage the patient perioperatively based on clinical criteria alone, (ii) obtain sleep studies, (iii) conduct a more extensive airway examination, and (iv) initiate indicated OSA treatment in advance of surgery. If this evaluation does not occur until the day of surgery, the surgeon and anesthesiologist together may elect for presumptive management based on clinical criteria or a last-minute delay of surgery.

In certain high risk populations, such as patients scheduled for weight-loss surgery, routine screening polysomnography should be performed before surgery (100).

Because of their propensity for airway collapse and sleep deprivation, patients at increased perioperative risk from OSA may be susceptible to the respiratory depressant and airway effects of anesthetics, particularly propofol (101,102). For superficial procedures, the use of local anesthesia or peripheral nerve blocks, with or without moderate sedation is recommended (103). CPAP or an oral appliance should be used during monitored anesthesia care in patients previously treated with these modalities. It has also been suggested that major conduction anesthesia (spinal/epidural) be used for peripheral procedures (104). Unless there is a medical or surgical contraindication, patients at increased perioperative risk from OSA should be extubated when fully awake. When possible, the semi-sitting or reverse Trendelenburg positions should be used during extubation and recovery. There are numerous effects of CPAP therapy that may be beneficial in the postoperative setting, and it may be useful to start CPAP therapy before surgery (105).

CONCLUSION

The preoperative evaluation of the severely obese patient requires meticulous preoperative, perioperative, and postoperative care. This involves a multidisciplinary approach, including the primary care physician, anesthesiologist, surgeon, and nursing staff. Since obese patients have a high incidence of hypertension, coronary artery disease, esophageal and laryngopharyngeal reflux disease, and deep vein thrombosis, medical professionals must make thorough evaluations to properly identify and address these medical comorbidities. Spirometric testing of pulmonary function is recommended in obese patients with additional risk factors of pulmonary dysfunction such as hypercapnia.

OSA is a common disorder with a prevalence linked to the obesity epidemic in Western society (44). OSA increases a patient's risk of perioperative respiratory complications. Prudence dictates that all effort should be taken not to miss the diagnosis of OSA before starting the case. Diagnosis OSA in morbidly obese patients will influence the anesthesia plan, perioperative monitoring of respiratory function, as well as postoperative treatment.

REFERENCES

1. Jackson BM, English SJ, Fairman RM, et al. Carotid artery stenting: identification of risk factors for poor outcomes. J Vasc Surg 2008; 48: 74–9.
2. Tait AR, Voepel-Lewis T, Burke C, et al. Incidence and risk factors for perioperative adverse respiratory events in children who are obese. Anesthesiology 2008; 108: 375–80.
3. Gendall KA, Raniga S, Kennedy R, et al. The impact of obesity on outcome after major colorectal surgery. Dis Colon Rectum 2007; 50: 2223–37.
4. Kucher N, Tapson VF, Goldhaber SZ. Risk factors associated with symptomatic pulmonary embolism in a large cohort of deep vein thrombosis patients. Thromb Haemost 2005; 93: 494–8.
5. Bamgbade OA, Rutter TW, Nafiu OO, et al. Postoperative complications in obese and nonobese patients. World J Surg 2007; 31: 556–60; discussion 561.
6. Malhotra A, Hillman D. Obesity and the lung: 3. Obesity, respiration and intensive care. Thorax 2008; 63: 925–31.
7. Forrest JB, Rehder K, Cahalan MK, et al. Multicenter study of general anesthesia. III. Predictors of severe perioperative adverse outcomes. Anesthesiology 1992; 76: 3–15.
8. Sjostrom L, Larsson B, Backman L, et al. Swedish obese subjects (SOS). Recruitment for an intervention study and a selected description of the obese state. Int J Obes Relat Metab Disord 1992; 16: 465–79.
9. Shnaider I, Chung F. Outcomes in day surgery. Curr Opin Anaesthesiol 2006; 19: 622–9.

10. Swinburn CR, Cooper BG, Mould H, et al. Adverse effect of additional weight on exercise against gravity in patients with chronic obstructive airways disease. Thorax 1989; 44: 716–20.
11. Sugerman HJ, Fairman RP, Sood RK, et al. Long-term effects of gastric surgery for treating respiratory insufficiency of obesity. Am J Clin Nutr 1992; 55: 597S–601S.
12. Thomas PS, Cowen ER, Hulands G, et al. Respiratory function in the morbidly obese before and after weight loss. Thorax 1989; 44: 382–6.
13. Schwab RJ, Gupta KB, Gefter WB, et al. Upper airway and soft tissue anatomy in normal subjects and patients with sleep-disordered breathing. Significance of the lateral pharyngeal walls. Am J Respir Crit Care Med 1995; 152: 1673–89.
14. Schwab RJ, Pasirstein M, Kaplan L, et al. Family aggregation of upper airway soft tissue structures in normal subjects and patients with sleep apnea. Am J Respir Crit Care Med 2006; 173: 453–63.
15. Thawley SE. Surgical treatment of obstructive sleep apnea. Med Clin North Am 1985; 69: 1337–58.
16. Carroll D. A peculiar type of cardiopulmonary failure associated with obesity. Am J Med 1956; 21: 819–24.
17. Bedell GN, Wilson WR, Seebohm PM. Pulmonary function in obese persons. J Clin Invest 1958; 37: 1049–60.
18. Rochester DF, Enson Y. Current concepts in the pathogenesis of the obesity-hypoventilation syndrome. Mechanical and circulatory factors. Am J Med 1974; 57: 402–20.
19. Leech J, Onal E, Aronson R, et al. Voluntary hyperventilation in obesity hypoventilation. Chest 1991; 100: 1334–8.
20. Zwillich CW, Sutton FD, Pierson DJ, et al. Decreased hypoxic ventilatory drive in the obesity-hypoventilation syndrome. Am J Med 1975; 59: 343–8.
21. Pedersen J, Torp-Pedersen E. Ventilatory insufficiency in extreme obesity. Acta Med Scand 1960; 167: 343–52.
22. Naimark A, Cherniack RM. Compliance of the respiratory system and its components in health and obesity. J Appl Physiol 1960; 15: 377–82.
23. Luce JM. Respiratory complications of obesity. Chest 1980; 78: 626–31.
24. Lazarus R, Sparrow D, Weiss ST. Effects of obesity and fat distribution on ventilatory function: the normative aging study. Chest 1997; 111: 891–8.
25. Remmers JE, Marttila I. Action of intercostal muscle afferents on the respiratory rhythm of anesthetized cats. Respir Physiol 1975; 24: 31–41.
26. Wadstrom C, Muller-Suur R, Backman L. Influence of excessive weight loss on respiratory function. A study of obese patients following gastroplasty. Eur J Surg 1991; 157: 341–6.
27. Robertson CH Jr, Pagel MA, Johnson RL Jr. The distribution of blood flow, oxygen consumption, and work output among the respiratory muscles during unobstructed hyperventilation. J Clin Invest 1977; 59: 43–50.
28. Fritts HW Jr, Filler J, Fishman AP, et al. The efficiency of ventilation during voluntary hyperpnea: studies in normal subjects and in dyspneic patients with either chronic pulmonary emphysema or obesity. J Clin Invest 1959; 38: 1339–48.
29. Kress JP, Pohlman AS, Alverdy J, et al. The impact of morbid obesity on oxygen cost of breathing (VO(2RESP)) at rest. Am J Respir Crit Care Med 1999; 160: 883–6.
30. Sharp JT, Henry JP, Sweany SK, et al. Effects of mass loading the respiratory system in man. J Appl Physiol 1964; 19: 959–66.
31. Sampson MG, Grassino K. Neuromechanical properties in obese patients during carbon dioxide rebreathing. Am J Med 1983; 75: 81–90.
32. Weiner P, Waizman J, Weiner M, et al. Influence of excessive weight loss after gastroplasty for morbid obesity on respiratory muscle performance. Thorax 1998; 53: 39–42.
33. Holley HS, Milic-Emili J, Becklake MR, et al. Regional distribution of pulmonary ventilation and perfusion in obesity. J Clin Invest 1967; 46: 475–81.

34. Pelosi P, Croci M, Ravagnan I, et al. Total respiratory system, lung, and chest wall mechanics in sedated-paralyzed postoperative morbidly obese patients. Chest 1996; 109: 144–51.

35. McClean KM, Kee F, Young IS, et al. Obesity and the lung: 1. Epidemiology. Thorax 2008; 63: 649–54.

36. Beuther DA, Sutherland ER. Overweight, obesity, and incident asthma: a meta-analysis of prospective epidemiologic studies. Am J Respir Crit Care Med 2007; 175: 661–6.

37. Jones RL, Nzekwu MM. The effects of body mass index on lung volumes. Chest 2006; 130: 827–33.

38. Shore SA. Obesity and asthma: implications for treatment. Curr Opin Pulm Med 2007; 13: 56–62.

39. Leslie WS, Hankey CR, Lean ME. Weight gain as an adverse effect of some commonly prescribed drugs: a systematic review. QJM 2007; 100: 395–404.

40. Welch KC, Foster GD, Ritter CT, et al. A novel volumetric magnetic resonance imaging paradigm to study upper airway anatomy. Sleep 2002; 25: 532–42.

41. Isono S, Remmers JE, Tanaka A, et al. Anatomy of pharynx in patients with obstructive sleep apnea and in normal subjects. J Appl Physiol 1997; 82: 1319–26.

42. Watanabe T, Isono S, Tanaka A, et al. Contribution of body habitus and craniofacial characteristics to segmental closing pressures of the passive pharynx in patients with sleep-disordered breathing. Am J Respir Crit Care Med 2002; 165: 260–5.

43. Isono S, Isono S, Tanaka A, et al. Anatomy of pharynx in patients with sleep-disordered breathing. J Appl Physiol 2002; 82: 260–5.

44. Schwartz AR, Patil SP, Laffan AM, et al. Obesity and obstructive sleep apnea: pathogenic mechanisms and therapeutic approaches. Proc Am Thorac Soc 2008; 5: 185–92.

45. Punjabi NM. The epidemiology of adult obstructive sleep apnea. Proc Am Thorac Soc 2008; 5: 136–43.

46. Young T, Palta M, Dempsey J, et al. The occurrence of sleep-disordered breathing among middle-aged adults. N Engl J Med 1993; 328: 1230–5.

47. Eikermann M, Jordan AS, Chamberlin NL, et al. The influence of aging on pharyngeal collapsibility during sleep. Chest 2007; 131: 1702–9.

48. Shinohara E, Kihara S, Yamashita S, et al. Visceral fat accumulation as an important risk factor for obstructive sleep apnoea syndrome in obese subjects. J Intern Med 1997; 241: 11–18.

49. Young T, Peppard PE, Gottlieb DJ. Epidemiology of obstructive sleep apnea: a population health perspective. Am J Respir Crit Care Med 2002; 165: 1217–39.

50. Schwartz AR, Gold AR, Schubert N, et al. Effect of weight loss on upper airway collapsibility in obstructive sleep apnea. Am Rev Respir Dis 1991; 144: 494–8.

51. Peiser J, Lavie P, Ovnat A, et al. Sleep apnea syndrome in the morbidly obese as an indication for weight reduction surgery. Ann Surg 1984; 199: 112–15.

52. Sundquist J, Li X, Friberg D, et al. Obstructive sleep apnea syndrome in siblings: an 8-year Swedish follow-up study. Sleep 2008; 31: 817–23.

53. Dempsey JA, Skatrud JB, Jacques AJ, et al. Anatomic determinants of sleep-disordered breathing across the spectrum of clinical and nonclinical male subjects. Chest 2002; 122: 840–51.

54. Sauerland EK, Mitchell SP. Electromyographic activity of the human Genioglossus muscle in response to respiration and to positional changes of the head. Bull Los Angeles Neurol Soc 1970; 35: 69–73.

55. Chamberlin NL, Eikermann M, Fassbender P, et al. Genioglossus premotoneurons and the negative pressure reflex in rats. J Physiol 2007; 579: 515–26.

56. Horner RL, Innes JA, Holden HB, et al. Afferent pathway(s) for pharyngeal dilator reflex to negative pressure in man: a study using upper airway anaesthesia. J Physiol 1991; 436: 31–44.

57. van Lunteren E. Muscles of the pharynx: structural and contractile properties. Ear Nose Throat J 1993; 72: 27–9, 33.

58. Orem J. The nature of the wakefulness stimulus for breathing. Respir Physiol 2000; 119: 113–21.
59. Mezzanotte WS, Tangel DJ, White DP. Waking genioglossal electromyogram in sleep apnea patients versus normal controls (a neuromuscular compensatory mechanism). J Clin Invest 1992; 89: 1571–9.
60. Horner RL, Innes JA, Morrell MJ, et al. The effect of sleep on reflex genioglossus muscle activation by stimuli of negative airway pressure in humans. J Physiol 1994; 476: 141–51.
61. Wheatley JR, Tangel DJ, Mezzanotte WS, et al. Influence of sleep on response to negative airway pressure of tensor palatini muscle and retropalatal airway. J Appl Physiol 1993; 75: 2117–24.
62. Lo YL, Jordan AS, Malhotra A, et al. Influence of wakefulness on pharyngeal airway muscle activity. Thorax 2007; 62: 799–805.
63. Badr MS, Skatrud JB, Dempsey JA. Effect of chemoreceptor stimulation and inhibition on total pulmonary resistance in humans during NREM sleep. J Appl Physiol 1994; 76: 1682–92.
64. Badr MS, Toiber F, Skatrud JB, et al. Pharyngeal narrowing/occlusion during central sleep apnea. J Appl Physiol 1995; 78: 1806–15.
65. Warner G, Skatrud JB, Dempsey JA. Effect of hypoxia-induced periodic breathing on upper airway obstruction during sleep. J Appl Physiol 1987; 62: 2201–11.
66. Ibrahim LH, Patel SR, Modarres M, et al. A measure of ventilatory variability at wake-sleep transition predicts sleep apnea severity. Chest 2008; 134: 73–8.
67. Van de Graaff WB. Thoracic influence on upper airway patency. J Appl Physiol 1988; 65: 2124–31.
68. Stanchina ML, Malhotra A, Fogel RB, et al. The influence of lung volume on pharyngeal mechanics, collapsibility, and genioglossus muscle activation during sleep. Sleep 2003; 26: 851–6.
69. Ballard RD, Irvin CG, Martin RJ, et al. Influence of sleep on lung volume in asthmatic patients and normal subjects. J Appl Physiol 1990; 68: 2034–41.
70. Kingshott RN, Sime PJ, Engleman HM, et al. Self assessment of daytime sleepiness: patient versus partner. Thorax 1995; 50: 994–5.
71. Lugaresi E, Cirignotta F, Coccagna G, et al. Some epidemiological data on snoring and cardiocirculatory disturbances. Sleep 1980; 3: 221–4.
72. Gottlieb DJ, Yao Q, Redline S, et al. Does snoring predict sleepiness independently of apnea and hypopnea frequency? Am J Respir Crit Care Med 2000; 162: 1512–17.
73. Deegan PC, McNicholas WT. Predictive value of clinical features for the obstructive sleep apnoea syndrome. Eur Respir J 1996; 9: 117–24.
74. Doherty LS, Kiely JL, Swan V, et al. Long-term effects of nasal continuous positive airway pressure therapy on cardiovascular outcomes in sleep apnea syndrome. Chest 2005; 127: 2076–84.
75. Nuckton TJ, Glidden DV, Browner WS, et al. Physical examination: mallampati score as an independent predictor of obstructive sleep apnea. Sleep 2006, 29: 903–8.
76. Stradling JR, Crosby JH. Predictors and prevalence of obstructive sleep apnoea and snoring in 1001 middle aged men. Thorax 1991; 46: 85–90.
77. Chung F, Yegneswaran B, Liao P, et al. STOP questionnaire: a tool to screen patients for obstructive sleep apnea. Anesthesiology 2008; 108: 812–21.
78. Sullivan CE, Berthon-Jones M, Issa FG. Remission of severe obesity-hypoventilation syndrome after short-term treatment during sleep with nasal continuous positive airway pressure. Am Rev Respir Dis 1983; 128: 177–81.
79. Kakkar RK, Berry RB. Positive airway pressure treatment for obstructive sleep apnea. Chest 2007; 132: 1057–72.
80. Won CH, Li KK, Guilleminault C. Surgical treatment of obstructive sleep apnoea in adults. Bmj 2008; 5: 44–5.

81. Carley DW, Olopade C, Ruigt GS, et al. Efficacy of mirtazapine in obstructive sleep apnea syndrome. Sleep 2007; 30: 35–41.

82. Heinzer RC, White DP, Jordan AS, et al. Trazodone increases arousal threshold in obstructive sleep apnoea. Eur Respir J 2008; 31: 1308–12.

83. Younes M, Park E, Horner RL. Pentobarbital sedation increases genioglossus respiratory activity in sleeping rats. Sleep 2007; 30: 478–88.

84. Younes M. Role of arousals in the pathogenesis of obstructive sleep apnea. Am J Respir Crit Care Med 2004; 169: 623–33.

85. Wellman A, Malhotra A, Jordan AS, et al. Chemical control stability in the elderly. J Physiol 2007; 581: 291–8.

86. Berry RB, Kouchi K, Bower J, et al. Triazolam in patients with obstructive sleep apnea. Am J Respir Crit Care Med 1995; 151: 450–4.

87. Hwang D, Shakir N, Limann B, et al. Association of sleep-disordered breathing with postoperative complications. Chest 2008; 133: 1128–34.

88. Ahmad S, Nagle A, McCarthy RJ, et al. Postoperative hypoxemia in morbidly obese patients with and without obstructive sleep apnea undergoing laparoscopic bariatric surgery. Anesth Analg 2008; 107: 138–43.

89. Eikermann MKJ, Dennehy K, Ortiz V, et al. Is obstructive sleep apnea a risk factor for difficult airway anatomy and desaturation? Anesthesiology 2008; 109: A227.

90. Hwang JC, St John WM, Bartlett D Jr. Respiratory-related hypoglossal nerve activity: influence of anesthetics. J Appl Physiol 1983; 55: 785–92.

91. Drummond GB. Influence of thiopentone on upper airway muscles. Br J Anaesth 1989; 63: 12–21.

92. Eastwood PR, Szollosi I, Platt PR, et al. Collapsibility of the upper airway during anesthesia with isoflurane. Anesthesiology 2002; 97: 786–93.

93. Eastwood PR, Platt PR, Shepherd K, et al. Collapsibility of the upper airway at different concentrations of propofol anesthesia. Anesthesiology 2005; 103: 470–7.

94. Norton JR, Ward DS, Karan S, et al. Differences between midazolam and propofol sedation on upper airway collapsibility using dynamic negative airway pressure. Anesthesiology 2006; 104: 1155–64.

95. Eikermann M, Vogt FM, Herbstreit F, et al. The predisposition to inspiratory upper airway collapse during partial neuromuscular blockade. Am J Respir Crit Care Med 2007; 175: 9–15.

96. Isono S, Tanaka A, Nishino T. Lateral position decreases collapsibility of the passive pharynx in patients with obstructive sleep apnea. Anesthesiology 2002; 97: 780–5.

97. Knill RL, Moote CA, Skinner MI, et al. Anesthesia with abdominal surgery leads to intense REM sleep during the first postoperative week. Anesthesiology 1990; 73: 52–61.

98. Chung F, Yegneswaran B, Liao P, et al. Validation of the Berlin questionnaire and American Society of Anesthesiologists checklist as screening tools for obstructive sleep apnea in surgical patients. Anesthesiology 2008; 108: 822–30.

99. Gupta RM, Parvizi J, Hanssen AD, et al. Postoperative complications in patients with obstructive sleep apnea syndrome undergoing hip or knee replacement: a case-control study. Mayo Clin Proc 2001; 76: 897–905.

100. O'Keeffe T, Patterson EJ. Evidence supporting routine polysomnography before bariatric surgery. Obes Surg 2004; 14: 23–6.

101. Zgleszewski SE, Zurakowski D, Fontaine PJ, et al. Is propofol a safe alternative to pentobarbital for sedation during pediatric diagnostic CT? Radiology 2008; 247: 528–34.

102. Eikermann MFP, Malhotra A, Jordan AS, et al. Differential effects of isoflurane and propofol on genioglossus muscle function and breathing. Anesthesiology 2008; 108: 897–906.

103. Meoli AL, Rosen CL, Kristo D, et al. Upper airway management of the adult patient with obstructive sleep apnea in the perioperative period—avoiding complications. Sleep 2003; 26: 1060–5.

104. Gross JB, Bachenberg KL, Benumof JL, et al. Practice guidelines for the perioperative management of patients with obstructive sleep apnea: a report by the American Society of Anesthesiologists Task Force on Perioperative Management of Patients with Obstructive Sleep Apnea. Anesthesiology 2006; 104: 1081–93; quiz 1117–18.
105. Lin CC. Effect of nasal CPAP on ventilatory drive in normocapnic and hypercapnic patients with obstructive sleep apnoea syndrome. Eur Respir J 1994; 7: 2005–10.

3 | Renal Changes in Obesity

William J. Benedetto

Instructor in Anesthesia, Harvard Medical School, Assistant in Anesthesia, Department of Anesthesia and Critical Care, Massachusetts General Hospital, Boston, Massachusetts, U.S.A.

INTRODUCTION

Research into the renal effects of obesity is at a relatively early stage compared to some of the other consequences of increased body weight. Emerging data, however, suggests that the renal implications of obesity are likely to have significant consequences for affected patients and bear consideration by the health care community.

PHYSIOLOGICAL RENAL CHANGES IN OBESITY

Obesity is associated with an increase in glomerular filtration rate (GFR), renal blood flow (RBF), and sodium reabsorption as well as microalbuminemia, and possibly proteinuria.

Mechanical Effects of Obesity on the Kidney

In the obese patient baseline intra-abdominal pressures can be as high 30 to 40 mmHg (1). These elevated pressures are transmitted to the kidneys and renal vasculature. In addition, the kidneys are encapsulated in adipose tissue, and observations in obese animals have demonstrated extension of this adipose tissue into the renal hilum and medullary sinuses, further increasing intrarenal pressure (1). This probably leads to dilatation of (primarily) the afferent arteriole and results in increased RBF and GFR (2). It has also been suggested that the increased intrarenal pressure causes histological changes in the nephron that impair the interdigitation of foot processes leading to increased filtration fraction and pressure natriuresis (3). This mechanical effect may be supported by the observation that renal impairment is worse in subjects with central as opposed to peripheral fat distribution patterns (4).

Metabolic Demand

Though obesity is associated with an absolute increase in filtration, it has been suggested that much of the change may be an adaptive response to the increased metabolic demands of obesity (5). Although not consistently shown in all studies, the changes in GFR have been demonstrated to parallel increases in body surface area. The absolute GFR in a given individual is greater in the obese state, but may be proportionally appropriate (5).

Sympathetic Tone

It is difficult to fully separate obesity related renal changes from those attributed to hypertension. Leptin expression associated with obesity is a sympathetic nervous system stimulant (6). This heightened sympathetic tone is implicated in the increased sodium reabsorption. Furthermore, it contributes to the dilatation of the afferent arteriole which leads to increased filtration (6). In fact, renal denervation in experimental animals markedly reduced the degree of sodium retention (1).

Renin–Angiotensin–Aldosterone System (RAAS)
The RAAS is involved in the obesity related alterations to renal physiology as well as in the development of renal impairment. Adipose tissue not only produces all components of the RAAS (renin, angiotensin, and aldosterone), but it also expresses receptors for these substances, acting as a local target for angiotensin II (3). Angiotensin II stimulates proliferation of adipose tissue, further increasing production of the components of the RAAS. These products, known contributors to the development of hypertension, are now linked to the development of obesity related renal impairment (5). Angiotensin II causes constriction of the efferent arteriole leading to increased filtration and proteinuria. It is also implicated in direct glomerular structural changes (7) and tissue damaging pathways (5).

Hyperlipidemia
Abnormal lipid profiles are common in patients with advanced obesity. Lipid deposition in glomerular and mesangial cells has been detected on biopsy. Whether or not this lipid deposition actually causes pathogenic changes is unclear (5). Although a role for "lipotoxicity" (inflammation and fibrosis related to this lipid deposition) has been proposed, little correlation with obesity related renal failure has been demonstrated (5). Further study is partly confounded by gross lipid abnormalities in one of the primary animal models used to study this disease.

Insulin
Insulin and insulin resistance are hallmarks of obesity related disease. Most, if not all, of the cell types in the kidney that are responsible for reabsorption of sodium express an insulin receptor (8). As a result, it has been proposed that the hyperinsulinemic state associated with obesity may be at least partially responsible for the increased sodium reabsorption.

STRUCTURAL CHANGES IN THE KIDNEYS RELATED TO OBESITY
The changes in the structure of the kidneys may correlate with the physiological alterations. A study of structural changes in humans, however, is difficult to carry-out in a truly scientific design, and so most investigations in this area are limited to animal data.

Gross Changes
In a study of healthy experimental animals with obesity induced by a high fat diet, the kidneys were significantly heavier after a relatively short period of time (7). This increase in kidney weight was most probably related to changes in the histology of the nephron (3).

Histological Changes
Results from the same study revealed significant changes in the histology of the nephron. Diffuse cell proliferation was noted in the mesangial and capillary endothelial cells. Bowman's space was also found to be consistently expanded in the obese animals (7). In addition, the tubular and glomerular basement membranes were significantly thickened. Further investigations noted deposition of hyaluronate

and an increase in intra-renal lipids (3). Transforming growth factor-β1 was also relatively over-expressed in their kidneys.

Hormonal Changes
In experimental animals fed the high-fat diet described above, there was a significant change in kidney-associated hormones after 24 weeks on the diet. Their plasma insulin concentration was almost twice that of the lean animals, a change noticeable as early as seven weeks after the diet change. Additionally, angiotensin I levels were significantly increased by the 24 week mark (7).

CONDITIONS ASSOCIATED WITH OBESITY RELATED RENAL PATHOLOGY
The pathophysiological consequences of obesity extend beyond any one organ system. The alterations in renal pathology and physiology associated with increased body mass index (BMI) have significant implications for systemic diseases.

Hypertension
It is becoming increasingly clear that hypertension and obesity are inexorably linked. The mechanism of the link and the role of the kidney in this linkage, however, remain somewhat elusive. Healthy experimental animals fed a high fat diet reproducibly show an increase in mean arterial pressure (7). There are several factors related to renal changes in obesity that contribute to this hypertension.

Sympathetic Activation
Increases in body weight are associated with increasing sympathetic activity, with significant effects on renal physiology particularly in the effects on sodium handling (9). The satiety hormone leptin probably plays a major role in this sympathetic activation, but the exact mechanism remains elusive. In experimental animals, obesity related hypertension can be significantly reduced through combined α and β adrenergic blockade (3,9).

Renin–Angiotensin–Aldosterone System
As noted previously, adipose tissue can actively produce components of the RAAS and there is evidence of RAAS activation in experimental animals with diet-induced obesity. The effect of the RAAS on the kidney is to cause increased sodium retention resulting in systemic hypertension. RAAS stimulation may also have direct toxic effects on the kidney by increasing the susceptibility of the nephron to hypertension induced damage (9).

Structural and Anatomic Changes in Obesity
The kidney is almost completely contained within a non-compliant capsule. As the mass of adipose tissue encircling it increases, along with the size of the kidney itself, pressures within this organ will increase. This increased renal pressure results in impaired pressure natriuresis, the ability of the kidney to compensate for increased MAP by excreting sodium (9). The end result is persistent arterial hypertension.

Diabetes Mellitus and the Metabolic Syndrome
Diabetes mellitus is a well recognized risk factor for chronic kidney disease (CKD). In 1988, the metabolic syndrome was described, which included hypertriglyceridemia, low HDL-cholesterol levels, hypertension, high fasting blood glucose, and perhaps most importantly, abdominal hypertension (10). These two processes

often overlap in their manifestations, implications, and may provide a link between obesity and kidney disease. In 2004 Chen et al. (11) published a cross-sectional study that demonstrated a significant correlation between the metabolic syndrome and CKD. Though it has been difficult to identify a specific pathological correlation between diabetes mellitus/metabolic syndrome and CKD, the tight association suggests that one probably exists and that obesity almost certainly plays a prominent role.

Chronic Kidney Disease
Obesity is a major risk factor for both hypertension and diabetes (5). These two illnesses account for up to 70% of all instances of chronic renal disease (5). With this in mind, the question before the U.S. medical profession confronted with an expanding obesity epidemic remains: Is obesity an independent risk factor for kidney disease?

Obesity as a Risk Factor
Given the confounders of diabetes and hypertension, it is difficult to separate obesity as a risk factor. Furthermore, the mechanisms that link obesity, independently, to renal disease are still being elucidated (12). Evidence is now emerging that obesity contributes to worsening renal dysfunction in patients with pre-existing renal disease (13). In a study of 73 patients without pre-existing renal disease who underwent unilateral nephrectomy, Praga et al.(14) noted a significant increase in the risk of developing renal insufficiency in patients with BMI > 30. A similar correlation was noted in patients suffering from IgA nephropathy. Although the exact mechanism of the worsening renal function remains obscure, some authors suggest the following (13):

1. *Insulin resistance:* This is a common finding in obesity, and has been associated with glomerular hypertension as well as histological changes in the kidney.
2. *Leptin:* Though the systemic role of leptin is not fully understood, there is animal evidence that exposure to elevated levels of leptin can result in proteinuria and glomerulosclerosis.
3. *Inflammation:* Adipose tissue is thought to produce C-reactive protein (CRP) plus an array of pro-inflammatory cytokines resulting in an obesity-induced systemic inflammatory state. Higher CRP levels have been associated with an elevated relative risk for impaired glomerular function.

Focal Segmental Glomerulosclerosis (FSGS) in Obesity
In the early 1970s an association was reported between massive obesity and nephritic-range proteinuria (15). Further investigation into this phenomenon found an association between obesity and the development of kidney lesions characteristic of FSGS. In 2001, Kambham et al. (15) published a clinicopathological study (based on renal biopsies) investigating glomerulosclerosis and glomerulomegaly in obese patients. Though the lesions were similar to those noted in idiopathic forms of FSGS, there were significant differences both in the histopathology and in the clinical course of the disease (15).

Obesity-related glomerulosclerosis was associated with fewer lesions of segmental sclerosis, more glomerulomegaly, and less extensive foot process effacement. Clinically, these patients had a lower incidence of nephrotic range proteinuria, a higher average serum albumin, lower serum cholesterol, and less edema than those with idiopathic FSGS. In addition, the patients with obesity related glomerulosclerosis were less likely to progress to end-stage renal disease (ESRD). Though the histological analysis of biopsy specimens revealed changes associated with FSGS, most authors suggest that the glomerulosclerosis in obesity is a related, but separate, entity from idiopathic FSGS (5,15).

ESRD and Obesity

Although directly relating obesity to renal disease is a challenge, at the very least obesity may be seen as the primary *reversible* risk factor for CKD (16). Once CKD progresses to ESRD, the role of obesity may become more clear. In a landmark study by Hsu et al. in 2006 (17), a strong correlation was found between increasing BMI and risk of ESRD. In this study, even after controlling for diabetes and hypertension, there was a direct relationship between increasing BMI and relative risk of ESRD. Subjects with Class I, II, and III obesity were shown to have a relative risk of 2.98, 4.68, and 4.99 for ESRD, respectively. Although the study relied on data from health screening check ups (some values were self-reported) scattered across 40 years, it is difficult to deny the correlation. As the rate of obesity continues to increase, this correlation may be at least partially responsible for the increase in the prevalence of ESRD in the U.S. population (16). Interestingly, despite obesity's strong correlation with the development of ESRD, there is some suggestion that obesity may actually reduce mortality in patients with ESRD. In a study by Johansen et al. (18) in 2004, increasing BMI in dialysis patients was associated with reduced risk of death by as much as 20%. The authors propose that increased BMI shelters the patient from the inflammatory and catabolic effects of ESRD. Obesity's protective effect extended through severe obesity (BMI > 37 kg/m^2), and included all ethnic groups except Asians.

Obesity in Kidney Transplantation

Kidney transplantation is a viable alternative to dialysis for patients with ESRD. The role of transplantation in the obese patient, however, remains somewhat controversial. Recently published practice guidelines recommended that obese patients with ESRD reduce their BMI to <30 kg/m^2 prior to undergoing transplantation (19). Indeed, most (but not all) transplant centers will not offer a kidney transplant to patients with a BMI > 35 kg/m^2 (16). Given the difficulty of achieving this goal and the likely protective effect of higher BMI in patients who do not receive a transplant and remain on dialysis, the decision to recommend weight loss to an obese patient is a difficult one. There have been multiple investigations into the overall morbidity and mortality, as well as graft survival and complication rates, associated with obesity and kidney transplantation. Unfortunately, the data are conflicting and range from significant increases in complications, to no change whatsoever (20). Several recent studies have shown that the obese transplant recipient is likely to suffer a higher rate of relatively minor, generally wound-related complications, but no change in long term survival or graft function.

Obese Donors

As the shortage of cadaveric kidney donors continues, more pressure is put upon the pool of living kidney donors. In light of the increasing BMI of the U.S. population and the increasing interest in expanding the criteria for organ donation, the safety and efficacy of the obese donor is becoming increasingly important. In 1999, Pesavento et al. (21) compared the outcomes of a group of living kidney donors with a BMI > 27 kg/m^2 to a group with a BMI < 27 kg/m^2 and found no increase in the rate of major complications. Minor complications such as incisional hernia or superficial wound infection were more common in the obese group. It is important to note, however, that the average BMI of 31 kg/m^2 in the obese donor group was relatively low. Clearly, further study is required as the pressure to expand the organ supply increases. Longer-term studies will also be important as the role of obesity in CKD becomes more apparent.

PERIOPERATIVE RENAL CONSIDERATIONS IN OBESITY

Changes in renal function associated with obesity tend to have long term or subtle effects on the kidney. There is little current data or literature specifically targeting the perioperative considerations surrounding renal changes in obesity. However, a few points bear keeping in mind regarding the renal changes in the obese patient presenting for surgery.

Intra-abdominal Pressure

As discussed above, the obese patient suffers from chronically increased intra-abdominal pressure. Use of pneumoperitoneum is known to cause oliguria (22). The degree of this oliguria is probably directly related to the level of pressure utilized, and is presumably due to the consequent reduction in RBF as demonstrated in an animal model (22). In a 2002 study by Nguyen et al. (23), obese patients who underwent laparoscopic procedures lasting an average of 232 minutes reported significantly lower urine output compared to a matched group having open procedures. Of note, there was no significant difference in creatinine or BUN levels between the two groups. Antidiuretic hormone, aldosterone, and renin levels were also investigated and were not significantly changed. This suggests that though transient oliguria is common in the obese patient undergoing laparoscopic surgery, the effects are probably transient and do not effect long-term renal function.

Perioperative Pharmacokinetics

The effects of obesity on renal function and the resulting impact on drug handling in the perioperative patient are not well documented. Given the increased RBF and GFR, renal clearance of drugs would be expected to be increased in the obese patient (24). Furthermore, some authors suggest that many of the commonly used estimates of creatinine clearance do not agree well with measured values in the critically ill obese patient (25). Although no specific guidelines exist at this time, caution should be used in dosing medications for the obese patient.

WEIGHT LOSS AND ITS EFFECT ON THE RENAL CHANGES IN OBESITY

On the basis of well established clinical and experimental data, obesity causes changes in renal function that lead to increased glomerular filtration, increased RBF, and albuminuria. The association between these changes and the proposed effects on important patient outcomes—such as chronic renal disease and its progression to end-stage—remains elusive but is gaining greater acceptance in the medical community (26). This association naturally leads to the question: Are these changes reversible? Several studies (26,27) have demonstrated that significant weight loss, brought about through diet modification (but not strictly protein restriction), can ameliorate the changes in renal function (GFR, RBF, albuminuria). A more recent study demonstrated similar effects in patients with severe obesity who underwent weight loss surgery (28). Furthermore, this study demonstrated that the changes were durable and the improvement in albuminuria continued over a two-year follow-up. Although the link between improving renal outcomes and weight loss has yet to be firmly established in the literature, the reports of improvement in the renal changes associated with obesity suggests that at least some component of disease progression may be averted.

REFERENCES

1. Hall JE, Errol D, Jones DW, et al. Mechanisms of obesity-associated cardiovascular and renal disease. Am J Med Sci 2002; 324: 127–37.
2. Chagnac A, Weinstein T, Korzets A, et al. Glomerular hemodynamics in severe obesity. Am J Physiol Renal Physiol 2000; 278: F817–F822.
3. Engeli S, Sharma A. Emerging concepts in the pathophysiology and treatment of obesity-associated hypertension. Curr Opin Cardiol 2002; 17: 355–9.
4. Pinto-Sietsma S-J, Navis G, Janssen WMT, et al. A central body fat distribution is related to renal function impairment, even in lean subjects. Am J Kidney Dis 2002; 41: 733–41.
5. Griffin KA, Kramer H, Bidani AK. Adverse renal consequences of obesity. Am J Physiol Renal Physiol 2008; 294: F685–F696.
6. Wolf G. After all those fat years: renal consequences of obesity. Nephrol Dial Transplant 2003; 18: 2471–4.
7. Henegar JR, Bigler SA, Henegar LK, et al. Functional and structural changes in the kidney in the early stages of obesity. J Am Soc Nephrol 2001; 12: 1211–17.
8. Tiwari S, Riazi S, Ecelbarger CA. Insulin's impact on renal sodium transport and blood pressure in health, obesity and diabetes. Am J Physiol Renal Physiol 2007; 293: F974–F984.
9. Hall JE. The kidney, hypertension, and obesity. Hypertension 2003; 41(Part 2): 625–33.
10. Locatelli F, Pozzoni P, Del Vecchio L. Renal manifestations in the metabolic syndrome. J Am Soc Nephrol 2006; 17: S81–S85.
11. Chen J, Muntner P, Hamm L, et al. The metabolic syndrome and chronic kidney disease in U.S. adults. Ann Intern Med 2004; 140: 167–74.
12. Eckel RH, Barouch WW, Ershow AG. Report of the National Heart, Lung, and Blood Institute-National Institute of Diabetes and Digestive and Kidney Diseases Working Group on the pathophysiology of obesity-associated cardiovascular disease. Circulation 2002; 105: 2923–8.
13. de Jong PE, Verhave JC, Pinto-Sietsma SJ, et al. Obesity and target organ damage: the kidney. Int J Obes 2002; 26(Suppl 4): S21–S24.
14. Praga M, Hernandez E, Herrero JC, et al. Influence of obesity on the appearance of proteinuria and renal insufficiency after unilateral nephrectomy. Kidney Int 2000; 58: 2111–18.
15. Kambham N, Markowitz GS, Valeri AM, et al. Obesity-related glomerulopathy: an emerging epidemic. Kidney International 2001; 59: 1498–509.
16. Kramer H, Luke A. Obesity and kidney disease: a big dilemma. Curr Opin Nephrol Hypertens 2007; 16: 237–41.
17. Hsu C-Y, McCulloch CE, Iribarren C, et al. body mass index and risk for end-stage renal disease. Ann Intern Med 2006; 144: 21–8.
18. Johansen KL, Young B, Kaysen GA, et al. Association of body size with outcomes among patients beginning dialysis. Am J Clin Nutr 2004; 80: 324–32.
19. Marks WH, Florence LS, Chapman PH, et al. Morbid obesity is not a contraindication to kidney transplantation. The American Journal of Surgery 2004; 187: 635–8.
20. Johnson DW, Isbel NM, Brown AM, et al. The effect of obesity on renal transplant outcomes. Transplantation 2002; 74: 675–80.
21. Pesavento TE, Henry ML, Falkenhain ME, et al. Obese living kidney donors: short-term results and possible implications. Transplantation 1999; 68: 1491–6.
22. Nguyen NT, Wolfe BM. The physiologic effects of pneumoperitoneum in the morbidly obese. Ann Surg 2005; 241: 219–26.

23. Nguyen NT, Perez RV, Fleming N, et al. Effect of prolonged pneumoperitoneum on intraoperative urine output during laparoscopic gastric bypass. J Am Coll Surg 2002; 195: 476–83.
24. Adams JP, Murphy PG. Obesity in anaesthesia and intensive care. Br J Anaesth 2000; 85: 91–108.
25. Snider RD, Kruse JA, Bander JJ, et al. Accuracy of estimated creatinine clearance in obese patients with stable renal function in the intensive care unit. Pharmacotherapy 1995; 15: 747–53.
26. Chagnac A, Weinstein T, Herman M, et al. The effects of weight loss on renal function in patients with severe obesity. J Am Soc Nephrol 2003; 14: 1480–6.
27. Morales E, Valero MA, Leon M, et al. Beneficial effects of weight loss in overweight patients with chronic proteinuric nephropathies. Am J Kidney Dis 2003; 41: 319–27.
28. Navarro-Diaz M, Serra A, Romero R, et al. Effect of drastic weight loss after bariatric surgery on renal parameters in extremely obese patients: long-term follow-up. J Am Soc Nephrol 2006; 17: S213–S217.

4 | Gastrointestinal and Hepatic Changes with Obesity

Mark A. Hoeft[1] and Vilma E. Ortiz[2]

[1]*Clinical Fellow in Anesthesia, Harvard Medical School, Resident, Department of Anesthesia and Critical Care, Massachusetts General Hospital, Boston, Massachusetts, U.S.A.*

[2]*Assistant Professor in Anesthesia, Harvard Medical School, Department of Anesthesia and Critical Care, Associate Anesthetist, Massachusetts General Hospital, Boston, Massachusetts, U.S.A.*

INTRODUCTION

The rising prevalence of overweight and obesity has brought about an epidemic of several pathologic conditions affecting the gastrointestinal and hepatic systems. From gastroesophageal reflux disease (GERD) to several cancers of the gut, just about every organ in the alimentary tract is affected by an increase in visceral adiposity.

GASTROINTESTINAL CHANGES
Esophageal
Gastroesophageal Reflux Disease

The prevalence of GERD in the general population is reported to range between 8% and 26%. In the obese population, it is purported to be anywhere from 39% to upwards of 61% (1). As the prevalence of GERD has increased with the obesity epidemic, many have attempted to identify obesity as the causal agent leading to reflux, but the relationship is complex and multifactorial (2,3). While both Swedish and Danish case control studies report no association between GERD and increasing weight (4,5), multiple other studies demonstrate the contrary. For example, frequency and severity of GERD symptoms in women have demonstrated a positive association with body mass index (BMI), particularly above the range of 20.0 to 22.4 kg/m^2 (6). El-Serag et al. demonstrated a strong positive association between obesity and frequency of GERD symptoms, as well as between obesity and erosive esophagitis (7). A recent meta-analysis also supports a consistent link between increasing BMI and the risk of GERD (8).

While diet and lifestyle may contribute to the pathogenesis of reflux, multiple factors have been proposed to explain the increased incidence of GERD in the obese population. These include (2,3,9,10):

1. Low basal or postprandial pressure of the lower esophageal sphincter (LES)
2. High gastroesophageal pressure gradient
3. Increased intra-abdominal pressure
4. Increase in the number of transient relaxations of the LES
5. Impaired esophageal motility
6. Increased output of bile and pancreatic enzymes
7. The presence of a hiatal hernia

Barrett's Esophagus

Barrett's esophagus is the metaplastic change of the normal esophageal squamous epithelium to columnar epithelium. GERD is postulated to be the inciting insult which leads to this pathologic differentiation. While BMI has not been shown to be correlated with the development of Barrett's esophagus, a case control study has demonstrated abdominal obesity (waist circumference) to be an independent risk factor for the development of this condition (8,11).

Adenocarinoma of the Esophagus

Barrett's esophagus is hypothesized to be the precursor to adenocarinoma of the esophagus. Individuals with Barrett's esophagus have a 30- to 40-fold increase in the risk of developing esophageal adenocarinoma. One trial demonstrated that obese individuals have a weight dependent increase in the risk of developing carcinoma with a multivariate-adjusted odds ratio of 7.6 among persons in the highest BMI quartile (>25.6 kg/m² for men; women >24.2 kg/m²) compared to those in the lowest (men <22.3 kg/m²; women <21.1 kg/m²) (12). These trends are also verified by a meta-analysis comparing obesity and adenocarinoma of the esophagus (8).

Gastric
Gastric Emptying and Incidence of Reflux

Obese patients have traditionally been considered to be at high risk for perioperative pulmonary aspiration given the potential for GERD and large gastric volumes with low·pH (13). However, among fasted, unmedicated preoperative patients with a BMI > 30 kg/m², Harter et al. found that the incidence of high volume, low pH was lower than in lean patients (14). Maltby et al. observed that healthy obese patients who drank 300 ml of a clear liquid 2 hours before scheduled surgery had similar range of residual gastric volume and pH than those who fasted for longer than 12 hours (15). Furthermore, gastric emptying of solids and liquids has not shown a correlation to body weight or body surface area (16). Thus, it seems that although the association between high BMI and GERD is substantiated, evidence points to normal gastric emptying in the otherwise healthy obese patient. In the perioperative period the likelihood of reflux and, thus, the potential for aspiration depends on factors such as (17):

1. Delayed gastric emptying as seen with conditions such as diabetic gastroparesis
2. Esophageal pathology
3. Impaired gastric emptying associated with certain medications (i.e., narcotics), intestinal obstruction, trauma, and pain
4. Distention of the stomach during (difficult) mask ventilation

Hiatal Hernia

Current research suggests that the risk of developing a hiatal hernia is related to increasing intragastric pressure, gastroesophageal pressure gradient, and BMI (3,18). Wilson et al. demonstrated a relationship between excessive body weight and the presence of hiatal hernia. When compared to thin (BMI < 20 kg/m²) and normal (BMI = 20–25 kg/m²) individuals, the risk of developing a hiatal hernia was 2.5 (CI 1.5–4.3) for overweight (BMI 25–30 kg/m²) and 4.2 (2.4–7.6) for obese (BMI > 30 kg/m²) individuals (19). Patients with hiatal hernias have lower esophageal pH readings and an increased incidence of esophagitis when compared to patients without hernias (1). Approximately 50% of patients undergoing bariatric surgery will have a hiatal hernia while only 15% will have symptoms of GERD (20).

Adenocarcinoma of the Gastric Cardia
Obesity is associated with an increased risk of adenocarcinoma of the gastric cardia (odds ratio, 2.3) (8,12).

Intestinal
Functional Disorders
Four studies analyzed the relationship between obesity and nonspecific functional gastrointestinal complaints such as diarrhea, vomiting, and abdominal pain. While all four publications found a statistical relationship between obesity and diarrhea, only two demonstrated an association between obesity and vomiting and abdominal pain (21–25). The increase in these symptoms in the obese population is unclear, but some of the leading hypotheses include:

1. Alteration in visceral sensation or motor function—increased colonic transit time has been demonstrated in the obese population (26)
2. Environmental factors that may induce osmotically driven diarrhea, such as the intake of an excessive amount of food with high carbohydrate and fat content
3. Effects of medications, such as lipase inhibitors or metformin
4. Comorbidities associated with obesity, such as cholelithiasis or even intestinal angina secondary to the atherosclerosis associated with obesity (26)

Colon Cancer
The increased risk of colon cancer has been well documented in obese men with a relative risk of 1.5 to 2.0 compared to men with a normal BMI. At the same time, BMI does not seem to be a significant determinant of colon cancer in females; however, a demonstrable risk is seen in obese females when an increase in waist-to-hip ratio is noted. In this instance, the relative risk for women (1.52) is similar to that in men (1.51). Diabetes mellitus, hyperglycemia, metabolic syndrome and hyperinsulinemia are all risk factors that appear to increase one's risk of developing colon cancer (27).

Pancreas
Pancreatic Changes in Obesity
The endocrine changes in obesity including glucose intolerance and diabetes have been well documented. Please refer to chapter 5 for a further discussion of this subject. In regards to anatomic changes, computed tomography scans have demonstrated an increase in pancreatic parenchymal and fat volume along with an increase in fat-to-parenchymal ratios in overweight and obese individuals (28).

Pancreatic Cancer
Just as development of pancreatic cancer has been associated with smoking and diabetes, obesity appears to confer an increased risk. Recent evidence supporting this finding refutes earlier studies that demonstrated no link between obesity and pancreatic cancer. A recent meta-analysis demonstrated a 19% increased risk of developing pancreatic cancer in individuals with a BMI $> 30\,\text{kg}/\text{m}^2$ compared to those with a BMI of $22\,\text{kg}/\text{m}^2$ (27,29).

HEPATIC CHANGES
Non-alcoholic Fatty Liver Disease and Non-alcoholic Steatohepatitis
Non-alcoholic fatty liver disease (NAFLD) is estimated to affect upwards of 90% of the morbidly obese population undergoing gastric bypass (30,31). The diagnosis of

NAFLD is a diagnosis of exclusion. It is defined by the accumulation of 5% to 10% fat within the liver by mechanisms that exclude pharmacotherapy, hypobetalipoproteinemia, viral hepatitis, autoimmune hepatitis, and significant alcohol consumption (>140 g per week in men, >70 g per week in women) (32).

On the more advanced spectrum of NAFLD lies *non-alcoholic steatohepatitis* (NASH). Along with the diagnosis of NAFLD, NASH requires the presence of lobular inflammation and hepatocellular ballooning. Advanced cases of NASH may progress to include cirrhosis, hepatocellular carcinoma, and end-stage liver disease (32). Among individuals diagnosed with NASH, 25% may progress to end-stage liver disease and 8% to liver related death over a 10-year period. While NASH many affect upwards of 30% of morbidly obese patients, the severity of NASH appears to be related to high BMI, presence of diabetes and initial fibrosis stage (30–32).

NAFLD is typically asymptomatic, but can present as non-specific right upper quadrant pain or fatigue in both pediatric and adults (typically fourth through sixth decade). Radiographic findings of fatty infiltration of the liver or abnormal serum aminotransferases, usually in the form of ALT levels (typically less than three times the upper limit of normal), can be some of the clinical findings suggestive of NAFLD (30–32).

Incidence of Gallstones
The relative risk of gallstone formation in the obese patient increases linearly with increasing BMI; this risk is noted to be greater in females compared to males. When compared with women of BMI < 24 kg/m², obese (BMI 30–35 kg/m²) and severely obese females (BMI > 45 kg/m²) have a 3.7 and 7.4 increased risk of gallstone formation, respectively. In males, central obesity and hyperinsulinemia have been better correlated with gallstone formation than BMI (33).

ANESTHETIC IMPLICATIONS STATUS POST-GASTRIC BYPASS
Altered Nutrient Absorption
Vitamin deficiencies are uncommon in compliant patients who dutifully take daily vitamin supplements, but individuals who are status post-gastric bypass may present with a variety of nutritional deficiencies. These may be divided into two categories: restricted intake (macro- and micronutrients) and bypass of absorptive and secretory areas of the stomach and small intestine. The most common long-term nutritional abnormalities include iron, vitamin B_{12}, calcium, folate, and thiamine deficiencies which may result in iron deficiency anemia, neurologic deficits, and osteopenia (34).

Rapid weight loss may predispose patients to protein depletion, copper, zinc, and vitamin K deficiencies. Copper deficiency may present as a demyelinating neuropathy that mimics vitamin B_{12} deficiency. Zinc deficiency may present with postprandial emesis or alopecia. Because of low levels of clotting factors II, VII, IX, and X, chronic vitamin K deficiency can lead to an abnormal prothrombin time with a normal partial thromboplastin time. Electrolyte and coagulation indices should be checked in poorly compliant and acutely ill patients as well as prior to surgery (34,35).

Ulceration Risk and the Use of Non-steroidal Anti-inflammatory Drugs (NSAIDs)
A recent report by Sasse et al. describes gastric perforation secondary to marginal ulcers in seven out of 1,670 patients who had undergone gastric bypass surgery.

A marginal ulcer is defined as a gastric ulcer of the jejunal mucosa near the site of a gastrojejunostomy. Of these patients with perforation, six were taking NSAIDs for arthritis, degenerative joint disease, or back pain. All perforations occurred between 24 and 42 months following the gastric bypass procedure. The authors recommend avoidance of NSAIDs in addition to a 12-week post-gastric bypass treatment regimen with proton pump inhibitors (36).

Wilson et al. describe their findings regarding NSAID use in a retrospective review of 1,001 patients' status post-Roux-en-Y laparoscopic gastric bypass (35). Two-hundred and twenty-six patients in this study required endoscopy secondary to gastrointestinal symptoms. NSAIDs use was present in 27% of the patients and accounted for an adjusted odds ratio of 11.5 for the risk of developing marginal ulcers and 10.1 adjusted odds ratio for staple-line dehiscence. The median time to presentation with a marginal ulcer was 2 months (interquartile range 1.0–103 months) while staple-line dehiscence occurred at a median time of 21.5 months (interquartile range 7.0–43 months). The authors recommended proton pump inhibitors for 12 months postoperatively in high risk patients (i.e., NSAID users).

GERD Symptoms and Aspiration Risk After Weight Loss Surgery

Many studies have analyzed the impact of laparoscopic adjustable gastric banding (LAGB), Roux-en-Y gastric bypass (RYBG), and vertical banded gastroplasty (VBG) on LES pressure and GERD symptoms. The data are conflicting as to whether or not GERD symptoms decrease after LAGB. However, improvements in esophageal manometry were noted in one study, though other trials have demonstrated an increase in LES pressure and LES length (1). VBG without an additional antireflux procedure does not appear to be an appropriate treatment for patients with GERD as trials have documented decreases in LES pressure and increases in reflux episodes. A recent retrospective review does demonstrate a decrease in reflux symptoms if a simultaneous crural repair is performed (20). RYBG appears to be the best option for obese patients with GERD as symptoms and need for antireflux medications have been demonstrated to decrease postoperatively (1).

Jean et al. reported on the risk of pulmonary aspiration—defined as "either the presence of bilious secretions or particulate matter in the tracheobronchial tree on direct examination, or presence of infiltrate on postoperative chest radiograph"—in patients who had previously undergone bariatric surgery and were scheduled for plastic or functional surgery (37). The bariatric procedures in this retrospective case control study included LAGB and VBG. A total of four episodes of aspiration were noted in the postbariatric group, none in the control group, a difference which was considered significant. The authors propose that physiologic changes after weight loss surgery may explain this finding: after LAGB, esophago-gastric peristalsis is altered; after VBG, basal LES pressure decreases and acid reflux increases.

REFERENCES

1. Sise A, Friedenberg F. A comprehensive review of gastroesophageal reflux disease and obesity. Obes Rev 2008; 9: 194–203.
2. Kaltenbach T, Crockett S, Gerson L. Are lifestyle measures effective in patients with gastroesophageal reflux disease? An evidence-based approach. Arch Int Med 2006; 166: 965–71.
3. Pandolfino J. The relationship between obesity and GERD: "big or overblown". Am J Gastroenterol 2008; 103: 1355–7.
4. Lagergren J, Bergström R, Nyrén O. No relation between body mass and gastro-oesophageal reflux symptoms in a Swedish population based study. Gut 2000; 47: 26–9.

5. Andersen LI, Jensen G. Risk factors for benign oesophageal disease in a random population sample. J Int Med 1991; 230: 5–10.
6. Jacobson BC, Somers SC, Fuchs CS, et al. Body-mass index and symptoms of gastroesophageal reflux in women. N Engl J Med 2006; 354: 2340–8.
7. El-Serag H, Graham D, Satia J, et al. Obesity is an independent risk factor for GERD symptoms and erosive esophagitis. Am J Gastroenterol 2005; 100: 1243–50.
8. Hampel H, Abraham NS, El-Serag HB. Meta-analysis: obesity and the risk for gastroesophageal reflux disease and its complications. Ann Int Med 2005; 143: 199–211.
9. Wu JC-Y, Mui L-M, Cheung CM-Y, et al. Obesity is associated with increased transient lower esophageal sphincter relaxation. Gastroenterology 2007; 132: 883–9.
10. Mejía-Rivas M, Herrera-López A, Hernández-Calleros J, et al. Gastroesophageal reflux disease in morbid obesity: the effect of Roux-en-Y gastric bypass. Obes Surg 2008; 18: 1217–24.
11. Corley D, Kubo A, Levin T, et al. Abdominal obesity and body mass index as risk factors for Barrett's esophagus. Gastroenterology 2007; 133: 34–41.
12. Lagergren J, Bergstrom R, Nyren O. Association between body mass and adenocarcinoma of the esophagus and gastric cardia. Ann Int Med 1999; 130: 883–90.
13. Vaughan R, Bauer S, Wise L. Volume and pH of gastric juice in obese patients. Anesthesiology 1975; 43: 686–9.
14. Harter R, Kelly W, Kramer M, et al. A comparison of the volume and pH of gastric contents of obese and lean surgical patients. Anesth Analg 1998; 86: 147–52.
15. Maltby J, Pytka S, Watson N, et al. Drinking 300 mL of clear fluid two hours before surgery has no effect on gastric fluid volume and pH in fasting and non-fasting obese patients Can J Anesth 2004; 51: 111–15.
16. Glasbrenner B, Pieramico O, Brecht-Krauss D, et al. Gastric emptying of solids and liquids in obesity. Clin Investig 1993; 71: 542–6.
17. Gal T. Airway management. In: Miller RD, ed. Miller's Anesthesia, 6th edn. Philadelphia, PA: Churchill Livingstone, 2005.
18. de Vries D, van Herwaarden M, Smout A, et al. Gastroesophageal pressure gradients in gastroesophageal reflux disease: relations with hiatal hernia, body mass index, and esophageal acid exposure. Am J Gastroenterol 2008; 103: 1349–54.
19. Wilson LJ, Ma W, I HB. Association of obesity with hiatal hernia and esophagitis. Am J Gastroenterol 1999; 94: 2840–4.
20. Frezza E, Barton A, Wachtel M. Crural repair permits morbidly obese patients with not large hiatal hernia to choose laparoscopic adjustable banding as a bariatric surgical treatment. Obes Surg 2008; 18: 583–8.
21. Levy R, Linde J, Feld K, et al. The association of gastrointestinal symptoms with weight, diet, and exercise in weight-loss program participants. Clin Gastroenterol Hepatol 2005; 3: 992–6.
22. Delgado-Aros S, Locke G, Camilleri M, et al. Obesity is associated with increased risk of gastrointestinal symptoms: a population-based study. Am J Gastroenterol 2004; 99: 801–6.
23. Moayyedi P. The epidemiology of obesity and gastrointestinal and other diseases: an overview. Dig Dis Sci 2008; 53: 2293–9.
24. Talley N, Howell S, Poulton R. Obesity and chronic gastrointestinal tract symptoms in young adults: a birth cohort study. Am J Gastroenterol 2004; 99: 1807–14.
25. Talley N, Quan C, Jones M, et al. Association of upper and lower gastrointestinal tract symptoms with body mass index in an Australian cohort. Neurogastroenterol Motil 2004; 16: 413–19.
26. Delgado-Aros S, Camilleri M, Garcia M, et al. High body mass alters colonic sensory-motor function and transit in humans. Am J Physiol Gastrointest Liver Physiol 2008; 295: G382–G388.
27. Giovannucci E, Michaud D. The role of obesity and related metabolic disturbances in cancers of the colon, prostate, and pancreas. Gastroenterology 2007; 132: 2208–25.

28. Saisho Y, Butler A, Meier J, et al. Pancreas volumes in humans from birth to age one hundred taking into account sex, obesity, and presence of type-2 diabetes. Clin Anat 2007; 20: 933–42.

29. Berrington de Gonzalez A, Sweetland S, Spencer E. A meta-analysis of obesity and the risk of pancreatic cancer. Br J Cancer 2003; 89: 519–23.

30. Beymer C, Kowdley K, Larson A, et al. Prevalence and predictors of asymptomatic liver disease in patients undergoing gastric bypass surgery. Arch Surg 2003; 138: 1240–4.

31. Torres D, Harrison S. Diagnosis and therapy of nonalcoholic steatohepatitis. Gastroenterology 2008; 134: 1682–98.

32. Boppidi H, Daram S. Nonalcoholic fatty liver disease: hepatic manifestation of obesity and the metabolic syndrome. Postgrad Med 2008; 120: E01–E07.

33. Mathus-Vliegen E, Van Ierland-Van Leeuwen M, Terpstra A. Determinants of gallbladder kinetics in obesity. Dig Dis Sci 2004; 49: 9–16.

34. Xanthakos S, Inge T. Nutritional consequences of bariatric surgery. Curr Opin Clin Nutr Metab Care 2006; 9: 489–96.

35. Ogunnaike BO, Jones SB, Jones DB, et al. Anesthetic considerations for bariatric surgery. Anesth Analg 2002; 95: 1793–805.

36. Sasse K, Ganser J, Kozar M, et al. Seven cases of gastric perforation in Roux-en-Y gastric bypass patients: what lessons can we learn? Obes Surg 2008; 18: 530–4.

37. Jean J, Compere V, Fourdrinier V, et al. The risk of pulmonary aspiration in patients after weight loss due to bariatric surgery. Anesth Analg 2008; 107: 1257–9.

5 | Endocrine Changes in Obesity

Gregory Ginsburg

*Instructor in Anesthesia, Harvard Medical School, Assistant in Anesthesia,
Department of Anesthesia and Critical Care, Massachusetts General Hospital,
Boston, Massachusetts, U.S.A.*

INTRODUCTION
Numerous hormonal abnormalities are associated with obesity. Some of these abnormalities are primary causes of obesity, while others occur as secondary manifestations of obesity and thus are reversible with weight loss.

DIABETES
Diabetes is a condition characterized by impairment of carbohydrate metabolism due to a deficiency of insulin activity.

Physiology
Insulin
Insulin, an important anabolic hormone involved in the synthesis of glycogen, protein, and fatty acids, acts to prevent catabolism and ketoacidosis. Pancreatic beta cells typically secrete 50 units of insulin per day. Insulin is metabolized by the liver and kidneys, so patients with hepatic or renal dysfunction may be prone to hypoglycemia. The rate of insulin release is normally *increased* in response to hyperglycemia, vagal (parasympathetic) stimulation, beta 1 blockade, and beta 2 agonism. The rate of insulin release is normally *decreased* in response to hypoglycemia, sympathetic stimulation, alpha agonists, beta 1 agonism, and somatostatin.

Etiology
Common causes of diabetes include obesity, autoimmune disease, pancreatitis, cystic fibrosis, pheochromocytoma, hemochromatosis, Cushing's syndrome, and acromegaly. Risk factors include family history and advancing age. There is a strong association between obesity and diabetes, and thus a full discussion of diabetes is presented.

Type I Diabetes Mellitus (Type I DM)
Type I DM, characterized by a failure to produce insulin, is commonly due to autoimmune pancreatic destruction. Patients are often diagnosed at a young age and may be thin. They require exogenous insulin and are susceptible to *diabetic ketoacidosis* (DKA).

DKA occurs in the setting of severe insulin deficiency, and may be triggered by infection or physiologic stress. Signs include nausea, vomiting, osmotic diuresis, hypovolemia, lethargy, anion gap metabolic acidosis, urinary ketones, abdominal pain, cardiac depression, and disordered breathing. The hallmarks of the management of this life-threatening condition include rehydration, exogenous insulin administration, and potassium replacement. Vigilant monitoring of fluid balance, electrolytes, and glucose levels is mandatory. Invasive (central) monitoring may be appropriate in patients who are unlikely to tolerate rapid fluid shifts or fluid overload, such as those with cardiopulmonary disease.

A typical treatment regimen consists of fluid replacement (normal saline at a rate of 10 ml/kg/hr) combined with initiation of an insulin infusion (0.1 unit/kg/hr) (1). The rate of the insulin infusion is to be adjusted based on plasma glucose levels. Once the glucose level falls below 250 mg/dL, a D_5W infusion should be initiated (1 ml/kg/hr) in order to facilitate continued insulin administration. Aggressive treatment should be pursued until the anion gap acidosis resolves. In DKA, total body potassium is depleted due to osmotic diuresis. However, serum potassium levels may be normal due to the shifting of potassium out of the cell as part of a compensatory mechanism to correct acidosis. As DKA is treated and the acidosis resolves, potassium will shift back into the cell, and hypokalemia may develop. The extremes of potassium levels seen in DKA are life-threatening, requiring close monitoring and prompt correction. Administration of bicarbonate, magnesium, and phosphate may also be necessary in some cases.

Type II Diabetes Mellitus (Type II DM)

Type II DM is the type of diabetes more commonly found in obese individuals. Diabetic obese patients can still produce endogenous insulin, but are resistant to its effects. High insulin levels are often present, yet hyperglycemia persists. These patients are susceptible to a complication called *nonketotic hyperglycemic hyperosmolar state* (NKHHS).

NKHHS classically occurs in dehydrated elderly patients. Triggers include sepsis, hyperalimentation, and pancreatectomy procedures. Patients may present with hyperglycemia, hyperosmolarity, and hypovolemia due to osmotic diuresis. These conditions, in turn, may lead to renal failure, thrombosis, lethargy, and seizures. Other signs include muscle cramps and visual changes. There is, however, enough endogenous insulin to preclude the formation of ketones. An acidosis may or may not be present. The management of NKHHS is similar to that of DKA, with primary emphasis on fluid replacement. Normal saline is typically the initial fluid of choice, followed by infusion of half-normal saline. Patients may have a body water deficit of 7 to 10 liters. A reasonable goal may be to replace half of the fluid deficit in the first 12 hours of treatment, and the remainder over 1 to 2 days (2). Potassium management is less problematic in NKHHS than in DKA due to the absence of acidosis-induced potassium shifts.

Manifestations of Diabetes in Obese Patients

Acute

Hyperglycemia.   Hyperglycemia is frequently asymptomatic. Severe hyperglycemia may be associated with DKA or NKHHS (see above). Perioperative hyperglycemia has been linked to compromised wound healing, higher infection rates, thromboembolic events, and worse outcomes in a variety of clinical scenarios (e.g., acute stroke) (3).

Hypoglycemia.   Acute signs include catecholamine discharge, tachycardia, hypertension, diaphoresis, and lightheadedness. Under general anesthesia, these signs may be absent or misinterpreted as light anesthesia. For this reason, it is generally prudent to err on the side of higher rather than lower blood glucose (4).

Chronic

Long-term manifestations of diabetes include retinopathy, nephropathy, neuropathy, coronary artery disease, peripheral vascular disease, stroke, autonomic dysfunction (characterized by orthostatic hypotension, gastroparesis, tachycardia, and intraoperative hemodynamic instability), immunocompromise, poor wound healing, stiff joints, and difficult airway.

Perioperative Management

Airway management may be problematic in the diabetic patient. Type II DM is associated with obesity, which itself may predispose to a difficult airway (difficult intubation, difficult ventilation, or difficult surgical airway) and obstructive sleep apnea, with its attendant perioperative respiratory complications. Chronic diabetes is associated with stiff joints and concomitant reductions in cervical spine and temporomandibular joint mobility. DM is also associated with gastroparesis, and therefore obese patients have an increased risk of aspiration due to "full stomach".

Blood glucose should be monitored and controlled throughout the perioperative period; this is particularly important for Type I diabetics who are at risk of hypoglycemia. Elective cases should be scheduled as the first case of the day. Regardless of fasting, insulin-dependent diabetics should receive insulin in order to prevent DKA, even if a simultaneous infusion of glucose is required to prevent hypoglycemia. The recommendation for the pre-operative management of a fasting insulin-dependent diabetic is to administer one-half to two-thirds of the total daily dose of insulin (NPH + regular) as NPH (5). Patients with Type II DM are generally advised to withhold oral hypoglycemic medications on the day of surgery so as to reduce the possibility of hypoglycemia in the preoperative fasting state. Insulin sensitizers and incretin mimetics are unlikely to cause hypoglycemia but, as a precaution, are nonetheless typically discontinued in the perioperative period (Table 1). Metformin should be discontinued perioperatively due to a risk of lactic acidosis (6).

Hyperglycemia is treatable by administration of insulin. In normal daily life, Type I diabetics self-administer subcutaneous insulin that is prepared in various formulations (Table 2). In the perioperative setting, intravenous administration of regular insulin is recommended as it has reliable absorption, an immediate onset, and a duration of action of approximately one hour. Although individual response to insulin is variable, blood glucose levels are typically reduced by 25 mg/dL per 1 unit of intravenous regular insulin. Insulin infusions are typically initiated at 1 unit/hour and titrated based on frequent blood glucose checks. Type 1 diabetics tend to be sensitive to insulin while type II diabetics are resistant to its effects. Electrolyte monitoring is prudent given that insulin administration predisposes to hypokalemia. Hyperglycemia may also lead to osmotic diuresis, for which fluid resuscitation is warranted.

Hypoglycemia is treatable by administration of D50 (50% dextrose in water). Each 1 ml of D50 raises blood glucose by approximately 2 mg/dL. Hypoglycemia may be prevented by an infusion of D5 (5% dextrose in water) at a starting rate of 1 ml/kg/hr (7). Frequent measurements of blood glucose are required in order to carefully titrate the infusion rate so as to avoid dangerous extremes of plasma glucose levels. It may be prudent to withhold beta 1 blockade therapy in hypoglycemic patients as it may exacerbate hypoglycemia.

Patients with *insulin pumps* may warrant a pre-operative consultation from the prescribing endocrinologist if the settings or management of the pump require clarification. In the perioperative period, it is reasonable to maintain a basal infusion rate while monitoring glucose levels hourly. A typical bolus may decrease blood glucose by 50 mg/dL (8). Postoperative diet disruptions, which may occur due to nausea or pain, mandate ongoing frequent glucose measurements.

Table 1 Classes (and Mechanism) of Oral Hypoglycemic Medications (1,2,29)

	Example	Onset	Duration
Alpha glucosidase inhibitor (decreases glucose absorption in gut)	Acarbose	Immediate	<20 min
	Miglitol	Immediate	<20 min
Biguanide (insulin sensitizer, reduces hepatic glucose release)	Metformin	1 hr	8–12 hrs
Dipeptidyl peptidase-4 inhibitors (promotes incretins)	Sitagliptin	1 hr	24 hrs
Meglitinide (increases insulin secretion)	Repaglinide	<15 min	6 hrs
Sulfonylurea (increases insulin secretion)	Glipizide	1 hr	6–12 hrs
	Glyburide	1 hr	6–24 hrs
	Chlorpropramide	1 hr	24–72 hrs
Thiazolidinedione (insulin sensitizer)	Pioglitazone	1 hr	24 hrs
	Rosiglitazone	1 hr	24 hrs

Table 2 Common Subcutaneous Insulin Preparations (1,2,5)

Class	Agent	Onset	Peak effect	Duration
Short	Glulisine	≤15 min	0.5–2 hrs	4–6 hrs
Short	Lispro	≤15 min	0.5–2 hrs	4–6 hrs
Short	Aspart	≤15 min	1–2 hrs	4–6 hrs
Short	Regular	≤15 min	2–4 hrs	6–10 hrs
Intermediate	NPH	1–4 hrs	6–12 hrs	12–18 hrs
Intermediate	Lente	1–4 hrs	6–15 hrs	18–28 hrs
Long	Ultralente	1–8 hrs	10–30 hrs	≥36 hrs
Long	Detemir	2–4 hrs	Lacks peak	Approx. 24 hrs
Long	Glargine	2–8 hrs	Lacks peak	Approx. 24 hrs

Hemodynamic instability is often present during the perioperative care of a diabetic patient. Patients often have chronic hypertension and may be hypovolemic due to antihypertensive medications, such as diuretics or angiotensin-converting enzyme inhibitors. Coronary artery disease, a propensity toward ischemia, and autonomic neuropathy can contribute to disturbances of blood pressure and heart rate. Invasive monitoring and utilization of vasoactive medications may be necessary.

Regional anesthesia may be problematic in diabetic patients with obesity because assessment of anatomical landmarks may be compromised. The hypotension that often occurs with neuraxial blocks (epidural, spinal) may be more extreme due to autonomic dysfunction. Peripheral nerve blocks are not contraindicated in patients with diabetes; however, preexisting peripheral neuropathies should be assessed prior to block placement. Furthermore, the effectiveness of techniques that utilize nerve stimulation may be compromised. The platelet dysfunction seen in diabetics with advanced renal failure may be a relative contraindication to regional anesthesia (9).

Intraoperative positioning of diabetic patients—especially patients with obesity, stiff joint syndrome, or preexisting neuropathies—requires special vigilance to padding and protection of vulnerable nerves.

Chronic renal insufficiency requires special attention to perioperative fluid management and judicious use of nephrotoxic agents (including intravenous contrast dye). Many medications (and/or their active metabolites) are eliminated via renal clearance, and therefore exhibit potentially prolonged effects. Medications in this category include, but are not limited to, certain muscle relaxants (e.g., pancuronium, vecuronium), opioids (e.g., morphine, meperidine), anticoagulants (e.g., dalteparin), and benzodiazepines (e.g., midazolam).

OBESITY AND SPECIFIC ENDOCRINE FACTORS
Thyroid Hormones
Thyroid hormones are involved in the regulation of metabolic rate and affect oxygen consumption, carbon dioxide production, minute ventilation, cardiac inotropy, and cardiac chronotropy. Levels of thyroid hormones are regulated by negative feedback mechanisms via the hypothalamic-pituitary axis. Plasma levels of thyroid-stimulating hormone, thyroxine, thyrotropin-releasing hormone, and thyroglobulin are all typically normal in obese patients. High caloric intake is associated with a rise in triiodothyronine (T3), while weight loss causes a decline. However, high BMI per se appears to be associated with normal T3 levels (10).

Parathyroid Hormones
Parathyroid hormone (PTH) is involved in the regulation of calcium homeostasis.

Obesity is a cause of secondary hyperparathyroidism; PTH levels are positively correlated with obesity. The underlying cause is thought to be obesity-associated deficiency of vitamin D, which in turn may be attributable to increased bone turnover rates. Alternatively, enhanced urinary calcium losses seen in obesity may be a trigger for hyperparathyroidism. The net result is that calcium levels in obese patients are typically normal, while ionized calcium levels are typically in the low to normal range (11).

Glucocorticoids
Cortisol is released from the adrenal gland in response to pituitary secretion of adrenocorticotropic hormone (ACTH), which in turn is stimulated by corticotropin releasing factor from the hypothalamus. Cortisol increases glucose levels and promotes vascular tone and responsiveness to catecholamines. It has anti-inflammatory properties, and is secreted in response to physiologic stress.

Obesity is characterized by increased rates of both cortisol production and cortisol metabolism; the net result is that basal levels of both cortisol and ACTH are normal (12). However, the hypothalamic-pituitary response to stress is altered in obesity. Specifically, patients with abdominal obesity demonstrate an increased release of ACTH and cortisol in response to stress (13). The significance of this hyperactive response to stress is unclear. Following weight loss, cortisol release in response to stress appears to normalize. Of note, the high cortisol level seen in Cushing's syndrome (hypercortisolism from any source) is itself a primary cause of "central" (abdominal) obesity in afflicted patients.

Catecholamines
Catecholamines, released via the sympathetic nervous system, exert wide ranging effects on a variety of body functions, including metabolism and hemodynamics.

In obese patients, epinephrine levels are usually low to normal, and epinephrine response to stress is diminished. However, norepinephrine levels are increased (14).

Overall, there is a chronic increase in sympathetic activity observed in obese patients. This phenomenon, thought to be a compensatory mechanism intended to limit further weight gain, may explain the high incidence of hypertension in obese patients.

Prolactin

Prolactin secretion from the pituitary gland regulates lactation in women.

In obese women, prolactin levels are normal. However, the circadian pattern of prolactin release is abnormal, as is the response to various stimuli. For example, prolactin response to hypoglycemia appears to be diminished in obese patients, a phenomenon which persists even after weight loss (15). This finding has been interpreted as evidence of underlying hypothalamic dysfunction in obesity.

Growth Hormone

Growth hormone (GH) is secreted from the anterior pituitary gland and promotes anabolic activity and growth. The effects of GH are, in part, mediated by insulin-like growth factor I (IGF-I), which also exerts a negative feedback effect on GH levels.

Obesity is characterized by a reduction in GH levels; the usual night-time peak of GH is markedly diminished. The etiology may be an increase in inhibition (somatostain) or some other source of suppression of the hypothalamic-pituitary axis. High endogenous insulin levels (observed in many obese patients) stimulate IGF-I production, which is postulated to inhibit GH (16). Furthermore, GH response to a variety of stimuli—including hypoglycemia and physiologic stress—is impaired. After weight loss, both the level and the responsiveness of GH appear to normalize.

Testosterone

Testosterone is an androgen steroid with anabolic and virilizing effects.

Obesity is correlated with low total testosterone levels, but normal levels of free testosterone. Consequently, obesity is generally not linked to symptoms of hypogonadism. The exception is extreme obesity (actual body weight more than double ideal body weight), in which both total and free testosterone levels fall.

Adipose tissue converts androgens to estrogens, and estrogen levels are positively correlated with obesity in men. Nevertheless, feminization does not occur in obese men (with the possible exception of cases of extreme obesity), and estrogen levels are generally reported to return to normal after weight loss (17).

Aldosterone

Aldosterone is a mineralocorticoid, secreted from the adrenal cortex, which promotes hypervolemia by means of sodium re-absorption. Aldosterone secretion is stimulated by the renin–angiotensin system and by ACTH from the pituitary gland.

Obese patients often have elevated aldosterone levels, which contribute to the high prevalence of hypertension in this population. Weight loss permits normalization of aldosterone levels (18).

Leptin

Leptin is a protein hormone derived from adipose tissue, an endocrine organ itself. Leptin mediates appetite, as well as energy intake and expenditure. Leptin levels are positively correlated with obesity, a paradoxical finding as leptin is thought to encourage the sensation of satiety. It is therefore speculated that obese patients have resistance to the effects of leptin, or some other dysfunction of leptin regulation (19).

POLYCYSTIC OVARY SYNDROME

Polycystic ovary syndrome (PCOS) is an endocrine disorder characterized by a complex and heterogeneous constellation of signs and symptoms. Currently, the diagnosis is made in patients who exhibit at least two of the following three disorders: menstrual irregularities (amenorrhea, oligomenorrhea), hyperandrogenism (hirsuitism, androgenic alopecia), and polycystic ovaries (typically visualized by ultrasonography) (20). Establishment of the diagnosis requires that other endocrine disorders be excluded, such as hyperprolactinemia, Cushing's syndrome, acromegaly, neoplasm, and congenital adrenal hyperplasia. PCOS is strongly correlated with obesity, insulin resistance, and infertility (21).

The etiology of PCOS is multifactorial and not fully established. Ovarian theca cells in affected women produce higher levels of testosterone than normal. This overproduction of testosterone may be secondary to imbalances in pituitary secretion of luteinizing hormone (LH) and follicle-stimulated hormone (FSH). Abnormalities of gonadotropin-releasing hormone secretion from the hypothalamus may alter LH and FSH levels.

In addition, high circulating insulin levels in women with PCOS contribute to insulin resistance and higher free testosterone levels. Adipose tissue in these women appears to contain a defect in the insulin signaling pathway (22). The causal relationship between obesity, insulin resistance, and PCOS is unclear. Weight loss—and its accompanying reduction in insulin resistance—improves but does not necessarily cure PCOS. The prevalence of Type II DM, hypertension, coronary disease, hyperlipidemia, vascular disease, and obstructive sleep apnea is higher in women with PCOS than would be expected in women with obesity alone.

The management of PCOS centers on treatment of the component disorders. Androgen excess and menstrual dysfunction may be treated with oral contraceptives and anti-androgens. Weight loss and oral hypoglycemic medications are effective in improving hyperandrogenemia and insulin resistance (i.e., glucose tolerance). Particularly helpful are the biguanides (e.g., metformin) and the thiazolidinediones (e.g., pioglitazone, rosiglitazone) (21).

METABOLIC SYNDROME

The definition, and even the existence, of an entity known as the metabolic syndrome is a source of ongoing controversy (23). The metabolic syndrome consists of a cluster of risk factors for cardiovascular disease and Type II DM, the overall effect of which is to foster a prothrombotic and proinflammatory state. Approximately 25% of the American population meets criteria for the diagnosis of metabolic syndrome. Most definitions are based on a combination of obesity, hyperlipidemia, hypertension, and glucose intolerance. Insulin resistance may be the crucial common factor that underlies the various components of the metabolic syndrome (24). There appears to be a genetic predisposition to the development of the metabolic syndrome, the details of which remain elusive (25).

Visceral obesity may constitute the cornerstone of the syndrome, and there is speculation that this type of excess adipose tissue—which is associated with abdominal (central) obesity—is more dangerous than other patterns of distribution of body fat. Specifically, waist circumference has been found to correlate more strongly than body mass index with risk of diabetes and cardio-vascular disease. The adipose tissue found in abdominal obesity may be dys-functional in its endocrine activity (producing a variety of hormones, cytokines, and growth factors), with particularly negative repercussions for insulin resis-tance. Obesity-associated adipocyte apoptosis, linked to various inflammatory mediators, may explain some of the insulin signaling pathway dysfunction which underlies insulin resistance (26).

Insulin resistance can progress from hyperinsulinemia to glucose intolerance, and ultimately to frank Type II diabetes. Many factors contribute to the emergence and subsequent worsening of insulin resistance, including diet, stress, smoking, and genetics. Progressive metabolic abnormalities, endothelial dysfunction, and inflammation exacerbate insulin resistance and hasten the development of diabetes and cardiovascular disease.

The usefulness of the diagnosis of metabolic syndrome has been the subject of much controversy. Some practitioners believe it is helpful to assign patients the diagnosis of metabolic syndrome, thus identifying high risk patients in order to educate them and to encourage risk factor modification and lifestyle change. Other practitioners believe that focusing on treatment of each component disorder is suf-ficient. However, various studies have found that metabolic syndrome is an inde-pendent risk factor for chronic renal failure, adverse vascular events including myocardial infarction and stroke, and deep venous thrombosis (27).

Perioperative management of metabolic syndrome focuses on glycemic con-trol. Many studies have shown that poor glucose control in the perioperative period is associated with worse outcomes (3). Lifestyle modification, including changes in diet and exercise, is considered to be the cornerstone of treatment. When feasible, patients are likely to benefit from preoperative optimization of existing hypertension, hyperlipidemia, and hyperglycemia (28).

REFERENCES

1. Longnecker DE. Anesthesiology. McGraw-Hill, 2008.
2. Dunn PF. Clinical Anesthesia Procedures of the Massachusetts General Hospital, 7th edn. Lippincott Williams & Wilkins, 2007.
3. Schricker T, Carvalho G. Tight perioperative glycemic control. J Cardiothorac Vasc Anesth 2005(19); 684–8.
4. Nunnally ME. Tight perioperative glycemic control: poorly supported and risky. J Car-diothorac Vasc Anesth 2005(19); 689–90.
5. Inzucchi SE. Glycemic control of diabetes in the perioperative setting. Int Anesthesiol Clin 2002; 40: 77–93.
6. Salpeter S, Greyber E, Pasternak G, et al. Risk of fatal and nonfatal lactic acidosis with metformin use in type 2 diabetes mellitus: systematic review and meta-analysis. Arch Intern Med 2003; 163: 2594–602.
7. Morgan GE, Mikhail MS, Murray MJ. Clinical Anesthesiology, 3rd edn. McGraw-Hill, 2002.
8. Ahmed Z, Lockhart C, Weiner M, et al. Advances in diabetic management: implications for anesthesia. Anesth Analg 2005; 100: 666–9.
9. Boccardo P, Remuzzi G, Galbusera M. Platelet dysfunction in renal failure. Semin Thromb Hemost 2004: 30; 579–89.
10. Kokkoris P. Obesity and endocrine disease. Endocrinol Metabol Clin North Am 2003; 32: 895–914.
11. Bell NH, Epstein S, Greene A, et al. Evidence for alteration of the vitamin D-endocrine system in obese subjects. J Clin Invest 1985; 76: 370–3.

12. Copinschi G, Cornil A, Leclercq R, et al. Cortisol secretion rate and urinary corticoid excretion in normal and obese subjects. Acta Endocrinol (Copenh) 1966; 51: 186–92.
13. Fok, AC, Tan KT, Jacob E, et al. Overnight (1 mg) dexamethasone suppression testing reliably distinguishes non-cushingoid obesity from Cushing's syndrome. Steroids 1991; 56: 549–51.
14. Young JB, Macdonald IA. Sympathoadrenal activity in human obesity: heterogeneity of findings since 1980. Int J Obes Relat Metab Disord 1992; 16: 959–67.
15. Kopelman PG, White N, Pilkington TR, et al. Impaired hypothalamic control of prolactin secretion in massive obesity. Lancet 1979; 1: 747–50.
16. Frystyk J, Vestbo E, Skajaerbaek C, et al. Free insulin-like growth factor in human obesity. Metabolism 1995; 44(10 Suppl 4): 37–44.
17. Strain GW, Zumoff B, Miller LK, et al. Effect of massive weight loss on hypothalamic-pituitary-gonadal function in obese men. J Clin Endocrinol Metab 1988; 66: 1019–23.
18. Tuck ML, Sowers J, Dornfeld L, et al. The effect if weight reduction on blood pressure, plasma renin activity, and plasma aldosterone levels in obese patients. N Engl J Med 1981; 304: 930–3.
19. Van Gaal LF, Wauters MA, Mertens IL, et al. Clinical endocrinology of human leptin. Int J Obes 1999; 23(Suppl 1): 29–36.
20. Rotterdam ESHRE/ASRM-Sponsored PCOS Consensus Workshop Group. Revised 2003 consensus on diagnostic criteria and long term health risks related to polycystic ovary syndrome (PCOS). Hum Reprod 2004; 19: 41–7.
21. Ehrmann DA. Polycystic ovary syndrome. N Engl J Med 2005; 352: 1223–36.
22. Dunaif A, Wu X, Lee A, et al. Defects in insulin receptor signaling in vivo in the polycystic ovary syndrome (PCOS). Am J Physiol Endocrinol Metab 2001; 281: E392–E399.
23. Mitka M. Does the metabolic syndrome really exist? JAMA 2005; 294: 2010–13.
24. Bagry HS, Raghavendran S, Carli F. Metabolic syndrome and insulin resistance: perioperative considerations. Anesthesiology 2008; 108: 506–23.
25. Grundy SM. What is the contribution of obesity to the metabolic syndrome. Endocrinol Metab Clin North Am 2004; 33: 267–82.
26. Martyn JAJ, Kaneki M, Yasuhara S. Obesity-induced insulin resistance and hypoglycemia. Anesthesiology 2008: 109: 137–48.
27. Gallagher EJ, LeRoith D, Karnieli E. The Metabolic Syndrome – from insulin resistance to obesity and diabetes. Endocrinol Metab Clin North Am 2008; 37: 559–79.
28. Ouattara A, Lecomte P, Le Manach Y, et al. Poor Intraoperative blood glucose control is associated with a worsened hospital outcome after cardiac surgery in diabetic patients. Anesthesiology 2005; 103: 687–94.
29. Yki-Jarvinen H. Thiazolidinediones. N Engl J Med 2004; 351: 1106–18.

6 | Hematological Considerations in the Obese Patient

Jonathan E. Charnin

Instructor in Anesthesia, Harvard Medical School, Assistant in Anesthesia, Department of Anesthesia and Critical Care, Massachusetts General Hospital, Boston, Massachusetts, U.S.A.

INTRODUCTION

Blood is a complex liquid organ that provides for transport of metabolic fuels and wastes, host defense, cell-to-cell signaling, and coagulation. Obesity causes important pro-inflammatory and pro-thrombotic changes in the blood and may also cause changes in red cell mass and platelet activation. Awareness of obesity related hematological considerations is important to optimize patient care in the perioperative period.

A STATE OF CHRONIC INFLAMMATION

Obesity is a complex state of diminished health and heightened inflammation. Obesity related pro-inflammatory molecules circulate in the blood, and their effects are often mediated by white blood cells. Inflammation contributes to the hypercoagulablity seen with obesity.

Mechanisms of Inflammation

Obesity is a state of nutritional excess where caloric intake and hormones regulating energy metabolism are usually in a pathologic state. Metabolic regulatory hormones like insulin, leptin, and resistin, circulate at abnormal levels in the plasma of obese individuals. These hormones influence the immune system and promote inflammation in the obese. Although a full explanation for the state of heightened inflammation caused by obesity is still being elucidated, some important contributors like insulin resistance have been identified.

Dietary contributions to inflammation: Ingestion of foods with high caloric density is common in obesity. Some of these food items are thought to be pro-inflammatory themselves. Which foods are pro-inflammatory is not clearly delineated, but foods high in saturated fat, cholesterol, and fructose are thought to be pro-inflammatory (1).

Insulin is the fundamental hormone that regulates blood glucose and energy balance. Obesity is associated with a state of insulin resistance, which often develops into Type II diabetes mellitus and the metabolic syndrome. Insulin resistance is associated with chronic inflammation (2). There is evidence from human cell culture that insulin itself exerts a pro-inflammatory effect (3).

Adipokines are cytokines that are produced primarily by fat cells, particularly white adipose tissue. It appears that visceral and abdominal fat produce more adipokines than fat located in other regions of the body.

Leptin is a 16 kDa protein hormone that is secreted by fat cells during states of positive energy balance. It affects the brain and endocrine system to regulate energy expenditure (4). Leptin levels rise in response to rising post-prandial insulin levels, and the elevated leptin reduces feeding and increases energy expenditure. Starvation reduces leptin production which promotes feeding (5). Leptin is important for thymic function, and it is a pro-inflammatory cytokine (4). Some obese individuals exhibit central resistance to the effects of leptin and have high circulating leptin levels.

Resistin is a cysteine-rich polypeptide that in both diet and genetically induced obesity promotes insulin resistance and raises blood glucose (5). It is thought to be produced in humans by macrophages, and in some studies is linked to obesity. Its exact role in regulation of glucose and fat metabolism is still under study. Resistin increases inflammation through tumor necrosis factor-α (TNF-α, interleukin-6 (IL-6), and SOCS3, and is linked to atherosclerosis (6).

Adiponectin is a hormone that circulates at very high levels in the blood stream (5–10 μg/mL of plasma). It sensitizes the body to insulin and exerts an anti-inflammatory effect. Adiponectin levels fall in obesity, contributing to insulin resistance and inflammation (7).

Cytokines like TNF-α and IL-6 are elevated in obese individuals. IL-6 has been found to be released directly from fat tissue. Consequently, it is thought that body fat itself can cause the production of this inflammatory cytokine (8).

Oxidative stress from excessive nutrient processing and the resulting increased metabolic load may contribute to inflammation (9).

Reduced Inflammation After Weight Loss
Weight loss achieved through bariatric surgery is associated with a decrease in some of the markers of systemic inflammation caused by obesity (9). It is likely that weight loss related to diet and exercise also reduces obesity associated inflammation.

OBESITY AND COAGULATION
The inflammatory state of obesity raises the blood concentration of the coagulation cascade proteins, and lowers the levels of the endogenous antifibrinolitics. Obesity significantly increases a person's pro-thrombotic risk. Central adiposity and the metabolic syndrome may contribute more to a pro-thrombotic state than fat in other locations.

Elevated Pro-coagulant Factors
Fibrinogen is converted by thrombin into fibrin, the tough polymer that binds platelets together and produces a blood clot. Fibrinogen is an acute phase reactant, and elevated fibrinogen levels may suggest inflammation. De Pergola found that fibrinogen was significantly elevated in obese women, and was correlated with body mass index (BMI) (10).

Von Willebrand factor is elevated in obesity. De Pergola found the von Willebrand antigen levels to be increased in association with waist to hip ratio (11).

Factor VII levels were also found to be directly proportional to waist to hip ratio (11).

Obesity Has Mixed Effects on Endogenous Anticoagulants
Plasminogen activator inhibitor-1 (PAI-1) is a potent inhibitor of plasminogen, the precursor of plasmin. Plasmin is the endogenous anti-thrombotic

enzyme that cleaves fibrin and dissolves blood clots. PAI-1 levels are increased in obesity and this leads to a reduction in the ability to dissolve unwanted thrombi (11).

Tissue plasminogen activator (TPA) is the proteolytic enzyme that cleaves plasminogen creating the activated enzyme plasmin. TPA levels in obese women are higher than in lean women. Obese men with visceral adiposity appear to have higher TPA levels than lean controls (12).

Protein C is an endogenous anticoagulant protein that when activated degrades Factor Va and VIIIa, thereby reducing the propagation of a clot (13). Obese individuals seem to have an increased level of protein C, but they demonstrate a relative resistance to its anti-thrombotic effects (12).

OBESITY AND ARTERIAL THROMBOSIS

Atherosclerosis is a degenerative disease of arteries that is associated with endothelial dysfunction and leads to the development of plaques that narrow the arterial lumen. Obesity itself may not be a significant contributor to atherosclerosis. Abdominal obesity and insulin resistance are strongly linked to coronary artery atherosclerosis and these risk factors are often seen in obesity. There is some evidence that childhood obesity is more tightly linked to early atherosclerosis than adult BMI (14).

Coronary artery disease and heart attack are more common in obese than in lean individuals. It is difficult to ascertain the risk attributable to obesity itself because obesity is associated with other risk factors like hyperlipidemia. In 1998, the American Heart Association issued a call to action, and named obesity as a major modifiable risk factor for heart disease (15). Studies in several large patient populations have suggested that the risk of cardiovascular disease rises even when the BMI is modestly elevated above normal (14).

Stroke probably occurs more frequently in obese individuals when compared to lean individuals. A 1983 analysis of data from the Framingham Heart Study showed that overweight women had an increased occurrence of stroke when compared to lean women (16). Investigators have recently examined the relationship of obesity related hormone changes, like insulin resistance or low leptin levels, and the relative risk of stroke. Weikert et al. looked at about 26,000 European subjects and found that elevated plasma resistin levels conferred a two-fold increased rate of myocardial infarction (MI), but not an increased rate of stroke (17). Lim et al. studied more than 300 Korean subjects with diabetes and found that low adiponectin levels were associated with an increased risk of stroke (18).

Peripheral arterial occlusive disease (PAOD) is associated with insulin resistance and the metabolic syndrome, but PAOD is not tightly correlated with obesity. Although some studies have found an inverse correlation between obesity and PAOD, it is unlikely that obesity has any protective effect on the peripheral vasculature (19). Obese individuals who have significant central obesity have an increased incidence of PAOD in association with the metabolic syndrome.

OBESITY AND VENOUS THROMBOSIS

Obesity is a risk factor for venous thrombotic disease. This condition encompasses deep vein thrombosis (DVT) and pulmonary embolism and is now called venous thromboembolism (VTE). VTE is a major cause of postoperative death in obese individuals.

Obese Individuals Are at Increased Risk for VTE

Using a large database from the Netherlands, Abdollahi analyzed individuals presenting with their first DVT. In a case-controlled study, they found a two-fold increase in the risk for spontaneous venous thrombosis in men and women who had a BMI > 30, and a 10-fold increase in DVT in women with a BMI > 30 who took oral contraceptive pills (20). A BMI > 60 may put post-operative patients at additional risk (21).

Stasis of Blood Contributes to VTE

Stasis of blood is one of three contributors to clotting described by Virchow.

1. Venous thrombosis is more frequent when individuals are sedentary for long periods of time. Obese individuals are perhaps more likely to be sedentary because of leptin resistance and a hypothalamic drive towards energy conservation.
2. Individuals with class III obesity may have other mechanical issues like elevated intra-abdominal pressures that foster venous stasis and result in thrombosis.
3. Intraoperative patient positioning may increase the risk of venous stasis. Abdominal insufflation and the reverse Trendelenburg position during laparoscopic surgery have both been found to slow the flow of blood through the femoral veins (22).

Hypercoagulation

Obesity itself, through the inflammatory changes previously outlined, is a hypercoagulable state and a risk factor for DVT. Some experts consider obesity a major risk factor, like malignancy, trauma, surgery and hospitalization, prolonged immobilization, pregnancy, and thrombophilias. On the other hand, Hirsh and Lee propose that obesity is a weaker risk factor, like smoking and long distance plane flights (23). It may be that a greater increase in the risk of thrombosis is seen in patients younger than age 40 (24). In some patients obesity can be a modifiable risk factor, although some require medical or surgical assistance with weight loss. Additional pro-thrombotic influences, like oral contraceptive pills, should be considered carefully in obese individuals because they place the patient at synergistically increased risk for thrombosis.

Inherited Thrombophilias

Although obese individuals are not immune from familial hypercoagulable states, it is not currently thought that a genetic predisposition for obesity is inherited concurrently with a thrombophilia. Factor V Leiden, the prothrombin gene mutation 20210A, protein C deficiency, protein S deficiency, and antithrombin deficiency are the most frequent familial thrombophilias. Acquired thrombophilias such as the lupus anticoagulant and the antiphospholipid antibody syndrome are also encountered, but are not familial. Obese individuals with thrombophilias are at substantially increased risk of thrombosis. Some centers choose to screen their bariatric surgery patients for thrombophilias pre-operatively.

Pulmonary Embolism and Death from VTE

Obese individuals are at high risk for pulmonary embolism (25). A review of national discharge databases was conducted by Stein et al. They found that both obese men and obese women were at increased risk for DVT and pulmonary embolism. They report that obese individuals have a relative risk of pulmonary embolism of about 2.2 in comparison to lean individuals (24). Podnos and his colleagues reviewed over 3,000 cases of open and laparoscopic gastric bypass and found that VTE was the cause of about half of the post-operative deaths (26).

Diagnosis of VTE May Be Difficult in Obese Patients
Currently, computed tomography of the pulmonary arteries and lower extremity veins is the test of choice to diagnose pulmonary embolism. Because of their size, some obese individuals will not be able to be accommodated on the CT scanner. For very large individuals, it may be impossible to diagnose pulmonary embolism. Sometimes, VTE can be diagnosed in obese individuals by using venous duplex ultrasound of the lower extremities.

DVT Prophylaxis Should Be Used for Hospitalized Obese Individuals
Mechanical DVT prophylaxis like graded compression stockings, intermittent compression devices, and pneumatic foot pumps can be used for obese individuals. Their use, however, may be limited by inadequate equipment size. Intermittent compression devices have been found to reduce the venous stasis associated with operative positioning and abdominal insufflation (27). In the absence of a contraindication, chemoprophylaxis for DVT is preferred as either the sole agent or in conjunction with mechanical prophylaxis (28).

Chemoprophylaxis for DVT involves using a low-dose anticoagulant to reduce the incidence of venous thrombosis. (Section IX).

Inferior vena cava filters (IVCFs) have been placed safely in obese individuals, especially using an intravascular ultrasound technique. Some reports suggest that obese individuals have higher complication rates during IVCF placement. There is a lack of consensus about the most appropriate use of IVCFs in obese individuals. Sapalla argues that because of the high mortality obese individuals experience from VTE, prophylactic IVCFs should be considered in patients with any of the following considerations: a BMI > 60 with truncal obesity or obstructive sleep apnea, severe venous stasis disease, a history of VTE, or a known hypercoagulable state (21). Prophylactic IVCF insertion is not usually undertaken in non-obese patients unless they have a known DVT and are unable to be anticoagulated or they have already experienced a pulmonary embolism. Because IVCF placement may have procedural complications, pro-thrombotic potential, and significant expense, these filters should not be placed without justification. Anticoagulation is the preferred treatment for VTE.

OBESITY AND THE BLOOD
Blood Volume
Standard estimates of blood volume for lean individuals suggest that blood comprises about 7% of the body weight, or a volume of 70 ml/kg of body weight. Some variation exists between men and women; women often have slightly less blood on a per-kilogram basis. Estimating blood volume in obese individuals requires additional calculation. Lemmens and colleagues have proposed an equation to estimate blood volume as indexed by the patient's body weight. They suggest the following equation be used from BMIs of 20 to >70 (29).

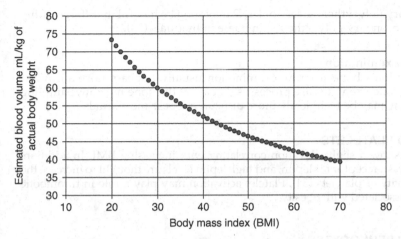

Figure 1 Estimating blood volume in obese individuals. Drawn using equation from Ref. 29.

$$\text{Indexed blood volume} = \frac{70}{\sqrt{\dfrac{\text{Patients's BMI}}{22}}}$$

Figure 1 shows this equation plotted out over a range of BMIs for quick reference.

Red Cell Mass
The red cell mass in obese individuals is usually normal considering their expanded blood volume in comparison to lean individuals. Either anemia or polycythemia should raise suspicion for a treatable cause. One study of obese women found that waist circumference was correlated with increased red cell mass, but BMI was not (30).

Anemia is frequently seen in individuals who have undergone weight reduction surgery.

Despite vitamin supplementation, *vitamin deficiencies* can be seen after weight reduction surgery, especially Roux-en-y gastric bypass. The most common anemia results from vitamin B_{12} deficiency, perhaps due to post-operative changes in intrinsic factor's ability to facilitate absorption of vitamin B_{12}. Folate deficiency can also cause anemia after Roux-en-y gastric bypass (31). Macrocytic anemia is the hallmark of B_{12} and folate deficiency.

Iron deficiency can occur commonly after Roux-en-y gastric bypass (31). A microcytic anemia should raise concern for this condition.

Polycythemia
Polycythemia is a disorder of increased red cell concentration. It can be primary (as a result of polycythemia vera), or secondary (as a result of lung disease, heart disease, or other pathologic states). Some obese individuals are at risk for obstructive sleep apnea, or obesity hypoventilation. These conditions are secondary inducers of polycythemia. In the past, tagged red blood cell scanning was the tool of choice for diagnosing polycythemia, but this test is difficult to interpret in the obese (32). It is now thought that mutations in the janus kinase 2 (JAK2) gene produce polycythemia

vera and primary polycythemia. Use of JAK2 may soon be helpful in differentiating primary from secondary polycythemia in obese individuals (33).

Bone Marrow Examination
In obese individuals bone marrow examination usually appears normal, unless there are other concurrent disease processes that affect the bone marrow. Sampling the bone marrow may be technically more difficult in obese individuals.

OBESITY AND PLATELETS
Platelet counts show a slight elevation correlating with increasing BMI. In addition, these cells express a receptor for leptin, and high leptin levels are thought to increase the thrombotic activity of platelets (34). Platelet activation may play a role in thrombotic complications associated with obesity.

OBESITY AND LEUKOCYTES
The effects of obesity on the immune system are complex. While it is thought that the inflammatory state of obesity produces a mild increase in white blood cell counts, not all reports concur. Some reports indicate that weight loss can facilitate a reduction in white blood cell count (35). The effects of obesity on specific types of white cells are still being determined.

ANTICOAGULATION IN OBESITY
Prophylactic Anticoagulation (Chemoprophylaxis for VTE)
Aspirin alone is not sufficient VTE prophylaxis for obese individuals. The 2008 guidelines from the American College of Chest Physicians recommends against the use of aspirin alone as chemoprophylaxis for VTE for any patient group (28).

    Low-dose unfractionated heparin (LDUH) given subcutaneously is better than mechanical prophylaxis, but less effective for chemoprophylaxis in obese individuals than low molecular weight heparins or fondaparinux. A three times per day dosing schedule of five thousand units or more is suggested (28). There is a low incidence of bleeding events with LDUH. Periodic monitoring of platelet count is indicated to screen for heparin induced thrombocytopenia (HIT).

    The ideal dosing of **low-molecular weight heparins** (LMWHs) in obese individuals remains an area of speculation. It is thought that obese individuals need more prophylactic LMWHs than lean individuals. The 2008 American College of Chest Physicians guidelines suggest that obese individuals having bariatric surgery should receive "higher than standard doses" of drugs used for DVT prophylaxis (28). While those guidelines intentionally do not suggest specific doses, certain assumptions can be made. Chemoprophylactic doses should, in most cases, be less than the dose used for full anticoagulation. Each drug used for chemoprophylaxis has its own dosing range for patients of different VTE risk and body size. Examples of dosing regimens for LMWHs are enoxaparin at the 40 mg subcutaneous (SC) twice daily dose or dalteparin at 7,500 to 10,000 units SC daily. The Matisse trial's comparison of therapeutic enoxaparin or therapeutic unfractionated heparin with therapeutic fondaparinux demonstrated a low rate of both bleeding and recurrence of VTE in obese subjects for all three treatment groups. The rate of major bleeding events was slightly over 1% for obese medical patients with therapeutic anticoagulation (32). It stands to reason that surgical patients are at higher risk of major bleeding events, but that choosing a dose that is higher than standard for usual chemoprophylaxis yet lower than therapeutic anticoagulation may be optimal.

Fondaparinux is a pentasaccharide anti-Xa drug used for anticoagulation. For lean individuals it is usually given at 2.5 mg subcutaneously as a daily injection for DVT prophylaxis. Obese individuals in the perioperative period should probably be given 5 mg of fondaparinux SC daily for VTE prophylaxis, as higher doses are more likely to produce therapeutic anticoagulation.

Therapeutic Anticoagulation

Intravenous unfractionated heparin should be started and titrated using a weight based nomogram (36). In severely obese patients, however, this regimen has been associated with supratherapeutic results. Yee has suggested using a weight based nomogram, but dosing the heparin based on ideal body weight plus 30% of the difference between actual and ideal body weight (37). The ease of monitoring intravenous heparin with the commonly available activated partial thromboplastin time (aPTT), along with its short half-life, makes it a frequently used anticoagulant in the perioperative period. Platelets should be monitored periodically to screen for HIT.

Coumadin and other oral or intravenous vitamin K antagonists should not be initiated in obese individuals without concurrent anticoagulation from a short-acting anticoagulant. Initiation of coumadin alone has been associated with a short lived pro-thrombotic state. Monitoring of coumadin's activity using the prothrombin time and its international normalized ratio is recommended. Dosing of coumadin is probably influenced more by a patient's diet and hepatic function than by their weight.

LMWHs can be used for therapeutic anticoagulation in obese patients. Several LMWHs are available including enoxaparin, tinzaparin, dalteparin, nadroparin, and others. Because they are produced by different processes, they have different properties. Data that applies to one kind of LMWH may not be generalized to other LMWHs. Because the aPTT does not reflect the activity of LMWHs, monitoring of LWMH is done using the anti-Factor Xa assay. LMWHs have renal clearance, and the doses must be adjusted for renal impairment. Questions remain regarding LMWHs' need to have dosing adjustments for Class III obesity. Different LMWHs will probably need to be considered on an individual basis. Enoxaparin is a commonly used LMWH which can be used in obese individuals at the 1 mg/kg SC twice daily dosing using the patient's actual body weight without adjustment (38). Al-Yaseen and others report that dalteparin has been used without significant side effects at a 200 unit per kg of actual body weight for individuals up to 190 kg (39). Consider consulting a pharmacist if you have questions about dosing LMWHs in individuals who weight more than 100 kg.

Fondaparinux is usually dosed therapeutically at 10 mg SC daily for patients over 100 kg. Activity can be measured using an anti-Factor Xa assay that has been calibrated for Fondaparinux.

Direct thrombin inhibitors include argatroban, lepirudin and bivalarudin. Argatroban has been used in obese patients up to a BMI of 50 with a starting infusion of 1 µg/kg of actual body weight per minute when the indication was treatment of HIT and the goal was an aPTT of 1.5 to 3 times the aPTT control value (40). A loading dose of 100 to 200 µg/kg of actual body weight may be appropriate.

Argatroban dosing is affected by hepatic dysfunction and hypoalbuminemia. Because of relative unfamiliarity of the direct thrombin inhibitors, consultation with a pharmacist is recommended.

Perioperative Cessation

Perioperative cessation of therapeutic anticoagulation when thoughtfully undertaken has a low incidence of complications. Mourelo et al. describe 25 patients who stopped their usual oral coumadin five days prior to Roux-en-y gastric bypass, and took SC enoxaparin until the night before surgery. There was a low incidence of both bleeding and thrombotic complications (41).

REFERENCES

1. Miller A, Adeli K. Dietary fructose and the metabolic syndrome. Curr Opin Gastroenterol 2008; 24: 204–9.
2. Tilg H, Moschen AR. Inflammatory mechanisms in the regulation of insulin resistance. Mol Med 2008; 14: 222–31.
3. Brundage SI, Kirilcuk NN, Lam JC, et al. Insulin increases the release of proinflammatory mediators. J Trauma 2008; 65: 367–72.
4. Lago R, Gomez R, Lago F, et al. Leptin beyond body weight regulation—current concepts concerning its role in immune function and inflammation. Cell Immunol 2008; 252: 139–45.
5. Burcelin R. Leptin and resistin: master enemy adipokines unified in brain to control glucose homeostasis. Endocrinology 2008; 149: 443–4.
6. Ahima RS, Lazar MA. Adipokines and the peripheral and neural control of energy balance. Mol Endocrinol 2008; 22: 1023–31.
7. Tilg H, Moschen AR. Role of adiponectin and PBEF/visfatin as regulators of inflammation: involvement in obesity-associated diseases. Clin Sci (Colch) 2008; 114: 275–88.
8. Mohamed-Ali V, Goodrick S, Rawesh A, et al. Subcutaneous adipose tissue releases interleukin-6, but not tumor necrosis factor-alpha, in vivo. J Clin Endocrinol Metab 1997; 82: 4196–200.
9. Vazquez LA, Pazos F, Berrazueta JR, et al. Effects of changes in body weight and insulin resistance on inflammation and endothelial function in morbid obesity after bariatric surgery. J Clin Endocrinol Metab 2005; 90: 316–22.
10. De Pergola G, De Mitrio V, Giorgino F, et al. Increase in both pro-thrombotic and antithrombotic factors in obese premenopausal women: relationship with body fat distribution. Int J Obes Relat Metab Disord 1997; 21: 527–35.
11. De Pergola G, De Mitrio V, Giorgino F, et al. Increase in both pro-thrombotic and antithrombotic factors in obese premenopausal women: relationship with body fat distribution. Int J Obes Relat Metab Disord 1997; 21: 527–35.
12. De Pergola G, Pannacciulli N. Coagulation and fibrinolysis abnormalities in obesity. J Endocrinol Invest 2002; 25: 899–904.
13. Cotran RS, Kumar V, Collins T, Robbins SL. Robbins Pathologic Basis of Disease, 6th edn. Philadelphia: Saunders, 1999.
14. Robinson MK, Thomas A. Obesity and Cardiovascular Disease. New York: Taylor & Francis, 2006.
15. Eckel RH, Krauss RM. American Heart Association call to action: obesity as a major risk factor for coronary heart disease. AHA Nutrition Committee [see comment]. Circulation 1998; 97: 2099–100.
16. Hubert HB, Feinleib M, McNamara PM, et al. Obesity as an independent risk factor for cardiovascular disease: a 26-year follow-up of participants in the Framingham Heart Study. Circulation 1983; 67: 968–77.
17. Weikert C, Westphal S, Berger K, et al. Plasma resistin levels and risk of myocardial infarction and ischemic stroke. J Clin Endocrinol Metab 2008; 93: 2647–53.

18. Lim S, Koo BK, Cho SW, et al. Association of adiponectin and resistin with cardiovascular events in Korean patients with type 2 diabetes: the Korean atherosclerosis study (KAS): a 42-month prospective study. Atherosclerosis 2008; 196: 398–404.

19. Creager MA, Loscalzo J, Dzau VJ. Vascular Medicine: A Companion to Braunwald's Heart Disease. Philadelphia, PA: W.B. Saunders, 2006.

20. Abdollahi M, Cushman M, Rosendaal FR. Obesity: risk of venous thrombosis and the interaction with coagulation factor levels and oral contraceptive use. Thromb Haemost 2003; 89: 493–8.

21. Sapala JA, Wood MH, Schuhknecht MP, et al. Fatal pulmonary embolism after bariatric operations for morbid obesity: a 24-year retrospective analysis. Obes Surg 2003; 13: 819–25.

22. Ido K, Suzuki T, Kimura K, et al. Lower-extremity venous stasis during laparoscopic cholecystectomy as assessed using color Doppler ultrasound. Surg Endosc 1995; 9: 310–13.

23. Hirsh J, Lee AY. How we diagnose and treat deep vein thrombosis. Blood 2002; 99: 3102–10.

24. Stein PD, Beemath A, Olson RE. Obesity as a risk factor in venous thromboembolism. Am J Med 2005; 118: 978–80.

25. Blaszyk H, Bjornsson J. Factor V. Leiden and morbid obesity in fatal postoperative pulmonary embolism [see comment]. Arch Surg 2000; 135: 1410–13.

26. Podnos YD, Jimenez JC, Wilson SE, et al. Complications after laparoscopic gastric bypass: a review of 3464 cases. Arch Surg 2003; 138: 957–61.

27. Schwenk W, Bohm B, Fugener A, et al. Intermittent pneumatic sequential compression (ISC) of the lower extremities prevents venous stasis during laparoscopic cholecystectomy. A prospective randomized study. Surg Endosc 1998; 12: 7–11.

28. Geerts WH, Bergqvist D, Pineo GF, et al. Prevention of venous thromboembolism: American College of Chest Physicians Evidence-Based Clinical Practice Guidelines (8th Edition). Chest 2008; 133: 381S–453S.

29. Lemmens HJ, Bernstein DP, Brodsky JB. Estimating blood volume in obese and morbidly obese patients. Obes Surg 2006; 16: 773–6.

30. Al-Hashem FH. Is it necessary to consider obesity when constructing norms for hemoglobin or when screening for anemia using hemoglobin levels? Saudi Med J 2007; 28: 41–5.

31. Vargas-Ruiz AG, Hernandez-Rivera G, Herrera MF. Prevalence of iron, folate, and vitamin B12 deficiency anemia after laparoscopic Roux-en-Y gastric bypass. Obes Surg 2008; 18: 288–93.

32. Leslie WD, Dupont JO, Peterdy AE. Effect of obesity on red cell mass results [see comment]. J Nucl Med 1999; 40: 422–8.

33. Tefferi A, Thiele J, Orazi A, et al. Proposals and rationale for revision of the World Health Organization diagnostic criteria for polycythemia vera, essential thrombocythemia, and primary myelofibrosis: recommendations from an ad hoc international expert panel. Blood 2007; 110: 1092–7.

34. Bhatt DL. What makes platelets angry: diabetes, fibrinogen, obesity, and impaired response to antiplatelet therapy? J Am Coll Cardiol 2008; 52: 1060–1.

35. Dixon JB, O'Brien PE. Obesity and the white blood cell count: changes with sustained weight loss. Obes Surg 2006; 16: 251–7.

36. Raschke RA, Reilly BM, Guidry JR, et al. The weight-based heparin dosing nomogram compared with a "standard care" nomogram. A randomized controlled trial [see comment]. Ann Intern Med 1993; 119: 874–81.

37. Yee WP, Norton LL. Optimal weight base for a weight-based heparin dosing protocol. Am J Health Syst Pharm 1998; 55: 159–62.

38. Spinler SA, Dobesh P. Dose capping enoxaparin is unjustified and denies patients with acute coronary syndromes a potentially effective treatment [comment]. Chest 2005; 127: 2288–9; author reply 9–90.

39. Al-Yaseen E, Wells PS, Anderson J, et al. The safety of dosing dalteparin based on actual body weight for the treatment of acute venous thromboembolism in obese patients [see comment]. J Thromb Haemost 2005; 3: 100–2.
40. Rice L, Hursting MJ, Baillie GM, et al. Argatroban anticoagulation in obese versus nonobese patients: implications for treating heparin-induced thrombocytopenia. J Clin Pharmacol 2007; 47: 1028–34.
41. Mourelo R, Kaidar-Person O, Fajnwaks P, et al. Hemorrhagic and thromboembolic complications after bariatric surgery in patients receiving chronic anticoagulation therapy. Obes Surg 2008; 18: 167–70.

7 | Preoperative Evaluation of the Obese Patient

Jean Kwo

Assistant Professor of Anesthesia, Harvard Medical School, Assistant Anesthetist, Department of Anesthesia and Critical Care, Massachusetts General Hospital, Boston, Massachusetts, U.S.A.

INTRODUCTION

Obesity is a complex chronic disease that results from social, behavioral, cultural, physiological, metabolic, and genetic factors. The most recent national health survey data puts the prevalence of obesity among U.S. adults as 33% (1). More than 66% of U.S. adults are overweight or obese. Obesity is a major risk factor for multiple co-morbidities. The National Institutes of Health (NIH) has issued evidence-based guidelines calling for weight loss in obese and overweight persons with two or more risk factors for obesity-related diseases (2).

CLASSIFICATION OF OBESITY
Body Mass Index

Body mass index (BMI) is a tool to estimate a healthy body weight based on how tall a person is. It is calculated by:

$$BMI = \frac{Weight(kg)}{Height^2(m^2)}$$

BMI is often used as an indicator of the amount of body fat because weight in excess of what is normal for a certain height is presumed to be due to adipose tissue. However, other factors such as muscularity, edema, muscle wasting, and stature can affect BMI significantly.

Classification

The World Health Organization (WHO) classification system for BMI is outlined in Table 1 (3). A BMI > 25 kg/m² is considered overweight and a BMI > 30 kg/m² is considered obese. The National, Heart, Lung and Blood Institute have also added waist circumference to their risk categories as central adiposity may be associated with greater risk (4). Men with waist circumferences > 40 inches and women with waist circumferences > 35 inches may be at increased risk of hypertension, type 2 diabetes mellitus (DM), and cardiovascular disease (5).

CRITERIA FOR BARIATRIC SURGERY

Criteria for the surgical treatment of obesity include a BMI ≥ 40 kg/m² or BMI ≥ 35 kg/m² with life-threatening cardiopulmonary problems or severe DM (2). Other medical complications of obesity that should be considered include weight-related degenerative joint disease, obstructive sleep apnea, and pulmonary hypertension. Patients should also have the ability to participate in treatment and long-term follow-up,

Table 1 International Classification of Adult Underweight, Overweight, and Obesity According to BMI (3)

Classification	BMI (kg/m²)
Underweight	<18.50
Severe thinness	<16.00
Moderate thinness	16.00–16.99
Mild thinness	17.00–18.49
Normal range	18.50–24.99
Overweight	≥25.00
Pre-obese	25.00–29.99
Obese	≥30.00
Obese class I	30.00–34.99
Obese class II	35.00–39.99
Obese class III	≥40.00

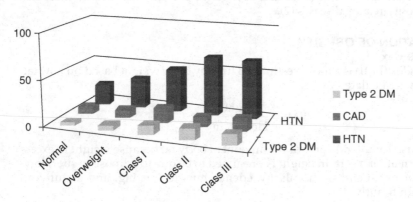

Figure 1 Prevalence of hypertension (HTN), type 2 diabetes mellitus (DM), and coronary artery disease (CAD) in different BMI categories (8).

and have an understanding of the operation and lifestyle changes that will need to be made.

MEDICAL CO-MORBIDITIES ASSOCIATED WITH OBESITY

Obesity is one of the leading causes of preventable death in the United States. It is associated with hypertension, dyslipidemia, type 2 DM, coronary artery disease, stroke, osteoarthritis, sleep apnea, and certain forms of cancers.

Cardiovascular

Hypertension

The age-adjusted prevalence of hypertension increases with increasing BMI (Fig. 1) (1). Hypertension may be the result of increased circulating blood volume, increased vascular constriction, decreased vascular relaxation, and increased cardiac output (6).

Dyslipidemia
The prevalence of high total cholesterol (defined as ≥ 240 mg/dL) is higher with increased BMI (7). Persons with predominantly abdominal obesity (defined as a waist-to-hip circumference ratio of ≥ 0.8 for women and ≥ 1.0 for men) have higher total cholesterol levels, higher low-density lipoprotein levels, and lower high-density lipoprotein levels than persons with smaller waist-to-hip circumference ratios (8).

Coronary Artery Disease (CAD)
Risk factors for CAD such as dyslipidemia, hypertension, type 2 DM, increased inflammatory markers, and a prothrombotic state are all associated with obesity. An increased waist-to-hip ratio, reflecting increased central adiposity, may be a better predictor of myocardial infarction than BMI (9).

Heart Failure
Because of increased metabolic demands, obesity results in an increase in total blood volume, stroke volume, left ventricular volume, and filling pressure, resulting in ventricular chamber dilation. This eventually leads to eccentric left ventricular hypertrophy and left ventricular diastolic dysfunction (10). A pattern of restrictive cardiomyopathy can develop due to fatty infiltration of the myocardium (6).

Arrhythmias
Obese patients have an increased risk of arrhythmias and sudden death. Cardiac conduction defects can result from accumulation of fat between cardiac muscle fibers of the sinus node, the atrioventricular node, and the right bundle branch. Eventually the entire myocardium of the atrioventricular region may be replaced by fat (6).

Respiratory
Obstructive Sleep Apnea (OSA)
Obesity is a risk factor for OSA. If untreated, OSA results in recurrent, prolonged arterial oxygen desaturation eventually leading to secondary cardiac and lung abnormalities including systemic and pulmonary hypertension, cardiac rhythm disturbances and, in extreme cases, right ventricular failure (11). OSA has also been associated with type 2 DM, stroke, automobile accidents, and death (12).

Endocrine
Diabetes Mellitus
Compared with normal weight individuals, those with a BMI ≥ 40 kg/m² are seven times more likely to be diagnosed with DM (13). Abdominal fat distribution, BMI, and weight gain are important risk factors for type 2 DM (Fig. 1).

Gastrointestinal
Gastroesophageal Reflux Disease (GERD)
Obesity is a risk factor for GERD, erosive esophagitis, and esophageal cancer. Overweight and obese individuals are respectively 1.5 and 2 times more likely to have symptoms of GERD as compared to non-obese individuals (14).

Hepatobiliary Disease
Obesity is associated with an increased risk of gallstone disease. Rapid weight loss is also associated with an increased risk of developing cholelithiasis (15).

Liver Disease

Nonalcoholic fatty liver disease (NAFLD) represents a range of liver damage, from steatosis to steatohepatitis (NASH), and can progress to cirrhosis and liver failure. The prevalence of NAFLD in obese individuals is almost 60% (16). Most patients with NAFLD have no signs or symptoms of liver disease at the time of diagnosis. Up to 25% of patients with NASH progress to cirrhosis (17). With the development of cirrhosis, the patient will have clinical and laboratory findings consistent with chronic liver disease. Diagnosis is made by exclusion of other causes of liver disease and liver biopsy.

Neurologic

While, obese patients often have co-morbidities that are risk factors for stroke including hypertension, diabetes, dyslipidemia, metabolic syndrome, and sleep-disordered breathing, obesity itself is also an independent risk factor for stroke (6). Obese patients have an increased risk of ischemic stroke, hemorrhagic stroke, and total stroke.

Renal

Obesity is associated with the two leading causes of end-stage renal disease—hypertension and diabetes—and is an independent risk factor for chronic renal disease (18). Glomerular changes associated with obesity include focal and segmental glomerulosclerosis and glomerulomegaly.

Oncology

Obese patients have higher death rates from cancer compared to normal weight patients (19). The higher death rates are mainly due to cancer of the esophagus, colon and rectum, liver, gallbladder, pancreas, kidney, as well as non-Hodgkin's lymphoma and multiple myeloma (19).

Osteoarthritis (OA)

The risk of OA increases 9% to 13% with each kilogram increase in body weight (20). Direct trauma due to excess body weight is a contributing factor. Leptin, a cytokine-like hormone secreted by adipose tissue, may play a role in cartilage and bone metabolism resulting in an increased risk of OA in the obese patient (21).

Psychiatric

Obesity is associated with increased risk of depression, bipolar disorder, and anxiety disorder. Approximately half of patients presenting for bariatric surgery are taking psychotropic medications (22).

Metabolic Syndrome

Metabolic syndrome refers to a cluster of metabolic abnormalities including central obesity, insulin resistance with or without type 2 DM, dyslipidemia, and hypertension. Central adiposity appears to play a key role in the development of metabolic syndrome (23). Patients with metabolic syndrome are at increased risk for cardiovascular events including myocardial infarction and stroke, and have increased mortality when compared to patients without metabolic syndrome (23).

MORTALITY ASSOCIATED WITH OBESITY

Obesity is a major cause of preventable death in the United States. When compared to normal weight individuals, those with a BMI $\geq 30\,mg/kg^2$ have a 1.6-fold greater risk of death (24). Obesity is associated with a greater risk of mortality from diabetes, cardiovascular disease, stroke, and certain types of cancers.

PREOPERATIVE ASSESSMENT OF THE OBESE PATIENT

Obesity can be associated with multiple co-morbidities. The incidence and severity of surgical complications are correlated more with co-morbidities and the type/ severity of the operative procedure than with BMI (25).

Cardiovascular

Cardiac complications occur in 1% to 1.4% of patients undergoing bariatric surgery (3).

Cardiac Evaluation

The American College of Cardiologists and the American Heart Association have published guidelines for the cardiac evaluation of patients undergoing non-cardiac surgery (26). Patients should be assessed for risk based on history, physical exam, and assessment of their functional status.

The Revised Cardiac Risk Index (RCRI) should be used to risk-stratify patients (27). The RCRI assigns 1 point for each of the following factors:

1. History of ischemic heart disease including history of myocardial infarction, electrocardiogram with abnormal Q waves, history of ischemia as demonstrated on stress testing, and history of angina or chest pain attributed to coronary ischemia
2. History of congestive heart failure
3. History of cerebrovascular disease including history of cerebrovascular accident or transient ischemic attack
4. History of DM requiring insulin
5. Preoperative serum creatinine >2.0 mg/dL

The risk of a perioperative cardiac event depends on the number of risk factors identified (Table 2). Perioperative beta-blockade should be considered in patients with one to two RCRI risk factors. Noninvasive cardiac stress testing can be considered in patients with three or more RCRI risk factors (26).

The patient's functional capacity should also be evaluated. The ability to perform > 4 metabolic equivalents (METs) of activity is associated with a low risk of perioperative cardiac events. Patients undergoing bariatric surgery with a functional capacity of < 4.5 METs as measured by exercise testing had a 16.7% complication rate

Table 2 Revised Cardiac Risk Index (RCRI) and the Rates of Major Cardiac Complications (27)

No. of RCRI risk factors	Rates of major cardiac complications (%)
0	0.5
1	0.9–1.3
2	3.6–6.6
≥3	9.1–11

as compared to a complication rate of 2.8% in those with a functional capacity > 4.5 METs (28). Thus, patients with good functional status can proceed to weight loss surgery without any further workup.

Cardiac Testing

Electrocardiogram. An electrocardiogram (ECG) should be obtained on the basis of age or concomitant cardiac disease. One study found ECG changes in 62% of patients undergoing bariatric surgery (29). These changes included left ventricular hypertrophy, right ventricular hypertrophy, short PR interval, bundle branch block, ST-T wave abnormalities, atrioventricular block, microvoltage, tachycardia, and atrial or ventricular ectopic beats. However, none of these changes were considered to be a contraindication for bariatric surgery.

Echocardiography. Indications for obtaining an echocardiogram include evaluation of ventricular function (both left and right) and evaluation of valvular heart disease. However, it may be difficult to obtain appropriate transthoracic echocardiography windows and high-quality two-dimensional images in the obese patient. The addition of contrast can improve identification of endocardial borders and assessment of ventricular wall motion (30).

Stress testing. Because of body habitus, the diagnostic value of stress tests may be limited. The exercise ECG test may be limited because of difficulty in getting an adequate tracing and decreased ability to exercise. One study showed that the accuracy of thallium scanning was diminished with a BMI > 30 kg/m^2 (31). Image quality can be improved by using a dual head camera, attenuation correction software and hardware, and higher tracer doses (32).

Echocardiography can also be used to image the heart during stress testing. Transesophageal echocardiography may provide superior quality images of the heart and has been used with dobutamine to detect myocardial ischemia in the obese patient.

Respiratory

Altered respiratory mechanics, OSA, pulmonary hypertension, and postoperative pulmonary embolism all contribute to poor pulmonary outcomes in the obese surgical patient. In the bariatric surgery population, the incidence of pulmonary complications ranges from 4% to 7% (3).

General Considerations

Risk factors associated with postoperative pulmonary complications (POPC) include a history of chronic obstructive pulmonary disease (COPD), age > 60 years, ASA class II or greater, functional dependence, and congestive heart failure (33). A low serum albumin (< 35 g/L) is also a strong marker for increased risk of POPC. While routine chest radiography and spirometry is not recommended, it may be appropriate in certain clinical conditions such as COPD or asthma.

Respiratory System Changes

Because increased amounts of metabolically active adipose tissue result in increased work of breathing, oxygen consumption and carbon dioxide production is increased in the obese individual. Obesity is also associated with a decrease in functional residual capacity, a decrease in both lung and chest wall compliance, and a lower oxygenation index (P_aO_2/P_AO_2). These changes are proportional to increasing BMI and are compounded by general anesthesia (34).

Obstructive Sleep Apnea

In a study of 40 consecutive patients evaluated for bariatric surgery, 71% were found to have OSA by polysomnogram (PSG) (35). Patients with OSA may be more sensitive to the respiratory depressant effects of anesthetic agents leading to postoperative oxygen desaturation and hypoxemia. Because of the high prevalence of OSA in obese patients, all patients presenting for bariatric surgery should be screened for OSA using one of the questionnaires currently available. Male gender, neck circumference >16 inches in females and >17 inches in males, hypertension, and high Mallampati score are all findings that are associated with OSA (11).

The Berlin Questionnaire is the most widely used questionnaire for OSA. It includes 11 questions in three categories. It has recently been validated in the surgical population with a sensitivity ranging from 68.9% to 87.2% depending on the severity of OSA (36).

The ASA Task Force on Perioperative Management of Patients with Obstructive Sleep Apnea has developed a consensus checklist for the routine OSA screening of surgical patients (37). Depending on the severity of OSA, the ASA checklist has been demonstrated to have a sensitivity of 72.1% to 87.2% (36).

The STOP questionnaire has recently been proposed as a screening tool for the preoperative clinic as it is easy to administer and score (38). Using an apnea hypopnea index (AHI) of 5 as the cutoff diagnosis of OSA, the sensitivity and specificity of the STOP questionnaire for detecting OSA was 65.6% and 60.0%. Increasing the AHI cutoff to 30 increased the sensitivity of the STOP questionnaire to 79.5%. An alternative scoring model (STOP-Bang, Fig. 2) incorporating BMI, age, gender, and neck circumference has been proposed to further improve the sensitivity of the STOP questionnaire. The sensitivities of the STOP-Bang questionnaire at AHI cutoffs of 5, >15, and >30 are 83.6%, 92.9%, and 100%, respectively.

---

1. Snoring

   Do you snore loudly?

2. Tired

   Do you often feel tired, fatigued, or sleepy during daytime?

3. Observed

   Has anyone observed you stop breathing during your sleep?

4. Blood Pressure

   Do you have or are you being treated for high blood pressure?

5. BMI > 35 kg/m²?

6. Age > 50 yrs?

7. Neck circumference > 40 cm?

8. Male Gender?

A "yes" answer to ≥3 questions is indicative of high risk of OSA.

Figure 2 STOP-Bang questionnaire for screening of obstructive sleep apnea (OSA) (38).

Scoring systems highlight the risk of OSA but are not diagnostic. Therefore, some groups have advocated that PSG be performed routinely on patients undergoing bariatric surgery. Small studies using PSG on all patients presenting for bariatric surgery have shown that up to 90% of these patients have OSA (39,40). Unfortunately, there are no studies looking at whether treatment should be instituted if OSA is diagnosed preoperatively and whether treatment affects perioperative outcomes. Thus, given the paucity of data, routine PSG before bariatric surgery cannot be recommended at this point.

Endocrine
Diabetes Mellitus
Patients with DM presenting for major surgery should have an assessment of their metabolic control. The stress associated with surgery and anesthesia elicits a neuroendocrine response resulting in peripheral insulin resistance, increased gluconeogenesis, impaired insulin secretion and potentially, hyperglycemia. Extreme hyperglycemia in type 2 DM is associated with hyperosmolarity and volume depletion. Hyperglycemia is also associated with impaired wound healing and decreased host defenses against infection.

Patients on insulin should be questioned about the type of insulin used, their insulin regimen, frequency and results of blood glucose monitoring, and frequency of hypoglycemic episodes. Long-acting basal insulin (glargine) is usually continued in the perioperative period. On the morning of surgery, the patient should be instructed to take one-half to two-thirds of his total daily insulin dose as intermediate insulin (NPH). Oral diabetes medications should be held on the day of surgery.

The complications of DM should also be assessed preoperatively. Patients with DM are more likely to have asymptomatic CAD. Autonomic neuropathy may be a predictor of silent myocardial disease and thus, patients with neuropathy, gastroparesis, and orthostatic hypotension may need additional screening for CAD.

Patients with DM are also at risk for diabetic nephropathy. Though an increased serum creatinine is a late sign of renal dysfunction, it may be used as a screening tool.

Gastrointestinal
Gastroesophageal Reflux Disease
Obese patients presenting for surgery should be evaluated for the presence of or symptoms of GERD. While GERD is common in the obese, aspiration is a relatively rare event in elective surgery.

Patients who have undergone bariatric surgery may be at increased risk for GERD and aspiration because of changes in gastric anatomy and physiology after weight loss surgery. In one small study, 6% of patients who had previously undergone bariatric surgery (gastric banding and gastroplasty) had an aspiration event on a subsequent general anesthetic (41). Compare this to the reported range of 1.5 to 9 clinically significant aspirations per 10,000 anesthetics in the general population (42).

Liver Disease
Obesity is associated with NAFLD. Risk factors for advanced liver disease include elevated preoperative liver function tests, hyperlipidemia, male gender, and increased waist-to-hip ratio (43,44). The preoperative assessment of obese patients should include liver function tests. If these are abnormal or there is a clinical suspicion of liver disease, then further investigation should be undertaken. Patients with cirrhosis

may need consultation with a gastroenterologist to optimize medical management, though there is no treatment for NASH-related cirrhosis other than weight loss.

Cholelithiasis
Gallstone formation is common following rapid weight loss due to bile stasis leading to sludge and formation of cholesterol stones in the gallbladder. Patients undergoing bariatric surgery should undergo a preoperative ultrasound to determine whether cholelithiasis is present as this may change the operative plan to include cholecystectomy.

Helicobacter pylori Infection
H. pylori infection in the bariatric surgery population is common. Because of paucity of data, routine preoperative detection of *H. pylori* infection and treatment cannot be recommended. However, treatment may result in a lower incidence of postoperative marginal ulcers. One small study showed a lower incidence of marginal ulcers in patients who had screening and preoperative *H. pylori* eradication, compared with patients who did not undergo screening (6.8% vs. 2.4%) (45).

Infection
Obesity is a risk factor for surgical site infections. Subcutaneous tissue oxygen tension has been demonstrated to be significantly lower in obese patients when compared with non-obese patients despite equivalent arterial oxygen tension (46). Increasing the oxygen concentration administered during anesthesia and maintaining euthermia (47) may be ways to decrease the risk of surgical wound infections.

Thromboembolism
Obesity is a risk factor for venous thromboembolism (48,49). All obese patients undergoing surgery should be considered at high risk for venous thromboembolism and should receive deep venous thrombosis prophylaxis.

The Role of Risk Assessment Indices
In general, obese surgical patients have multiple co-morbidities that increase the risk of surgery. The study of co-morbidities and complications, and risk scoring systems may help identify patients at high risk for postoperative complications.

One study using health insurance claims data found that the two co-morbidities most predictive of post-surgical complications are GERD and sleep apnea (50). Another study looking at in-hospital complications after bariatric surgery found an overall complication rate of 6.8% (51). Factors associated with an increased risk of complications include age $\geq$ 50 years, male gender, Hispanic ethnicity, a history of congestive heart failure, cardiac arrhythmia, other neurological disorders, and peptic ulcer disease.

One proposed risk-scoring system is the Obesity Surgery Mortality Risk Score (OS-MRS) (52). This system assigns 1 point to each of 5 preoperative variables: (i) BMI $\geq$ 50 kg/m^2, (ii) male gender, (iii) hypertension, (iv) known risk factors for pulmonary embolism (previous thromboembolism, preoperative vena cava filer, hypoventilation, pulmonary hypertension), and (v) age $\geq$ 45 years. Patients with scores of 0 to 1 were considered low-risk, 2 to 3 moderate-risk, and 4 to 5 high-risk. Using this scoring system, the mortality rate in low-risk, moderate-risk, and high-risk patients were 0.2%, 1.2%, and 2.4%, respectively.

CONCLUSIONS

With the increased prevalence of obesity in the general population, more obese patients are presenting for surgery. A careful preoperative evaluation serves to ensure that the patient is medically optimized for the procedure. In addition, it may serve to identify risks for postoperative adverse events such that measures may be implemented preoperatively to mitigate these complications.

REFERENCES

1. Flegal KM, Carroll MD, Ogden CL, et al. Prevalence and trends in obesity among US adults, 1999–2000. JAMA 2002; 288: 1723–7.
2. NIH Conference. Gastrointestinal surgery for severe obesity. Consensus Development Conference Panel. Ann Intern Med 1991; 115: 956–61.
3. World Health Organization: Global Database on Body Mass Index. [Available from: http://apps.who.int/bmi/index.jsp?introPage=intro_3.html] (accessed September 2008).
4. Watson K. Managing cardiometabolic risk. An evolving approach to patient care. Crit Pathw Cardiol 2007; 6: 5–14.
5. National Heart Lung and Blood Institute. Classification and risks of overweight and obesity. [Available from: http://www.nhlbi.nih.gov/health/public/heart/obesity/lose_wt/bmi_dis.htm] (accessed September 2008).
6. Poirier P, Giles TD, Bray GA, et al. Obesity and cardiovascular disease: pathophysiology, evaluation, and effect of weight loss. An update of the 1997 American Heart Association scientific statement on obesity and heart disease from the Obesity Committee of the Council on Nutrition, Physical Activity, and Metabolism. Circulation 2006; 113: 898–918.
7. Brown CD, Higgins M, Donato KA, et al. Body mass index and the prevalence of hypertension and dyslipidemia. Obes Res 2000; 8: 605–19.
8. Canoy D, Wareham N, Luben R, et al. Serum lipid concentration in relation to anthropometric indices of central and peripheral fat distribution in 20,021 British men and women: results from the EPIC-Norfolk population-based cohort study. Atherosclerosis 2006; 189: 420–7.
9. Yusuf S, Hawken S, Ounpuu S, et al. and INTERHEART Study Investigators. Obesity and the risk of myocardial infarction in 27,000 participants from 52 countries: a case-control study. Lancet 2005; 366: 1640–9.
10. Alpert MA. Obesity cardiomyopathy: pathophysiology and evolution of the clinical syndrome. Am J Med Sci 2001; 321: 225–36.
11. Cartagena R. Preoperative evaluation of patients with obesity and obstructive sleep apnea. Anesthesiology Clin N Am 2005; 23: 463–78.
12. Patil SP, Schneider H, Schwartz AR, et al. Adult obstructive sleep apnea: pathophysiology and diagnosis. Chest 2007; 132: 325–37.
13. Mokdad A, Ford ES, Bowman BA, et al. Prevalence of obesity, diabetes, and obesity-related health risk factors, 2001. JAMA 2003; 289: 76–9.
14. Hampel H, Abraham NS, El-Serag HB. Meta-analysis: obesity and the risk for gastroesophageal reflux disease and its complications. Ann Int Med 2005; 143: 199–211.
15. Everhart JE. Contributions of obesity and weight loss to gallstone disease. Ann Int Med 1993; 119: 1029–35.
16. Angulo P. Non-alcoholic fatty liver disease. New Engl J Med. 2002; 346: 1221–31.
17. Sachdev MS, Riely CA, Madan AK. Nonalcoholic fatty liver disease of obesity. Obes Surg 2006; 16: 1412–19.
18. Praga M. Morales E. Obesity, proteinuria and progression of renal failure. Curr Opin Nephrol Hypertens 2006; 15: 481–6.
19. Calle EE, Rodriguez C, Walker-Thurmond K, et al. Overweight, obesity, and mortality from cancer in a prospectively studied cohort of U.S. adults. New Engl J Med 2003; 348: 1625–38.

20. Cicuttini FM, Baker JR, Spector TD. The association of obesity with osteoarthritis of the hand and knee in women: a twin study. J Rheumatol 1996; 23: 1221–6.
21. Van Saasa JL, Vandenbroucke JK, van Romunde LK, et al. Osteoarthritis and obesity in the general population. A relationship calling for an explanation. J Rheumatol 1988; 15: 1152–8.
22. Collazo-Clavell ML, Clark MM, McAlpine DE, et al. Assessment and preparation of patients for bariatric surgery. Mayo Clin Proc 2006; 81(10 suppl): S11–S17.
23. Watson K. Managing cardiometabolic risk. An evolving approach to patient care. Crit Pathw Cardiol 2007; 6: 5–14.
24. Adams KF, Schatzkin A, Harris TB, et al. Overweight, obesity, and mortality in a large prospective cohort of persons 50 to 71 years old. New Engl J Med 2006; 355: 763–78.
25. Buchwald H, Avidor Y, Braunwald E, et al. Bariatric surgery: a systematic review and meta-analysis. JAMA 2005; 293: 1724–37.
26. Fleisher LA, Beckman JA, Brown KA, et al. ACC/AHA 2007 guidelines on perioperative cardiovascular evaluation and care of noncardiac surgery: executive summary. A report of the American College of Cardiology/American Heart Association Task Force on Practice Guidelines (Writing Committee to revise the 2002 guidelines on perioperative cardiovascular evaluation for noncardiac surgery). Circulation 2007; 116: 1971–96.
27. Lee TH, Marcantonio ER, Mangione CM, et al. Derivation and prospective validation of a simple index for prediction of cardiac risk of major noncardiac surgery. Circulation 1999; 100: 1043–9.
28. McCullough PA, Gallagher MJ, deJong AT, et al. Cardiorespiratory fitness and complications after bariatric surgery. Chest 2006; 130: 517–25.
29. Catheline JM, Bihan H, Quang TL, et al. Preoperative cardiac and pulmonary assessment in bariatric surgery. Obes Surg 2008; 18: 271–7.
30. Hundley WG, Kizilbash AM, Afridi I, et al. Effect of contrast enhancement on transthoracic echocardiographic assessment of left ventricular regional wall motion—a comparison with invasive techniques. Am J Cardiol 1999; 84: 1365–8.
31. Hansen CL, Woodhouse S, Kramer M. Effect of patient obesity on the accuracy of thallium-201 myocardial perfusion imaging. Am J Cardiol 2000; 85: 749–52.
32. Duvall WL, Croft LB, Corriel JS, et al. SPECT myocardial perfusion imaging in morbidly obese patients: image quality, hemodynamic response to pharmacologic stress, and diagnostic and prognostic value. J Nucl Cardiol 2006; 13: 202–9.
33. Qaseem A, Snow V, Fitterman N, et al. Risk assessment for and strategies to reduce perioperative pulmonary complications for patients undergoing noncardiothoracic surgery: a guideline from the American College of Physicians. Ann Int Med 2006; 144: 575–80.
34. Pelosi P, Croci M, Ravagnan I, et al. The effects of body mass on lung volumes, respiratory mechanics, and gas exchange during general anesthesia. Anesth Analg 1998; 87: 654–60.
35. Frey WC, Pilcher J. Obstructive sleep-related breathing disorders in patients evaluated for bariatric surgery. Obes Surg 2003; 13: 676–83.
36. Chung F, Yegneswaran B, Liao P, et al. Validation of the Berlin Questionnaire and the American Society of Anesthesiologists checklists as screening tools for obstructive sleep apnea in surgical patients. Anesthesiology 2008; 108: 822–30.
37. Gross JB, Bachenberg KL, Benumof JL, et al. Practice guidelines for the perioperative management of patients with obstructive sleep apnea: a report by the American Society of Anesthesiologists Task Force on Perioperative Management of Patients with Obstructive Sleep Apnea. Anesthesiology 2006; 104: 1081–93.
38. Chung F, Yegneswaran B, Liao P. STOP questionnaire: a tool to screen patients for obstructive sleep apnea. Anesthesiology 2008; 108: 812–21.
39. O'Keeffe T, Patterson EJ. Evidence supporting routine polysomnography before bariatric surgery. Obes Surg 2004; 14: 23–6.
40. Daltro C, Gregorio PB, Alves E, et al. Prevalence and severity of sleep apnea in a group of morbidly obese patients. Obes Surg 2007; 17: 809–14.

41. Jean J, Compere V, Fourdrinier V, et al. The risk of pulmonary aspiration in patients after weight loss due to bariatric surgery, Anesth Analg 2008; 107: 1257–59.

42. Warner MA, Warner ME, Weber JG. Clinical significance of pulmonary aspiration during the perioperative period. Anesthesiology 1993; 78: 56–62.

43. Kroh M, Liu R, Chand B. Laparoscopic bariatric surgery: what else are we uncovering? Liver pathology and preoperative indicators of advanced liver disease in morbidly obese patients. Surg Endosc 2007; 21: 1957–60.

44. Ong, JP, Elariny H, Collantes R, et al. Predictors of nonalcoholic steatohepatitis and advanced fibrosis in morbidly obese patients. Obes Surg 2005; 15: 310–15.

45. Schirmer B, Cengiz E, Miller A. Flexible endoscopy in the management of patients undergoing Roux-en-Y gastric bypass. Obes Surg 2002; 12: 634–8.

46. Kabon B, Nagele A, Reddy D, et al. Obesity decreases perioperative tissue oxygenation. Anesthesiology. 2004; 100: 274–80.

47. Kurz A, Sessler DI, Lenhardt R for the Study of Wound Infection and Temperature Group. Perioperative normothermia to reduce the incidence of surgical-wound infection and shorten hospitalization. N Engl J Med 1996; 334: 1209–15.

48. Goldhaber SZ, Grodstein F, Stampfer MJ, et al. A prospective study of risk factors for pulmonary embolism in women. JAMA 1997; 277: 642–5.

49. Stein PD. Beemath A. Olson RE. Obesity as a risk factor in venous thromboembolism. Am J Med 2005; 118: 978–80.

50. Cawley J, Sweeney MJ, Kurian M, et al. Predicting complications after bariatric surgery using obesity-related co-morbidities. Obes Surg 2007; 17:1451–6.

51. Weller WE, Rosati C, Hannan EL. Predictors of in-hospital postoperative complications among adults undergoing bariatric procedures in New York State, 2003. Obes Surg 2006; 16: 702–8.

52. DeMaria EJ, Murr M, Byrne K, et al. Validation of the Obesity Surgery Mortality Risk Score in a multicenter study proves it stratifies mortality risk in patients undergoing gastric bypass for morbid obesity. Ann Surg 2007; 246: 578–84.

8 | Psychological Considerations for Patients with Severe Obesity Presenting for Surgery

Stephanie Sogg

Staff Psychologist, MGH Weight Center, Boston, Massachusetts, U.S.A.

PSYCHOLOGICAL CHARACTERISTICS OF INDIVIDUALS WITH SEVERE OBESITY

In general, patients with obesity are not psychologically different from patients without obesity (1).

1. There is no "psychological profile" common to patients with obesity.
2. Patients are not obese because of a mental deficiency or mental illness, character flaw, or personality disorder.
3. Thus, in the psychological realm, there is little reason to vary perioperative care for patients with obesity.

However, research does suggest that severely obese individuals are at higher risk than individuals without obesity for certain types of psychiatric problems (1,2). Patients seeking treatment for obesity, particularly weight loss surgery (WLS) (3), have higher rates of such problems than patients who are not seeking treatment for their obesity. In one study, 66% of a sample of individuals seeking WLS was found to have a lifetime history of an Axis I psychiatric disorder (4). In particular, patients with obesity appear to have a higher risk of experiencing depression, anxiety disorders, and binge eating disorder (BED) at some point in their lives.

Population studies have shown that individuals with severe obesity are at greatly elevated risk for lifetime and/or current depression (2,5,6), and this seems to be more true of women with severe obesity than it is for men (7). Studies of patients presenting for WLS have found lifetime prevalence rates of depression up to 50% (4,8).

Similarly, individuals with obesity are at increased risk for anxiety disorders (6). In a large population study, Petry et al. (2) found that the likelihood of having an anxiety disorder increased with BMI and that patients with moderate or severe obesity were at significantly increased risk for current and lifetime history of an anxiety disorder.

Many authors have noted a high prevalence of BED among patients with obesity, particularly among those presenting for WLS. However, due to methodological issues, estimates of the prevalence of BED in patients seeking WLS vary tremendously, from 2% (9) to 57.5% (10).

For any surgery where depression, anxiety, or BED is relevant, it is important to be aware that patients with obesity are at increased risk for these problems. For instance, patients with depression may be less adherent to post-surgical self-care, which may increase the risk of poor outcomes (11).

It should be noted, however, if a psychological condition is present in a surgical patient with obesity, it is the condition itself (e.g., major depression) that is relevant, rather than the obesity per se, and the appropriate interventions should not differ according to weight status. For instance, an obese patient with an anxiety disorder may be particularly anxious about undergoing general anesthesia. In such a case, the patient's anxiety, rather than his or her weight, would be the relevant factor.

OBESITY AND QUALITY OF LIFE

One reason that patients with obesity may be at higher risk for depression and other mental health problems is the greatly compromised quality of life that is likely to accompany severe obesity (7).

Obesity is related to numerous comorbidities, including but not limited to obstructive sleep apnea, hypertension, type II diabetes, osteoarthritis and other musculoskeletal pain, hypercholesterolemia, and infertility. Thus, it is not surprising that the health-related quality of life of individuals with obesity tends to be significantly poorer than for those without obesity (12,13).

In addition to its impact on health-related quality of life, obesity can affect almost every aspect of an individual's everyday life and functioning (14). People with obesity face numerous practical limitations, such as low energy, reduced mobility and stamina, poor availability of affordable, attractive clothing, and being unable to fit into the seats at restaurants, doctors' offices, entertainment venues, and on airplanes.

BIAS AND STIGMA

Another reason that patients with obesity may be at higher risk for mental health difficulties is that they are subjected to a significant amount of stigma and discrimination (7,15–18).

Research shows there is pervasive, fairly universal stigma and discrimination against people with obesity, even among healthcare professionals (19–21). This seems to be directly related to a widespread but inaccurate belief that all individuals have 100% control over their weight, and that obesity is attributable solely to laziness and other undesirable personality traits or bad habits (20,22,23). It has been empirically established that the etiology of obesity is heavily influenced by genetics (24,25). The heritability of weight is almost equivalent to that of height (23), and has been estimated to be between 45% and 75% (26). In addition, obesity may be the result of other physiological causes, such as weight-promoting medications, and/or specific medical conditions that make individuals susceptible to weight gain and impede weight loss (e.g., polycystic ovary syndrome).

Bias and stigma may be among the factors contributing to poorer medical care of patients with obesity. Patients with obesity may face barriers to accessing healthcare, such as impaired mobility, limited ability to travel, lack of medical equipment that can accommodate individuals with obesity, etc. (27). Patients with obesity are less likely to undergo routine, preventive healthcare and screening (28,29). This may be partly due to the lack of appropriate equipment, as noted above, and partly due to aversive interactions with medical providers. Research suggests that medical providers may be less likely to recommend thorough testing and routine screenings for patients with obesity (28,30). Patients with obesity frequently report that medical providers have been insensitive when discussing their weight (27,31). Additionally, patients with obesity report that medical providers tend to dismiss many presenting complaints as being attributable solely to weight, without thorough evaluation of the reported symptoms.

The medical professional can do a great deal to work against his or her own biases toward patients with obesity. Become aware of your own biases, and work to control the extent to which they affect your interactions with patients who have obesity. Be careful to use nonstigmatizing, nonperjorative language; research has shown that patients prefer the use of terms such as "weight" or "BMI" to ones like "fat" and "obesity" (31). In addition, it is beneficial to maintain an office environment that is comfortable for patients of all sizes (27):

1. Make sure that the chairs in your waiting room are large enough, and preferably without arms
2. Make sure doorways and corridors are wide enough for patients with obesity
3. Obtain a scale with a high upper limit
4. Weigh patients in a private area
5. Train ancillary staff to discuss weight in a sensitive manner

WEIGHT LOSS SURGERY

WLS is currently the only treatment for obesity that yields substantial and long-lasting results. It is also one of the few types of surgery for which patient adjustment to surgery and safe, effective outcome depend so much on patient behaviors. Therefore, psychosocial factors play an important role during all phases of the WLS process.

The 1991 NIH Guidelines regarding WLS recommend psychosocial evaluation for WLS patients (32). This type of evaluation tends to examine such aspects as the patient's weight history, eating patterns, eating pathology, knowledge about WLS and post-surgical regimen, motivating factors, outcome expectations, psychosocial history, and current psychosocial functioning (8,33–35).

The mental health professional on the WLS surgery team can also play a role in preparing the patient for WLS. This role may include such elements as educating the patient about the types of behavior changes that will be necessary after surgery, and helping the patient to anticipate and practice these changes; helping the patient to anticipate post-surgery challenges and develop strategies to manage them; intervening with cognitive restructuring techniques to address the shame that some patients feel about undergoing WLS; helping the patient to cope with fears about surgery; and ensuring that patients who need psychosocial treatment to prepare for surgery are given appropriate referrals (35).

The mental health professional on the WLS surgery team can also play a role in helping the patient with post-surgery adjustment. This role may include such elements as providing behavioral problem-solving support to enhance patient adherence to post-operative regimens; helping the patient adjust psychologically and emotionally to the significant changes in eating; helping the patient to adjust to changes in his or her body image; and assisting in the adjustment to the types of changes in interpersonal functioning that may occur after WLS.

REFERENCES

1. Stunkard AJ, Wadden TA. Psychological aspects of severe obesity. Am J Clin Nutr 1992; 55: 524S–532S.
2. Petry NM, Barry D, Pietrzak RH, et al. Overweight and obesity are associated with psychiatric disorders: results from the national epidemiologic survey on alcohol and related conditions. Psychosom Med 2008; 70: 288–97.
3. Wadden TA, Butryn ML, Sarwer DB, et al. Comparison of psychosocial status in treatment-seeking women with class III vs. class I-II obesity. Obesity 2006; 14: 90S–98S.

4. Kalarchian MA, Marcus MD, Levine MD, et al. Psychiatric disorders among bariatric surgery candidates: relationship to obesity and functional health status. Am J Psychiatry 2007; 164: 328–34.
5. Onyike CU, Crum RM, Lee HB, et al. Is obesity associated with major depression? Results from the third national health and nutrition examination survey. Am J Epidemiol 2003; 158: 1139–47.
6. Scott KM, McGee MA, Wells JE, et al. Obesity and mental disorders in the adult general population. J Psychosom Res 2008; 64: 97–105.
7. Berkowitz RI, Fabricatore AN. Obesity, psychiatric status, and psychiatric medications. Psychiatr Clin North Am 2005; 28: 39–54, 7–8.
8. Wadden TA, Sarwer DB. Behavioral assessment of candidates for bariatric surgery: a patient-oriented approach. Obesity 2006; 14(Suppl 2): 53S–62S.
9. Burgmer R, Grigutsch K, Zipfel S, et al. The influence of eating behavior and eating pathology on weight loss after gastric restriction operations. Obes Surg 2005; 15: 684–91.
10. Hsu LK, Betancourt S, Sullivan SP. Eating disturbances before and after vertical banded gastroplasty: a pilot study. Int J Eat Disord 1996; 19: 23–34.
11. Pignay-Demaria V, Lesperance F, Demaria RG, et al. Depression and anxiety and outcomes of coronary artery bypass surgery. Ann Thorac Surg 2003; 75: 314–21.
12. de Zwaan M, Lancaster KL, Mitchell JE, et al. Health-related quality of life in morbidly obese patients: effect of gastric bypass surgery. Obes Surg 2002; 12: 773–80.
13. Kolotkin RL, Meter K, Williams GR. Quality of life and obesity. Obes Rev 2001; 2: 219–29.
14. Livingston EH, Fink AS. Quality of life: cost and future of bariatric surgery. Arch Surg 2003; 138: 383–88.
15. Ashmore JA, Friedman KE, Reichmann SK, et al. Weight-based stigmatization, psychological distress, & binge eating behavior among obese treatment-seeking adults. Eat Beh 2008; 9: 203–9.
16. Chen E, Bocchieri-Ricciardi L, Munoz D, et al. Depressed mood in class III obesity predicted by weight-related stigma. Obes Surg 2007; 17: 673–75.
17. Friedman KE, Reichmann SK, Costanzo PR, et al. Weight stigmatization and ideological beliefs: relation to psychological functioning in obese adults. Obes Res 2005; 13: 907–16.
18. Kasen S, Cohen P, Chen H, et al. Obesity and psychopathology in women: a three decade prospective study. Int J Obes 2007; 32: 558–66.
19. Crandall CS. Prejudice against fat people: ideology and self-interest. J Pers Soc Psychol 1994; 66: 882–94.
20. Hilbert A, Rief W, Braehler E. Stigmatizing attitudes toward obesity in a representative population-based sample. Obesity 2008; 16: 1529–34.
21. Teachman BA, Brownell KD. Implicit anti-fat bias among health professionals: is anyone immune? Int J Obes Relat Metab Disord 2001; 25: 1525–31.
22. Chambliss HO, Finley CE, Blair SN. Attitudes toward obese individuals among exercise science students. Med Sci Sports Exerc 2004; 36: 468–74.
23. Friedman JM. Modern science versus the stigma of obesity. Nat Med 2004; 10: 563–9.
24. Bouchard C. The biological predisposition to obesity: beyond the thrifty genotype scenario. Int J Obes 2007; 31: 1337–9.
25. Bouchard C, Tremblay A, Despres JP, et al. The response to long-term overfeeding in identical twins. N Engl J Med 1990; 322: 1477–82.
26. Farooqi IS, O'Rahilly S. Genetic factors in human obesity. Obes Rev 2007; 8(Suppl 1): 37–40.
27. Puhl R, Brownell KD. Bias, discrimination, and obesity. Obes Res 2001; 9: 788–805.
28. Adams CH, Smith NJ, Wilbur DC, et al. The relationship of obesity to the frequency of pelvic examinations: do physician and patient attitudes make a difference? Wom Health 1993; 20: 45–57.

29.   Wee C, McCarthy E, Davis R, et al. Obesity and breast cancer screening. J Gen Intern Med 2004; 19: 324–31.
30.   Hebl MR, Xu J. Weighing the care: physicians' reactions to the size of a patient. Int J Obes 2001; 25: 1246–52.
31.   Wadden TA, Didie E. What's in a name? Patients' preferred terms for describing obesity. Obes Res 2003; 11: 1140–6.
32.   Panel NCDC. Gastrointestinal surgery for severe obesity. Consensus Development Conference Panel. Ann Intern Med 1991; 115: 956–61.
33.   Fabricatore AN, Crerand CE, Wadden TA, et al. How do mental health professionals evaluate candidates for bariatric surgery? Survey results. Obes Surg 2006; 16: 567–73.
34.   Sogg S, Mori DL. The Boston interview for gastric bypass: determining the psychological suitability of surgical candidates. Obes Surg 2004; 14: 370–80.
35.   Sogg S, Mori DL. Revising the Boston interview: incorporating new knowledge and experience. Surg Obes Relat Dis 2008; 4: 455–63.

SUGGESTED READING

Friedman JM. Modern science versus the stigma of obesity. Nat Med 2004; 10: 563–9.
Puhl R, Brownell KD. Bias, discrimination, and obesity. Obes Res 2001; 9: 788–805.
Wadden TA, Didie E. What's in a name? Patients' preferred terms for describing obesity. Obes Res 2003; 11: 1140–6.
Wadden TA, Sarwer DB. Behavioral assessment of candidates for bariatric surgery: a patient-oriented approach. Obesity 2006; 14S2: 53S–62S.
Wadden TA, Sarwer DB, Womble LG, et al. Psychosocial aspects of obesity and obesity surgery. Surg Clin North Am 2001; 81: 1001–24.

9 | Anesthetic Drug Administration

John L. Walsh

Assistant Professor of Anesthesia, Harvard Medical School, Assistant Anesthetist,
Department of Anesthesia and Critical Care, Massachusetts General Hospital,
Boston, Massachusetts, U.S.A.

INTRODUCTION

As noted by Buillon and Shafer (1), many package inserts provide per-kilogram adult-dosing guidelines for the drugs which are used in anesthetizing patients. For the morbidly obese patient, dosing in this manner often leads to gross over-dosing. Physiologically, obese patients have been observed to have an increased blood volume (2), cardiac output (2–4), adipose mass (5), lean-body mass (5), hepatic blood flow (2), α_1-acid glycoprotein concentration (6), CYP450 2A1 activity (7), glucuronidation rate (8), glomerular filtration rate (9), and renal tubular secretion (10). At the same time, the activities of CYP450 3A4 and CYP450 2B6 (7), and renal tubular reabsorption (11) are decreased. While at first blush it would appear that knowledge of these factors would enable an intuitive prediction of drug distribution in the obese patent, in practice, the intuitive predictions are often not correct. This has led to the view that drug dosing should be based on published studies for each drug considered, not on extrapolation of first principles (5). The application of the results of published studies, however, is most accurate when the drug is administered in the manner in which the study was carried out, and extrapolation from them is itself prone to misinterpretation. Finally, it should be pointed out that the predicted concentrations from pharmacokinetic studies may be grossly inaccurate for any particular individual and so the derived doses should only serve as a starting estimate until a better measure of effect may be relied upon.

The next section describes an interpretation of dosing schemes for select drugs used in anesthesia based on the data from published studies. The third section discusses the pharmacokinetics and dynamics of inhaled anesthetics in obesity. The final section provides a lexicon of the abbreviations used in these discussions.

INDIVIDUAL DRUGS
Antibiotics
Vancomycin

Volume of distribution (Vd). The results of three studies demonstrate the Vd of vancomycin to increase in the obese subject by 13% to 49% (12). The average weights of the patients in these studies ranged from 94 to 165 kg; however, there was no simple linear relationship between the weight and the increased Vd.

Clearance (CL). In the two studies in which CL was reported, a direct correlation between total body weight and clearance was seen (12).

Dosage adjustment. Assuming a single compartment model of distribution, the initial dose of vancomycin given to an obese patient should be increased by 13% to 49% over that given to a lean patient to obtain the same peak concentration seen in a lean patient. To maintain the trough concentration above the minimum inhibitory concentration, the time to repeat the dose should be adjusted by the shortened half-life. The new re-dosing time would be:

t = (IBW/TBW) × (Adjusted dose/Lean dose) × (Lean dosing interval)

where IBW is the ideal body weight and TBW is the total body weight.

Aminoglycosides (12)

Volume of distribution. The results of six studies demonstrate the Vd of gentamicin to increase in the obese subject by 30% to 55%. Three studies demonstrate the Vd of tobramycin to increase in the morbidly obese by 37% to 58%. Two studies demonstrate the Vd of amikacin to increase by 38% to 42% in the morbidly obese.

Clearance. The values of clearance for the aminoglycosides are higher in the obese subject than their controls (115–160%). However, the increase appears to be matched by the increase in Vd so that the elimination half-life remains constant.

Dosage adjustment. Bearden and Rodvold (12) suggest using a correction factor of 40% for the Vd of aminoglycosides. Consequently, they suggest that the adjusted weight used for calculating a loading dose be the IBW plus 40% of the weight above IBW. Since the increase in clearance matches the increase in Vd, the dosing interval should remain the same.

Cefazolin

Obesity changes such pharmacokinetic determinants as albumin binding, cardiac output, and regional blood flow. Lagneau et al. (13) account for these changes in a physiologically based pharmacokinetic model to predict the time-course of cefazolin distribution in the extracellular fluid of an obese (100 kg) subject. Their predictions suggest that giving 2 g prior to skin incision followed by 1 g four hours later will maintain the extracellular cefazolin concentration above a minimum inhibitory concentration of 2 µg/mL for at least six hours. Edmiston et al. (14) studied cefazolin levels in the plasma and tissues of morbidly obese patients with BMIs from 40 to >60 and suggested that in these patients 2 g of cefazolin pre-incision followed by 2 g at three hours may not be enough. However, since cefazolin distributes only in the extracellular fluid (13), it is probable that the concentration in Edmiston's tissue homogenates underestimates the extracellular concentration, where cefazolin exerts its effect. Consequently, a loading dose of 2 g of cefazolin seems appropriate for a range of body weights, but no re-dosing strategy is definitive.

Ciprofloxacin

Volume of distribution. In a study by Allard et al. (15), the investigators found that the steady-state Vd of ciprofloxacin in obese patients (269 L, mean weight of 111 kg) was greater than that in the control subjects (219 L, mean weight of 72 kg).

Clearance. The calculated clearance was proportionally higher for the obese patients vs. their lean controls (897 mL/min vs. 744 mL/min) so that the terminal half-life for each group was roughly equal.

Dosage adjustment. Dosing obese patients by their IBW plus 45% of the weight above IBW should produce concentration-time profiles that are similar to those of their lean counterparts during the terminal phase of distribution following a bolus.

Sedatives
Midazolam
Volume of distribution. In a study by Greenblatt et al. (16), the investigators found that the Vd of midazolam in obese subjects (114 L, mean weight of 117 kg) determined by venous samples greatly exceeded that measured in lean subjects (31 L, mean weight of 66 kg). This observation led to the conclusion that "midazolam should be increased at least in proportion to total weight and possibly more." The calculation of Vd is, however, heavily weighted by the terminal elimination phase and consequently not clinically relevant to the purpose of preoperative anxiolysis. In fact, a perusal of the concentration-time curves indicates that dosing in proportion to body weight would increase the concentration in the obese subject above that in the lean subject at all measured time points (>5 min), and in the early phase would increase the concentration by over 100%.

Clearance. The CL of midazolam in obese subjects tended to be slightly lower than in lean subjects (472 mL/min vs. 530 mL/min). However, this trend did not reach statistical significance.

Dosage adjustment. Consistent with the Greenblatt paper report of a "central compartment volume" for midazolam approximately 50% higher in the obese subjects, dosing by a weight about 50% of the way between LBM and TBW is probably reasonable from a pharmacokinetic viewpoint. From a pharmacodynamic point of view, however, it must be realized that obese patients are often sleep deprived and may be more sensitive to the effects of benzodiazepines.

Hypnotics
Propofol
The pharmacokinetics of propofol change depending upon how the drug is administered (bolus vs. infusion) (17). The discussion below is divided along those lines.

Bolus. Two studies comment on the dependence of the induction dose of propofol on LBM (or lean tissue mass), but the subjects of these studies were thin so that extrapolation to the obese patient is unproven (18,19). Similarly, in thin patients, Adachi et al. (20) showed that the hypnotic dose of propofol per kilogram TBW was less in the heavier patients than in the lean patients.

Support for a recommendation of a dosing scheme may be sought from first principles: Krejcie and Avram (21) point out that it is the "front-end" kinetics of mixing within the vascular volume, flow, and the diffusion of the drug that determine the anesthetic induction dose, not the total volume of distribution, elimination clearance and elimination half-life. This concept is supported by the ovine model of Ludbrook and Upton (22) which shows that cardiac output and cerebral blood flow play a large role in the induction dose, whereas tissue distribution plays a relatively minor role. If we assume that the dose needed to yield an equivalent effect is inversely proportional to the cardiac output (23), using the relationship described by Divitiis et al. (3) between weight and cardiac output, an appropriate induction dose for the obese patient would appear to be:

$$\text{Adjusted dose} = \text{IBW dose} \times (1 + 0.007(\text{TBW} - \text{IBW}))$$

Infusion. In a study in thin patients, Hirota et al. (24) showed that dosing propofol infusions by TBW yielded steady-state propofol concentrations that increased with weight and concluded that dosing for infusions should be based on a weight less than TBW. Gepts et al. (25), as well, showed an increase in propofol concentration associated with an increase in weight and suggested dosing by a fixed dose plus a body weight-related dose.

In a study done in obese patients, Servin et al. (26) determined the pharmacokinetic parameters for eight obese patients and ten controls. By taking the ratio of the averages of the steady-state concentrations determined from the parameters for each group, we can determine that the infusion rate for the obese group would have had to be about 50% higher than that in the control group in order to achieve the same steady-state concentration. Coincidentally, that translates to dosing by the IBW plus 50% of the difference between the IBW and the TBW. It should be noted that owing to the time-varying nature of the pharmacokinetics, the initial adjustment ends up being less than 50% and grows to 50% as the infusion progresses.

Thiopental
Using a physiological pharmacokinetic model, Wada et al. (27) determined that bolus doses of thiopental should be dosed by LBM in order to achieve a defined peak plasma concentration. Analysis of the effect of body weight by this model showed that it was the associated change in cardiac output which caused the change in pharmacokinetics.

Opioids
Sufentanil
Bolus. Gepts et al. (28), in a group of relatively thin patients (47–94 kg), were unable to show a significant influence of weight on the parameters in their pharmacokinetic model and suggested that "within the weight range studied, sufentanil dosing need not be adjusted for weight." Schwartz et al. (29), on the other hand, looked for a difference in slightly heavier groups (control 70.1 ± 13 kg; obese 94.1 ± 14 kg) and found that when dosed by TBW the plasma concentrations of the obese subject were still less than those of the control subjects for most of the first two hours after the bolus. They suggested that for these patients loading doses should "account for" TBW.

Infusion. Slepchenko et al. (30) used the weight-independent pharmacokinetic model of Gepts et al. (28) to run a target-controlled infusion of sufentanil in morbidly obese patients. They discovered that the plasma concentrations achieved by the infusion were approximately those predicted (the median error within 20–30%) with a bias toward the model over-predicting the actual concentrations. The bias (~10%) appeared to increase with increasing weight.

Remifentanil
Egan et al. (31) developed a pharmacokinetic model for the distribution of remifentanil in a study of 12 obese patients and 12 matched lean controls. The model, based on data from one-minute infusions, predicted that infusions in obese patients should be based on LBM since the plasma concentrations resulting from infusions based on TBW dosing grossly exceeded those experienced by the matched lean controls. The concentrations resulting from LBM dosing closely approximated those experienced by the matched lean controls.

Fentanyl
Shibutani et al. (32), in a study of 39 severely and morbidly obese patients, determined that two weight-independent pharmacokinetic models of fentanyl over-predicted the actual plasma concentrations sampled during infusions. They developed a "pharmacokinetic mass" (PK mass) which could be used to adjust the infusion rates

of these previous models (i.e., dose proportionally to the PK mass) to minimize the predicted error. Their formulation was approximately:

- For 52 kg < TBW < 100 kg: PK mass = 52 kg + 0.65 (TBW – 52 kg)
- For 100 kg < TBW < 140 kg: PK mass = 83 kg + 0.4 (TBW – 83 kg)
- For TBW > 140 kg: Choose a PK mass between 100 and 108 kg.

Muscle Relaxants
Succinylcholine
Lemmens et al. (33) studied the effects of three dosing schemes for succinylcholine in 45 morbidly obese patients (BMI > 40 kg/m^2). Following 2 mg of midazolam, 2.5 mg/kg LBW of propofol, and 3 µg/kg LBW of fentanyl, the patients received a bolus dose of succinylcholine at 1 mg/kg; 15 subjects were dosed by IBW, 15 by 130% IBW, and 15 by TBW. All patients were successfully intubated on the first or second try, but the intubating conditions were judged increasingly better in the groups receiving the higher doses of succinylcholine (five of the patients in the low-dose group had poor intubating conditions; none of the patients in the high-dose group did; 13 out of 15 patients in the high-dose group had intubating conditions that were judged excellent). On the other hand, the time to 50% recovery increased from 299 seconds to 435 seconds.

In a study of 30 obese adolescents, Rose et al. (34) determined that calculation of dose by either body weight or body surface area yielded a better correlation with the effect of the drug than dosing by BMI. The ED$_{95}$ for succinylcholine, dosed by TBW, was 0.344 mg/kg.

Vecuronium
Weinstein et al. (35) showed that if obese patients (80 kg vs. controls of 60 kg) are dosed with vecuronium by TBW, the time to 75% recovery of twitch strength and the times from 5% to 25% and from 25% to 75% recovery of twitch strength are prolonged significantly. As demonstrated by Schwartz et al. (36), part of the prolongation appears to be due to an increase in distribution and elimination half-lives of vecuronium in the obese subjects (93.4 kg). [Note: The elimination half-life for the controls estimated from their figure (70 min) matches that previously described by Rupp et al. (37)]. That the Vd appears smaller in the obese population in Schwartz's study may be an artifact of eliminating four late data points from the concentration averages. Although Schwartz recommends dosing vecuronium by IBW, it is unclear to what goal that recommendation is directed. In fact, using Schwartz's pharmacokinetic parameters, the differences of which were not statistically significant, we would conclude that obese patients should be dosed by less than IBW.

Rocuronium
Leykin et al. (38) studied the effect of 0.6 mg/kg of rocuronium administered to morbidly obese patients (BMI > 40) and normal body weight controls (BMI < 25). The differences in onset (normal weight controls faster than obese subjects) and difference in duration of block between the normal weight subjects (25.4 min) and the obese subjects dosed by IBW (22.3 min) did not reach statistical significance. When the morbidly obese were dosed by TBW, the duration of the block until 25% twitch recovery was significantly longer than that of the normal weight controls (55.6 min vs. 25.4 min). Consequently, if a similar duration of action is being sought, the morbidly obese should receive a bolus dosed by IBW.

Cisatracurium
Leykin et al. (39) studied the effect of 0.2 mg/kg of cisatracurium administered to morbidly obese patients (BMI > 40) and normal body weight controls (BMI < 25). When the morbidly obese were dosed by TBW they had a similar onset of action as the normal body weight controls (132 sec vs. 135 sec), and both had a much faster onset of action than the morbidly obese dosed by IBW (182 sec). When dosed by TBW, the morbidly obese had a longer duration of action (until return of 25% twitch height) than the normal body weight controls (74.6 min vs. 59.1 min), who in turn had a longer duration of action than the morbidly obese dosed by IBW (59.1 min vs. 45 min). Consequently, to achieve the same onset in a morbidly obese patient as in a lean patient, the obese patient should receive a bolus dosed by TBW; to obtain a similar duration of action, the obese patient should be dosed by IBW plus 50% of the weight above IBW.

INHALATIONAL ANESTHETICS
Obese Vs. Non-Obese
Obesity decreases the functional residual capacity, increases the cardiac output, and increases the size of the fat group. As described by Eger, these actions should theoretically serve to delay the rates of inhalational anesthetic wash-in (the rise in the end-tidal anesthetic concentration) and wash-out (the decline in the end-tidal anesthetic concentration) in the obese relative to those of the non-obese (40).

Wash-In
Despite the argument given above, any differences in wash-in are relatively minor with the wash-in curves for both desflurane and sevoflurane showing little difference between obese and non-obese subjects (41,42).

When desflurane, sevoflurane, and isoflurane are compared in the morbidly obese, their rates of wash-in are inversely related to their blood:gas partition coefficients: desflurane washing in faster than sevoflurane; sevoflurane washing in faster than isoflurane (43,44). The differences in wash-in rates may be overcome by "overpressure," however, and thus do not confer a benefit to one agent over another (40).

Wash-Out
As more procedures are being performed on an outpatient basis, the need for agents with quick recovery profiles and fewer side effects is becoming increasingly important (45).

Sevoflurane Vs. Desflurane
When compared to desflurane, the rate of emergence from sevoflurane in the morbidly obese appears to depend markedly upon the specifics of the study; the rate of emergence is greatly dependent on how the agents are titrated, especially toward the end of the case (46). The concept is similar to that of the context-sensitive half-life observed in intravenous anesthetics. In studies in which the inhaled concentrations have been titrated down while the surgeon is closing to a minimum alveolar concentration of 0.5 or a targeted bispectral index of 60, most studies show a fairly short time to emergence and time to cognitive and

psychomotor recovery in morbidly obese patients receiving either desflurane or sevoflurane, with the edge leaning toward desflurane (47,48).

With respect to post-operative nausea and vomiting, two studies were unable to demonstrate differences in incidence between sevoflurane and desflurane (47,49).

Isoflurane

Desflurane and sevoflurane have much lower blood:gas partition coefficients than isoflurane; consequently, their pharmacokinetic on-set and off-set rates are quicker than those of isoflurane (43,44). Despite these kinetic differences, Brodsky notes that there are no studies demonstrating a clear-cut reason to choose any of the above three anesthetic agents over the others on clinical grounds (45). On the other hand, this lack of evidence may simply reflect the rarity of adverse events, and should be interpreted in that context.

Halothane

Obesity has been shown to be a risk factor for death from hepatitis following administration of halothane (50). Because of this, the use of halothane in obese patients is best avoided.

ABBREVIATIONS

BMI (Body mass index)

$$BMI = \frac{Body\ weight\ (kg)}{(Height\ (m))^2}$$

CL (Clearance)

Clearance is a pharmacokinetic parameter intended to relate plasma drug concentration to the rate of drug elimination (51). For drugs with first-order kinetics, the rate of elimination equals the clearance times the concentration.

IBW (Ideal body weight) (8)

A calculation based on height and gender derived from mortality data reported in the Statistical Bulletin of the Metropolitan Life Insurance Company in 1970.

• For males: IBW = 110 lbs ± 5 lb/inch above or below 5 ft height
• For females: IBW = 100 lbs ± 5 lb/inch above or below 5 ft height

Translated into the metric system, this becomes:

• For males: IBW = 49.9 kg ± 0.89 kg/cm above or below 152.4 cm
• For females: IBW = 45.4 kg ± 0.89 kg/cm above or below 152.4 cm

LBM (Lean body mass) (1)

A calculation based on height, gender and weight, purported to be how much a person would weigh if he/she did not have any body fat.

• For males: LBM = 1.1 (weight (kg)) − 128 (weight (kg)/height (cm))^2
• For females: LBM = 1.07 (weight (kg)) − 148 (weight (kg)/height (cm))^2

It should be noted that these formulae yield parabolas and consequently start to decrease after a certain weight. After this point the LBM should be considered to be the maximum value for the equation. The nomogram in Figure 1 provides a visual reference relating LBM to weight, height and gender (1).

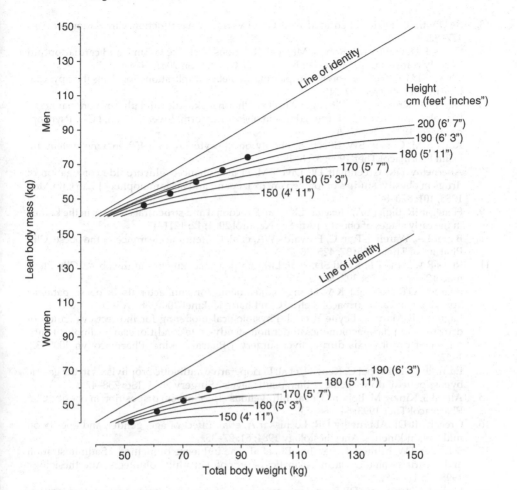

Figure 1 Nomogram relating lean body mass to total body weight, height, and gender. The solid dots represent the values for IBW. *Source*: From Ref. 1.

TBW (Total body weight)	The patient's actual body weight.
Vd (Volume of distribution)	The volume of distribution is an abstraction intended to relate the concentration of drug in the plasma to the total amount of drug in the body (51). The intended interpretation is that if a given dose of drug were to instantaneously equilibrate throughout the body, the concentration seen in the plasma times this volume would equal the dose given.

REFERENCES

1. Bouillon T, Shafer SL. Does size matter? Anesthesiology 1998; 89: 557–60.
2. Alexander JK, Dennis EW, Smith WG, et al. Blood volume, cardiac output, and distribution of systemic blood flow in extreme obesity. Cardiovasc Res Cent Bull 1962; 1: 39–44.

3. de Divitiis O, Fazio S, Petitto M, et al. Obesity and cardiac function. Circulation 1981; 64: 477–82.
4. Collis T, Devereux RB, Roman MJ, et al. Relations of stroke volume and cardiac output to body composition: the strong heart study. Circulation 2001; 103: 820–5.
5. Cheymol G. Effects of obesity on pharmacokinetics implications for drug therapy. Clin Pharmacokinet 2000; 39: 215–31.
6. Derry CL, Kroboth PD, Pittenger AL, et al. Pharmacokinetics and pharmacodynamics of triazolam after two intermittent doses in obese and normal-weight men. J Clin Psychopharmacol 1995; 15: 197–205.
7. Kotlyar M, Carson SW. Effects of obesity on the cytochrome P450 enzyme system. Int J Clin Pharmacol Ther 1999; 37: 8–19.
8. Abernethy DR, Greenblatt DJ, Divoll M, et al. Enhanced glucuronide conjugation of drugs in obesity: studies of lorazepam, oxazepam, and acetaminophen. J Lab Clin Med 1983; 101: 873–80.
9. Henegar JR, Bigler SA, Henegar LK, et al. Functional and structural changes in the kidney in the early stages of obesity. J Am Soc Nephrol 2001; 12: 1211–17.
10. Bauer LA, Wareing-Tran C, Edwards WA, et al. Cimetidine clearance in the obese. Clin Pharmacol Ther 1985; 37: 425–30.
11. Reiss RA, Haas CE, Karki SD, et al. Lithium pharmacokinetics in the obese. Clin Pharmacol Ther 1994; 55: 392–8.
12. Bearden DT, Rodvold KA. Dosage adjustments for antibacterials in obese patients: applying clinical pharmacokinetics. Clin Pharmacokinet 2000; 38: 415–26.
13. Lagneau F, Marty J, Beyne P, et al. Physiological modeling for indirect evaluation of drug tissular pharmacokinetics under non-steady-state conditions: an example of antimicrobial prophylaxis during liver surgery. J Pharmacokinet Pharmacodyn 2005; 32: 1–32.
14. Edmiston CE, Krepel C, Kelly H, et al. Perioperative antibiotic prophylaxis in the gastric bypass patient: do we achieve therapeutic levels? Surgery 2004; 136: 738–47.
15. Allard S, Kinzig M, Boivin G, et al. Intravenous ciprofloxacin disposition in obesity. Clin Pharmacol Ther 1993; 54: 368–73.
16. Greenblatt DJ, Abernethy DR, Locniskar A, et al. Effect of age, gender, and obesity on midazolam kinetics. Anesthesiology 1984; 61: 27–35.
17. Schnider TW, Minto CF, Gambus PL, et al. The influence of method of administration and covariates on the pharmacokinetics of propofol in adult volunteers. Anesthesiology 1998; 88: 1170–82.
18. Leslie K, Crankshaw DP. Lean tissue mass is a useful predictor of induction dose requirements for propofol. Anaesth Intensive Care 1991; 19: 57–60.
19. Chassard D, Berrada K, Bryssine B, et al. Influence of body compartments on propofol induction dose in female patients. Acta Anaesthesiol Scand 1996; 40: 889–91.
20. Adachi YU, Watanabe K, Higuchi H, et al. The determinants of propofol induction of anesthesia dose. Anesth Analg 2001; 92: 656–61.
21. Krejcie TC, Avram MJ. What determines anesthetic induction dose? It's the front-end kinetics, doctor! Anesth Analg 1999; 89: 541–4.
22. Ludbrook GL, Upton RN. A physiological model of induction of anaesthesia with propofol in sheep. 2. Model analysis and implications for dose requirements. Br J Anaesth 1997; 79: 505–13.
23. Upton RN, Ludbrook GL, Grant C, et al. Cardiac output is a determinant of the initial concentrations of propofol after short-infusion administration. Anesth Analg 1999; 89: 545–52.
24. Hirota K, Ebina T, Sato T, et al. Is total body weight an appropriate predictor for propofol maintenance dose? Acta Anaesthesiol Scand 1999; 43: 842–4.
25. Gepts E, Camu F, Cockshott ID, et al. Disposition of propofol administered as constant rate intravenous infusions in humans. Anesth Analg 1987; 66: 1256–63.

26. Servin F, Farinotti R, Haberer JP, et al. Propofol infusion for maintenance of anesthesia in morbidly obese patients receiving nitrous oxide. A clinical and pharmacokinetic study. Anesthesiology 1993; 78: 657–65.

27. Wada DR, Bjorkman S, Ebling WF, et al. Computer simulation of the effects of alterations in blood flows and body composition on thiopental pharmacokinetics in humans. Anesthesiology 1997; 87: 884–99.

28. Gepts E, Shafer SL, Camu F, et al. Linearity of pharmacokinetics and model estimation of sufentanil. Anesthesiology 1995; 83: 1194–204.

29. Schwartz AE, Matteo RS, Ornstein E, et al. Pharmacokinetics of sufentanil in obese patients. Anesth Analg 1991; 73: 790–3.

30. Slepchenko G, Simon N, Goubaux B, et al. Performance of target-controlled sufentanil infusion in obese patients. Anesthesiology 2003; 98: 65–73.

31. Egan TD, Huizinga B, Gupta SK, et al. Remifentanil pharmacokinetics in obese versus lean patients. Anesthesiology 1998; 89: 562–73.

32. Shibutani K, Inchiosa MA Jr, Sawada K, et al. Accuracy of pharmacokinetic models for predicting plasma fentanyl concentrations in lean and obese surgical patients: derivation of dosing weight ("pharmacokinetic mass"). Anesthesiology 2004; 101: 603–13.

33. Lemmens HJ, Brodsky JB. The dose of succinylcholine in morbid obesity. Anesth Analg 2006; 102: 438–42.

34. Rose JB, Theroux MC, Katz MS. The potency of succinylcholine in obese adolescents. Anesth Analg 2000; 90: 576–8.

35. Weinstein JA, Matteo RS, Ornstein E, et al. Pharmacodynamics of vecuronium and atracurium in the obese surgical patient. Anesth Analg 1988; 67: 1149–53.

36. Schwartz AE, Matteo RS, Ornstein E, et al. Pharmacokinetics and pharmacodynamics of vecuronium in the obese surgical patient. Anesth Analg 1992; 74: 515–18.

37. Rupp SM, Castagnoli KP, Fisher DM, et al. Pancuronium and vecuronium pharmacokinetics and pharmacodynamics in younger and elderly adults. Anesthesiology 1987; 67: 45–9.

38. Leykin Y, Pellis T, Lucca M, et al. The pharmacodynamic effects of rocuronium when dosed according to real body weight or ideal body weight in morbidly obese patients. Anesth Analg 2004; 99: 1086–9, table of contents.

39. Leykin Y, Pellis T, Lucca M, et al. The effects of cisatracurium on morbidly obese women. Anesth Analg 2004; 99: 1090–4, table of contents.

40. Eger EI, 2nd, Saidman LJ. Illustrations of inhaled anesthetic uptake, including intertissue diffusion to and from fat. Anesth Analg 2005; 100: 1020–33.

41. Casati A, Marchetti C, Spreafico E, et al. Effects of obesity on wash-in and wash-out kinetics of sevoflurane. Eur J Anaesthesiol 2004; 21: 243–5.

42. La Colla G, La Colla L, Turi S, et al. Effect of morbid obesity on kinetic of desflurane: wash-in wash-out curves and recovery times. Minerva Anestesiol 2007; 73: 275–9.

43. Torri G, Casati A, Comotti L, et al. Wash-in and wash-out curves of sevoflurane and isoflurane in morbidly obese patients. Minerva Anestesiol 2002; 68: 523–7.

44. La Colla L, Albertin A, La Colla G, et al. Faster wash out and recovery for desflurane vs sevoflurane in morbidly obese patients when no premedication is used. Br J Anaesth 2007; 99: 353–8.

45. Brodsky JB, Lemmens HJ, Saidman LJ. Obesity, surgery, and inhalation anesthetics—is there a "drug of choice"? Obes Surg 2006; 16: 734.

46. Eger EI 2nd, Shafer S. The complexity of recovery from anesthesia. J Clin Anesth 2005; 17: 411–12.

47. Vallejo MC, Sah N, Phelps AL, et al. Desflurane versus sevoflurane for laparoscopic gastroplasty in morbidly obese patients. J Clin Anesth 2007; 19: 3–8.

48. Arain SR, Barth CD, Shankar H, et al. Choice of volatile anesthetic for the morbidly obese patient: sevoflurane or desflurane. J Clin Anesth 2005; 17: 413–19.

49. De Baerdemaeker LE, Jacobs S, Den Blauwen NM, et al. Postoperative results after desflurane or sevoflurane combined with remifentanil in morbidly obese patients. Obes Surg 2006; 16: 728–33.
50. Walton B, Simpson BR, Strunin L, et al. Unexplained hepatitis following halothane. Br Med J 1976; 1: 1171–6.
51. Rowland M, Tozer TN. Clinical Pharmacokinetics: Concepts and Applications, 3rd edn. Baltimore: Williams & Wilkins, 1995.

10 | Airway Management in the Obese

Torin D. Shear

Instructor in Anesthesia, Harvard Medical School, Assistant in Anesthesia, Department of Anesthesia and Critical Care, Massachusetts General Hospital, Boston, Massachusetts, U.S.A.

INTRODUCTION

Paramount to the practice of anesthesia is the successful management of the airway. The failure to do so is a major factor in anesthesia related morbidity and mortality (1). Review of the American Society of Anesthesiologists (ASA) Closed Claims database shows that claims for death/brain damage associated with induction of anesthesia have decreased in recent years. Strategic and technological advances in managing the difficult airway undoubtedly have played a significant role in this improvement (2,3).

The obese patient presents unique challenges; both physiologic and anatomic changes occur that affect the airway. Despite conflicting evidence, several authors have suggested an increased incidence of difficult airway in the obese population (4,5,6).

ANATOMY OF THE AIRWAY
Basic Anatomy

The pharynx is divided into three areas: the nasopharynx, oropharynx, and laryngopharynx.

1. The *nasopharynx* extends from the base of the skull and includes the nares, nasal septae, and adenoids
2. The *oropharynx* includes the oral cavity, tongue, and teeth
3. The *laryngopharynx* lies posterior to the oropharynx at the confluence of the nasal and oral cavity. Supported by a cartilage skeleton, pharyngeal muscles control laryngopharyngeal function and tone. Important innervation to this area is provided by the glossopharyngeal and vagus nerves.

Anatomic Variation of Obesity

In obese patients the deposition of adipose tissue in the pharynx leads to a decrease in pharyngeal area (7,8). Specifically, visceral fat and adiposity are inversely associated with pharyngeal cross-sectional area (7). Fatty deposition of the tongue, uvula, tonsils, and aryepiglottic folds can decrease the patency and alter the appearance of the glottis and surrounding structures (9,10). Additionally, lateral parapharyngeal fat deposition can result in large submandibular skin folds making mask ventilation difficult (10).

Pharyngeal muscles used to dilate the pharynx include the hyoid, genioglossus, and tensor palatine. These muscles are located anterior to the pharynx and dilate the pharyngeal aperture by pulling the anterior wall forward. With increasing adiposity, the shape of the pharynx changes making the dilating action of this muscle group less effective (10).

Increased fatty tissue in the anterior cervical region increases external pressure on the pharynx which may lead to collapse and obstruction of the airway. Indeed, the effects of mass loading on the upper airway have been well studied in both animals and humans (11). Consistent increases in airway resistance and decrease in airway diameter are seen with increased extraluminal pressure. This is believed to play a role in obstructive sleep apnea and has implications in the sedated or anesthetized patient. The outward manifestation of fat deposition in this area is increased neck circumference which has been correlated with obstructive sleep apnea and difficult mask ventilation (10,12,13).

While upper airway patency is partially maintained by the pharyngeal dilating muscles discussed, the thorax also plays a role. Caudal traction by the trachea and thorax during inspiration acts to dilate the pharynx and decrease airway resistance. Obesity decreases lung volumes, specifically functional residual capacity, and thus decreases the caudal traction on the upper airway provided by the thorax. This leads to a decrease in airway patency (14).

EVALUATION OF THE AIRWAY
History
A complete medical history and airway evaluation are essential in formulating the anesthetic plan for the obese patient. First, a history of difficult intubation should be sought, including review of prior anesthetic records. A history of snoring is important as it indicates partial airway obstruction, and has been associated with difficult mask ventilation (15). Additionally, symptoms such as apnea during sleep and daytime somnolence may indicate the presence of obstructive sleep apnea, which has been correlated with difficult intubation (16). A simple four question screening tool, the STOP questionnaire, has been validated for perioperative screening of obstructive sleep apnea (17). Comorbid disease states associated with difficult intubation include conditions characterized by diminished cervical range of motion, limited mouth opening, and distorted airway anatomy. Examples include rheumatoid arthritis, scleroderma, and thyroid goiter.

Physical Exam
Predicting the Difficult Mask
Multiple factors have been associated with difficult mask ventilation. Those specific to obesity include a body mass index (BMI) >26 kg/m² and a large neck circumference (13,16). Large submandibular fat pads or jowels may prevent jaw-lift and chin-thrust during mask ventilation. Edentulous patients and those with facial hair may also present a challenge.

Predicting Difficult Intubation
Each individual airway exam finding is of limited value in predicting the difficult intubation (18). However, a thorough exam of the airway combining multiple findings may increase sensitivity and specificity in terms of predicting difficulties (18).

The standard airway exam as recommended by the ASA is shown in Table 1 (3). It includes the relative approximation of the maxilla and mandible, the shape of the palate, the length and thickness of the neck and its range of motion, the Mallampati class, and the thyromental distance.

A large meta-analysis found the Mallampati classification to be of limited predictive value in the general population (19). However, a modified Mallampati class greater than or equal to class 3 was associated with problematic intubation in obese patients (20).

Table 1 Airway Physical Exam as Recommended by the American Society of Anesthesiologists

1. Length of upper incisors
2. Relation of maxillary and mandibular incisors during normal jaw closure
3. Relation of maxillary and mandibular incisors during voluntary protrusion
4. Interincisor difference
5. Visibility of uvula (Mallampati classification)
6. Shape of palate
7. Compliance of mandibular space
8. Thyromental distance
9. Length of neck
10. Thickness of neck
11. Range of motion of head and neck

Source: Adapted from Ref. 3.

Table 2 Safe Apnea Time in Obese Patients: Reverse Trendelenburg vs. Supine

	25° Head up (sec)	Supine (sec)	P-value
Safe apnea period (SaO_2 > 92%)	201 ± 56	155 ± 70	0.02

Source: Adapted from Ref. 24.

Although data is conflicting, several studies indicate that BMI per se is not a predictor of difficult intubation (21,22). A large neck circumference, however, has been associated with difficult intubation (21,23). Gonzalez et al. found a neck circumference >43 cm to have a sensitivity of 92% (20).

Summary
A thorough airway exam, including neck circumference, should be performed on every obese patient. As the predictive value of the physical exam is limited, the practitioner must always be prepared for the unanticipated difficult airway.

PREOXYGENATION
Positioning
Proper positioning of the obese patient prior to the induction of general anesthesia is critical. A decrease in functional residual capacity leads to faster oxygen desaturation during apnea (23). Prolonging non-hypoxic apnea time through adequate preoxygenation is a key component of safe airway management.

The reverse Trendelenburg position (approximately 20–25°) has been shown to increase the safe apnea period (24,25) (Table 2; Fig. 1). A foot board applied to the operating room bed will prevent the patient from sliding downward. A stand is often needed for the anesthetist as the patient's head will be elevated in this position. Some have advocated achieving a 20° to 25° incline by stacking blankets to create a ramp. While a suitable alternative, this technique may create uneven positioning of the patient and can be cumbersome as the blankets often have to be removed for proper surgical positioning, leaving the patient in a suboptimal position should airway difficulties arise during emergence.

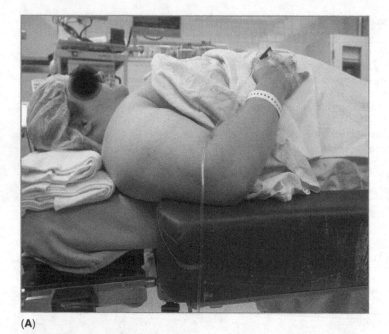

(A)

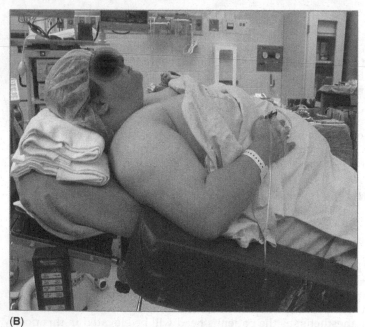

(B)

Figure 1   (A) This figure demonstrates the patient in the supine position. Reverse Trendelenburg of 20–25° as shown in (B) increases the safe apnea period, allowing for safer manipulation of the airway. A footboard (not shown) is necessary to prevent the patient from sliding down the operating table. *Source*: Pictures courtesy of Vilma E. Ortiz, MD.

Methods of Preoxygenation

The goal of preoxygenation is to displace nitrogen gas in the lungs with oxygen thereby increasing the oxygen stores available during apnea. A tight mask seal is needed to prevent the entrainment of room air and allow for adequate denitrogenation.

Fractional inspired oxygen of 1.0 should be instituted. High fresh gas flows of 10 L/min are needed for maximal preoxygenation, specifically when deep breath techniques are used (26).

Both vital capacity and tidal volume breathing preoxygenation techniques have been extensively studied (27–32). Tidal volume breathing for 3 to 5 minutes or 8 vital capacity breaths over 60 seconds is recommended. Only one study has evaluated the relative effectiveness of these techniques in the obese patient and found no difference between them (33).

The use of positive end-expiratory pressure (PEEP) during preoxygenation and mask ventilation prevents atelectasis and improves oxygenation (34). In addition, it may prolong time to desaturation (safe apnea period) by attenuating the reduction in FRC that occurs with the induction of general anesthesia. Its routine use during induction may depend in part on patient comfort.

Endpoints of Preoxygenation

The goal of preoxygenation is denitrogenation, as indicated by an end-tidal oxygen concentration >90% or end-tidal nitrogen concentration <5%. Most commonly, failure to achieve these endpoints is the result of improper mask seal or inadequate fresh gas flow.

MASK VENTILATION

Assuming no contraindications such as full stomach or gastro-esophageal reflux, mask ventilation is the initial technique employed in most instances of airway management. The supine obese patient provides a challenge in this regard as increased pressure is required to move the diaphragm caudad and increased fatty tissue can make securing a tight mask seal difficult. Early placement of an oral airway is often needed to prevent airway closure as pharyngeal tone is decreased during induction.

Two-hand mask ventilation may be required when large neck circumference or submandibular fat deposits are encountered. Care must be taken to avoid overinflating the stomach, particularly when mask ventilation is challenging. Proper positioning in the "sniffing" position can help align the major airway axes and create a patent airway. In addition, placing the patient in reverse Trendelenburg position can facilitate diaphragmatic excursion.

LARYNGEAL MASK AIRWAY

The laryngeal mask airway (LMA) has become a mainstay in airway management, securing a place as both a routine airway management device and a rescue device. Advantages include easy, quick placement with reliable results. Additionally, its use as a conduit to provide endotracheal intubation has been well documented. Limitations include a lack of protection against pulmonary aspiration, inadequate seal at high inflation pressures, and risk of laryngospasm.

Elective Use of LMA

Routine use of the LMA in the anesthetic management of obese patients is controversial. Some do not recommend its use secondary to a presumed increased risk of aspiration (35). Severe obesity is associated with gastro-esophageal reflux and motility disorders (36). However, the risk of pulmonary aspiration compared to lean patients is not well defined. Furthermore, no data defines a BMI beyond which aspiration risk is clearly increased. The incidence of aspiration associated with LMAs is estimated at 0.02% in all patients (37). Given the serious nature of this complication, it may be prudent to limit the use of LMAs in the severely obese to airway emergencies.

Obesity increases resistance of the respiratory system such that higher peak inspiratory pressures are required for ventilation (38). Higher pressures can cause leaking around the LMA, potentially causing hypoventilation and gastric insufflation. Nonetheless, positive pressure ventilation of the mildly obese with an LMA is feasible, although as discussed above, its safety is ill defined (39).

A new device, the ProSeal LMA (PLMA), involves a modification of the traditional LMA that includes an esophageal drain tube through which a gastric tube can be inserted. The PLMA has a higher leak pressure allowing higher peak inspiratory pressures to be used (39). Additionally, the esophageal vent may be used to drain regurgitated fluid. Both of these features may make this a better option for obese patients. However, a comparison of the LMA and PLMA devices did not show a demonstrable benefit of the PLMA (39).

Conduit for Intubation

The use of an LMA to provide a conduit for intubation is well described and can be an integral part of the difficult airway algorithm. The technical feasibility and safety of this maneuver in the obese has been studied. Frappier et al. demonstrated the effectiveness of the intubating LMA (ILMA) in 118 consecutive morbidly obese patients (BMI 45 kg/m^2) revealing 96.3% success rate (40). No adverse events were noted in this population; however, patients needing a rapid sequence induction (i.e., reflux symptoms) were excluded. Caution must be taken with this technique as at least one report describes an aspiration event upon manipulation of the LMA for intubation during emergent airway management (41).

LMA as a Rescue Device

The LMA is a well established airway rescue device and plays an integral role in the management of the difficult airway (3) (Appendix). While the obese population may be at increased risk for aspiration, the establishment of an airway is of obvious priority. To that end, the LMA can be a valuable tool to the practitioner and should be a part of every difficult airway cart (3).

Conclusion

The LMA is an invaluable tool for management of the difficult airway in lean and obese patients alike. The routine use of the LMA in the severely obese is controversial because of a presumed increased risk of aspiration. In addition, if positive pressure ventilation is needed, higher peak airway pressures may cause a leak around the LMA leading to gastric insufflation.

The ILMA provides another means by which the airway can be secured. It is well studied in obese patients and maybe useful as part of an algorithmic approach to airway management.

DIRECT LARYNGOSCOPY
Position
As discussed in detail already (See Preoxygenation section), correct patient positioning is imperative. Optimal position for laryngoscopy involves either reverse Trendelenburg or elevation of the back of the bed with the head in a sniffing position to align the oral, pharyngeal and laryngeal axes of the airway.

Equipment
The choice of laryngoscope blade has not been prospectively evaluated in the obese. However, newer devices allowing indirect laryngoscopy have been compared to traditional blades. A randomized trial comparing the Airtraq™ laryngoscope and Macintosh blades in the morbidly obese demonstrated a shorter intubation time and higher minimum oxygen saturation using the Airtraq™ device (42). Nonetheless, user preference and expertise remain the most significant factors when choosing a blade. A short handle maybe helpful as the large chest wall of some obese patients can interfere with placement of the blade in the mouth.

VIDEO-ASSISTED INTUBATION
Newer technologies allowing indirect visualization of the glottic opening by rigid and flexible fiberoptic devices can be useful given the higher probability of difficult intubation in the obese.

Rigid Fiberoptic Laryngoscopy
Video-laryngoscopy has been shown to improve the visualization of the larynx in severely obese patients and thus provides a useful technique in this population (43).

The LMA CTrach, a modified ILMA with continuous video has also been shown to be an efficient airway tool in severely obese patients (44). This technique is subject to the limitations, advantages, and disadvantages previously discussed in the section on LMAs.

Flexible Fiberoptic Laryngoscopy
Anatomic variation of the airway that may make intubation of the obese patient more difficult can be obviated with the use of a flexible fiberscope. Advantages include the ability to maneuver through difficult, redundant, hypertrophied soft tissue, and the relative ease of performing an awake intubation with this device. Disadvantages include the shorter safe apnea period in the anesthetized obese patient necessitating skillful, expeditious use of the fiberscope. Additionally, secretions and blood in the airway can preclude its use.

Other Specialized Equipment
Additional equipment such as the Bullard laryngoscope and lighted stylette are well described and prescribed techniques, though studies in obese patients are lacking. Thus their use in this population is largely dependent on user preference and experience. Table 3 lists a number of basic and more advanced techniques for airway management.

DIFFICULT AIRWAY ALGORITHM
As with any anesthetic, planning and preparing for a difficult airway is imperative when caring for the obese patient. This includes availability of a dedicated difficult

Table 3 Techniques for Difficult Airway Management[a]

Alternative laryngoscope blades
Awake intubation
Blind intubation
Fiberoptic intubation
Tube changer or stylette
Laryngeal mask airway alone or as conduit for intubation
Lighted stylette
Retrograde intubation
Surgical invasive airway
Rigid bronchoscopy with ventilation
Two person mask ventilation

Source: Adapted from Ref. 3.
[a]Additional techniques exist; this list is not intended to be comprehensive.

airway cart and extra personnel skilled in airway management. The ASA has published an algorithm to aid the care provider in this task (Appendix).

EXTUBATION

Factors such as ease of mask ventilation and intubation, length of surgery, and intra-operative fluid shifts play a role in the decision to extubate. Because obesity shortens the safe apnea period, maximizing both FRC volume and oxygen content may help prevent oxygen desaturation upon extubation. To this end, the patient should be placed in the semi-recumbent or reverse Trendelenburg position and allowed to breathe 100% oxygen prior to extubation. Given that these patients are prone to airway obstruction, a fully awake patient will help maintain a patent airway. One can also consider the placement of a nasopharyngeal airway prior to extubation. Additionally, the clinician must ensure a full recovery of neuromuscular function. Care should be taken not to interpret non-purposeful movement as a sign of wakefulness. Spontaneous respiration at a rate >12 to 14 is ideal. A rate <12 may suggest narcosis necessitating opioid reversal or delay in extubation.

In those patients with obstructive sleep apnea, extubation directly to non-invasive positive pressure ventilation may be needed (10).

Lastly, equipment and personnel must be available for reintubation. This is of particular concern in those patients with a history of obstructive sleep apnea. In this patient population, the risk of life-threatening post-extubation obstruction requiring reintubation was 5% in one review (10).

APPENDIX

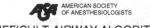

AMERICAN SOCIETY
OF ANESTHESIOLOGISTS

DIFFICULT AIRWAY ALGORITHM

1. Assess the likelihood and clinical impact of basic management problems:
   A. Difficult ventilation
   B. Difficult intubation
   C. Difficult with patient cooperation or consent
   D. Difficult tracheostomy
2. Actively pursue opportunities to deliver supplemental oxygen throughout the process of difficult airway management
3. Consider the relative merits and feasibility of basic management choices:

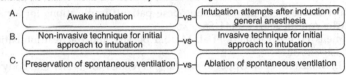

A. Awake intubation —vs— Intubation attempts after induction of general anesthesia

B. Non-invasive technique for initial approach to intubation —vs— Invasive technique for initial approach to intubation

C. Preservation of spontaneous ventilation —vs— Ablation of spontaneous ventilation

4. Develop primary and alternative strategies:

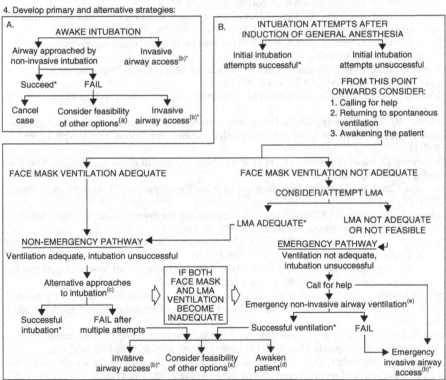

* Confirm ventilation, tracheal intubation, or LMA placement with exhaled CO_2

a. Other options include (but are not limited to): surgery utilizing face mask or LMA anesthesia, local anesthesia infiltration or regional nerve blockade. Pursuit of these options usually implies that mask ventilation will not be problematic. Therefore, these options may be of limited value if this step in the algorithm has been reached via the emergency pathway.
b. Invasive airway access includes surgical or percutaneous tracheatomy or cricothyrotomy

c. Alternative non-invasive approaches to difficult intubation include (out are not limited to): use of different laryngoscope blades, LMA as an intubation conduit (with or without fiberoptic guidance), fiberoptic intubation, inbating stylet or tube changer, light wand, retrograde intubation, and blind oral or nasal intubation.
d. Consider re-preparation of the patient for awake intubation or canceling surgery.
e. Options for emergency non-invasive airway ventilation include (but are not limited to): rigid bronchoscope, esophageal-tracheal combitube ventilation, or transtracheal jet ventialtion.

Source: From Ref. 3.

REFERENCES

1. Caplan RA, Posner KL, Ward RJ, et al. Adverse respiratory events in anesthesia: a closed claims analysis. Anesthesiology 1990; 72: 828–33.
2. Peterson GN, Domino KB, Caplan RA, et al. Management of the difficult airway: a closed claims analysis. Anesthesiology 2005; 103: 33–9.
3. Practice guidelines for the management of the difficult airway: an updated report by the American Society of Anesthesiologists Task Force on Management of the Difficult Airway. Anesthesiology 2003; 98: 1269–77.
4. Voyagis GS, Kyriakis KP, Dimitriou V, et al. Value of oropharyngeal Mallampati classification in predicting difficult laryngoscopy among obese patients. Eur J Anaesthesiol 1998; 15: 330–4.
5. Benumof JL. Obstructive sleep apnea in the obese patient: implications for airway management. J Clin Anesth 2001; 13: 144–56.
6. Brodsky J, Lemmens H, Brock-Utne J, et al. Morbid obesity and tracheal intubation. Anesth Analg 2002; 94: 732–6.
7. Busetto L, Calo E, Mazza M, et al. Upper airway size is related to obesity and body fat distribution in women. Eur Arch Otorhinolaryngol 2008.
8. White DP, Lombard RM, Cadieux RJ, et al. Pharyngeal resistance in normal humans: an influence of gender, age and obesity. J App Phys 1985; 58: 365–71.
9. Shelton KE, Woodson H, Gay S, et al. Pharyngeal fat in obstructive sleep apnea. Am Rev Respir Dis 1993; 148: 462–6.
10. Benumof JL. Obstructive sleep apnea in the adult obese patient: implications for airway management. J Clin Anesth 2001; 13: 145–56.
11. Koenig JS, Thach BT. Effects of mass loading on the upper airway. J App Phys, 1988; 64: 2294–9.
12. Davies RJ, Stradling JR. The relationship between neck circumference, radiographic pharyngeal anatomy and the obstructive sleep apnea syndrome. Eur Respir J 1990; 3: 509–14.
13. Langeron O, Masso E, Huraux C, et al. Prediction of difficult mask ventilation. Anesthesiology 2000; 92: 1229–36.
14. Van de Graaf W. Thoracic influence on upper airway patency. J App Phys 1988; 65: 2124–31.
15. Hiremath AS, Hillman DR, James AL, et al. Relationship between difficult tracheal intubation and obstructive sleep apnea. Br J Anaesth 1998; 80: 606–11.
16. Kheterpal S. Han R. Tremper K, et al. Incidence and predictors of difficult and impossible mask ventilation. Anesthesiology 2006; 105: 885–91.
17. Chung F, Yegneswaran B, Liao P, et al. STOP questionnaire: a tool to screen patients for obstructive sleep apnea. Anesthesiology 2008; 108: 812–21.
18. Shiga T, Wajima Z, Inoue T, et al. Predicting difficult intubation in apparently normal patients: a meta-analysis of bedside screening test performance. Anesthesiology 2005; 103: 429–37.
19. Lee A, Fan LT, Gin T, et al. A systematic review (meta-analysis) of the accuracy of the Mallampati tests to predict the difficult airway. Anes Analg 2006; 102: 1867–78.
20. Gonzalez H, Minville V, Delanoue K, et al. The importance of increased neck circumference to intubation difficulties in obese patients. Anes Analg 2008; 106: 1132–6.
21. Ezri T, Medalion B, Weisenberg M, et al. Increased body mass index is not a predictor of difficult laryngoscopy. Can J Anes 2002; 50: 179–83.
22. Brodsky J, Lemmens H, Brock-Utne J, et al. Morbid obesity and tracheal intubation. Anes Analg 2002; 94: 732–6.
23. Jense H, Dubin S, Silverstein P, et al. Effect of obesity on safe duration of apnea in anesthetized humans. Anes Analg 1991; 72: 89–93.
24. Dixon B, Dixon J, Carden J, Burn A, et al. Preoxygenation is more effective in the 25° head-up position than in the supine position in severely obese patients. Anesthesiology 2005; 102: 1110–15.

25. Lane S, Saunders D, Schofield A, et al. A prospective, randomized controlled trial comparing the efficacy of pre-oxygenation in the 20° head-up vs supine position. Anesthesiology 2005; 60: 1064–7.

26. Nimmagadda U, Chiravuri S, Salem R, et al. Preoxygenation with tidal volume and deep breathing techniques: the impact of duration of breathing and fresh gas flow. Anes Analg 2001; 92: 1337–41.

27. Gold MI, Durate I, Muravchick S. Arterial oxygenation in conscious patients after 5 minutes and after 30 seconds of oxygen breathing. Anesth Analg 1981; 60: 313–15.

28. Goldberg ME, Norris MC, Laryani GE, et al. Preoxygenation in the morbidly obese: a comparison of two techniques. Anesth Analg 1989; 68: 520–2.

29. Norris MC, Dewan DM. Preoxygenation for cesarean section: a comparison of two techniques. Anesthesiology, 1985; 62: 827–9.

30. Gambee AM, Hertzka R, Fisher D. Preoxygenation techniques: comparison of three minutes and 4 breaths. Anesth Analg 1987; 66: 468–70.

31. Valentine SJ, Marjot R, Monk CR. Preoxygenation in the elderly: a comparison of the 4-maximal breath and 3-minute techniques. Anesth Analg 1990; 71: 516–19.

32. McCarthy G, Elliott P, Mirakhur K, et al. A comparison of different preoxygenation techniques in the elderly. Anaesth 1991; 46: 824–7.

33. Rapapot S, Joannes-Boyau O, Bazin R, et al. Comparison of eight deep breaths and tidal volume breathing preoxygenation techniques in morbid obese patients. Ann Fr Anesth Reanim 2004; 23: 1155–9.

34. Coussa M, Proietti S, Schnyder P, et al. Prevention of atelectasis formation during the induction of general anesthesia in morbidly obese patients. Anes Analg 2004; 98: 1491–5.

35. Brimacombe J, Brain AIJ, Berry A. The Laryngeal Mask Airway: Review and Practical Guide. London: WB Saunders, 1997.

36. Suter M, Dorta G, Giusti V, et al. Gastro-esophageal reflux and esophageal motility disorders in morbidly obese patients. Obesity Surgery. 2004; 14: 959–66.

37. Brimacombe J, Berry A. The incidence of aspiration associated with the laryngeal mask airway —a meta-analysis of published literature. J Clin Anesth. 1995; 7: 297–305.

38. Pelosi P, Croci M, Ravagnan I, et al. The effects of body mass on lung volumes, respiratory mechanics, and gas exchange during general anesthesia. Anesth Analg 1998; 87: 654–60.

39. Natalini G, Franceschetti M, Pantelidi M, et al. Comparison of the standard laryngeal mask airway and the ProSeal laryngeal mask airway in obese patients. Br J Anaesth 2003; 90: 323–6.

40. Frappier J, Guenoun T, et al. Airway management using the intubating laryngeal mask airway for the morbidly obese patient. Anesth Analg 2003; 96: 1510–15.

41. Abdi W, Ndoko S, Amathieu R, et al. Evidence of pulmonary aspiration during difficult airway management of a morbidly obese patient with the LMA CTrach™. Br J Anaesth 2008; 100: 275–7.

42. Ndoko S, Amathieu R, Tual L, et al. Tracheal intubation of morbidly obese patients: a randomized trial comparing performance of Macintosh and Airtraq™ laryngoscopes. Br J Anaesth 2008; 100: 263–8.

43. Marrel J, Blanc C, Frascarolo P, et al. Videolaryngoscopy improves intubation condition in morbidly obese patients. Eur J Anesth. 2007; 24: 1045–9.

44. Dhonneur G, Ndoko S, Yavchitz A, et al. Tracheal intubation of morbidly obese patients: LMA CTrach vs direct laryngoscopy. Br J Anaesth 2006; 97: 742–5.

11 | Perioperative Monitoring of the Obese Patient

Hovig V. Chitilian

Instructor in Anesthesia, Harvard Medical School, Assistant in Anesthesia, Department of Anesthesia and Critical Care, Massachusetts General Hospital, Boston, Massachusetts, U.S.A.

INTRODUCTION
The ASA (American Society of Anesthesiologists) standards of monitoring require the presence of a qualified anesthesia provider as well as the continual evaluation of a patient's oxygenation, ventilation, circulation, and temperature (1). These standards apply to all patients who are undergoing an anesthetic. Although obesity is associated with a greater number of comorbidities, the presence of obesity, in and of itself, is not an indication for additional monitoring (2). This chapter will address some of the unique considerations that apply to obese patients for intraoperative and postoperative monitoring.

MONITORING OXYGENATION
Pulse oximetry is used for the intraoperative and postoperative monitoring of oxygenation. The reported incidence of obstructive sleep apnea (OSA) in the obese patient population ranges from 40% to 90% (3). However, even in the absence of polysomnographically confirmed OSA, morbidly obese patients are at increased risk for postoperative hypoxemia (4). The ASA practice guidelines for the perioperative management of patients with OSA (2006) recommend continuous pulse oximetry monitoring of hospitalized patients who are at risk for OSA following their discharge from the recovery room (5). Continuous monitoring with pulse oximetry in the postoperative period should be maintained as long as patients remain at increased risk for airway compromise (5).

MONITORING VENTILATION
Capnography is used to monitor ventilation intraoperatively. Ventilation–perfusion mismatch in severely obese patients may reduce the accuracy with which end-tidal carbon dioxide ($ETCO_2$) reflects arterial carbon dioxide tension ($PaCO_2$) (6).

Transcutaneous CO_2 ($TcCO_2$) pressure monitoring has been shown to accurately estimate $PaCO_2$ in patients with BMI > $40\,kg/m^2$ (7). One study of 30 severely obese patients (BMI > $35\;kg/m^2$) showed $TcCO_2$ to be more accurate than $ETCO_2$ at estimating $PaCO_2$. However, the reported differences were small and of questionable clinical significance (6).

MONITORING CIRCULATION
Arterial Pressure
Arterial blood pressure is used as a surrogate measure of organ perfusion. A properly sized blood pressure cuff is essential for accurate measurements. The bladder length should be approximately 80% of the upper arm circumference. The bladder width

should be approximately 40% of the upper arm circumference (8). The American Heart Association recommends the following cuff sizes based on arm circumference (8):

Arm circumference (cm)	Cuff size (cm × cm)
27–34	16 × 30
35–44	16 × 36
45–52	16 × 42

In the instance where a patient's upper arm is either conically shaped or too short to accommodate the appropriate cuff size, blood pressure measurements may be taken using a forearm cuff, a wrist-mounted blood pressure measuring device, or an intra-arterial catheter (9). One study comparing arterial blood pressure monitoring methods in overweight intensive care unit patients found that oscillometric blood pressure measurements underestimate intra-arterial blood pressure readings (10).

Central Venous and Intracardiac Pressures
The use of invasive cardiac monitoring should be guided by the clinical circumstances. Obesity, in and of itself, is not an indication for central venous or intracardiac pressure monitoring. Central venous catheters and introducers must be of sufficient length to insure that all lumens are positioned intravascularly (11). Obesity has been associated with an increased risk of mechanical complications during internal jugular vein cannulation (12). The use of ultrasound-guidance should be considered to aid in central venous cannulation (2).

AWARENESS
Analysis of the ASA Closed Claims Project data has identified morbid obesity as a factor associated with recall during general anesthesia (13). However, other studies have not found an association between increased BMI and intraoperative awareness (14,15). Two studies describing the use of the bispectral index (BIS) monitor in the care of obese patients have suggested that BIS-targeted dosing of anesthetic agents results in shorter emergence and extubation times (16,17). According to the ASA practice advisory for intraoperative awareness and brain function monitoring, routine brain function monitoring is not indicated for patients receiving general anesthesia (18).

NEUROMUSCULAR FUNCTION
The dosing of neuromuscular blocking agents based on actual body weight results in a prolongation of action in obese patients (19). As obese patients are at increased risk for postoperative respiratory complications (20), full reversal of neuromuscular blockade should be verified prior to extubation. Murphy et al. suggest the superiority of acceleromyography to qualitative train-of-four assessment; however, no studies to date have specifically examined monitoring of neuromuscular blockade in obese patients (21).

TEMPERATURE
No studies have specifically looked at the effects of general anesthesia on thermoregulation in obese patients compared to controls. Intraoperative hypothermia has been associated with surgical wound infection, coagulopathy, myocardial infarction, and delayed postanesthetic recovery (22). Given the morbidity associated with

intraoperative hypothermia, body temperature should be measured in all patients receiving general anesthesia for greater than 30 minutes. Core temperature can be measured in the distal esophagus, nasopharynx, tympanic membrane, or pulmonary artery (23).

REFERENCES

1. ASA. Standards for basic anesthetic monitoring. 2005. [Available from: http://www.asahq.org/publicationsAndServices/standards/02.pdf].
2. Passannante AN, Rock P. Anesthetic management of patients with obesity and sleep apnea. Anesthesiol Clin North America 2005; 23: 479–91.
3. Lopez PP, Stefan B, Schulman CI, et al. Prevalence of sleep apnea in morbidly obese patients who presented for weight loss surgery evaluation: more evidence for routine screening for obstructive sleep apnea before weight loss surgery. Am Surg 2008; 74: 834–8.
4. Ahmad S, Nagle A, McCarthy RJ, et al. Postoperative hypoxemia in morbidly obese patients with and without obstructive sleep apnea undergoing laparoscopic bariatric surgery. Anesth Analg 2008; 107: 138–43.
5. Gross JB, Bachenberg KL, Benumof JL, et al. Practice guidelines for the perioperative management of patients with obstructive sleep apnea: a report by the American society of anesthesiologist task force on perioperative management of patients with obstructive sleep apnea. Anesthesiology 2006; 104: 1081–93.
6. Griffin J, Terry BE, Burton RK, et al. Comparison of end-tidal and transcutaneous measures of carbon dioxide during general anesthesia in severely obese adults. Br J Anaesth 2003; 91: 498–501.
7. Maniscalco M, Zedda A, Faraone S, et al. Evaluation of a transcutaneous carbon dioxide monitor in severe obesity. Intensive Care Med 2008; 34: 1340–4.
8. Pickering TG, Hall JE, Appel LJ, et al. Recommendations for blood pressure measurement in humans and experimental animals. Part 1: Blood pressure measurement in humans: a statement for professionals from the Subcommittee of Professional and Public Education of the American Heart Association Council on High Blood Pressure Research. Circulation 2005; 111: 697–716.
9. de Senarclens O, Feihl F, Giusti V, et al. Brachial or wrist blood pressure in obese patients: which is best? Monit 2008; 13: 149–51.
10. Araghi A, Bander JJ, Guzman JA. Arterial blood pressure monitoring in overweight critically ill patients: invasive or noninvasive? Crit Care 2006; 10: R64.
11. Ottestad E, Schmiessing C, Brock-Utne JG, et al. Central venous access in obese patients: a potential complication. Anesth Analg 2006; 102: 1293.
12. Karakitsos D, Labropoulos N, De Groot E, et al. Real-time ultrasound-guided catheterisation of the internal jugular vein: a prospective comparison with the landmark technique in critical care patients. Crit Care 2006; 10: 162–9.
13. Domino KB, Posner KL, Caplan RA, et al. Awareness during anesthesia: a closed claims analysis. Anesthesiology 1999; 90: 1053–61.
14. Wennervirta J, Ranta S and Hynynen M. Awareness and recall in outpatient anesthesia. Anesth Analg 2002; 95: 72–7.
15. Sandin RH, Enlund G, Samuelsson P, et al. Awareness during anaesthesia: a prospective case study. Lancet 2000; 355: 707–11.
16. Pandazi A, Bourlioti A and Kostopanagiotou G. Bispectral index (BIS) monitoring in morbidly obese patients undergoing gastric bypass surgery: experience in 23 patients. Obes Surg 2005; 15: 58–62.
17. Ibraheim O, Alshaer A, El-Dawlaty A, et al. Effect of bispectral index (BIS) monitoring on postoperative recovery and sevoflurane consumption among morbidly obese patients undergoing laparoscopic gastric banding. Middle East J Anesthesiol 2008; 19: 819–30.

18. Apfelbaum JL, Arens JF, Cole DJ, et al. Practice advisory for intraoperative awareness and brain function monitoring: a report by the American Society of Anesthesiologists Task Force on Intraoperative Awareness. Anesthesiology 2006; 104: 847–64.
19. Casati A, Putzu M. Anesthesia in the obese patient: pharmacokinetic considerations. J Clin Anesth 2005; 17: 134–45.
20. Rose DK, Cohen MM, Wigglesworth DF, et al. Critical respiratory events in the postanesthesia care unit. Patient, surgical, and anesthetic factors. Anesthesiology 1994; 81: 410–18.
21. Murphy GS, Szokol JW, Marymont JH, et al. Intraoperative acceleromyographic monitoring reduces the risk of residual neuromuscular blockade and adverse respiratory events in the postanesthesia care unit. Anesthesiology 2008; 109: 389–98.
22. Hannenberg AA, Sessler DI. Improving perioperative temperature management. Anesth Analg 2008; 107: 1454–57.
23. Sessler DI. Temperature monitoring and perioperative thermoregulation. Anesthesiology 2008; 109: 318–38.

12 | Physiologic Changes with Pneumoperitoneum in the Obese Patient

Lorenzo Berra[1] and William R. Kimball[2]

[1]Clinical Fellow in Anesthesia, Harvard Medical School, Resident, Department of Anesthesia and Critical Care, Massachusetts General Hospital, Boston, Massachusetts, U.S.A.

[2]Assistant Professor of Anesthesia and Critical Care, Harvard Medical School, Associate Anesthetist, Department of Anesthesia and Critical Care, Massachusetts General Hospital, Boston, Massachusetts, U.S.A.

INTRODUCTION

Initial studies of physiologic changes during laparoscopy addressed normal females undergoing gynecologic surgery, while subsequent studies investigated laparoscopic cholecystectomy. Such studies are not directly comparable because of body position differences (Trendelenburg vs. reverse Trendelenburg). Other differences included patient age, medical comorbidities, and factors such as preoperative hydration. More recently, the ability to insufflate gas outside the peritoneal cavity has extended such techniques to other operations. Most studies of physiologic changes during pneumoperitoneum in obese subjects are recent. This chapter will address changes during laparoscopy while emphasizing specific impacts on obese subjects. Most of these data relate to weight loss operations.

RESPIRATORY SYSTEM

During inspiration, either spontaneous or via positive pressure ventilation, both the lungs and the chest wall expand leading to expansion of both the rib cage and abdomen. The pressure change within the rib cage and abdomen is identical, but each structure's volumetric expansion will be proportional to its individual compliance, presuming the amount of blood within these structures remains constant.

Insufflating gas into the abdomen (pneumoperitoneum) increases intra-abdominal pressure. The incremental pressure rise for an identical volumetric increase becomes progressively larger (the abdomen becomes less compliant). Assessing changes in lung function during pneumoperitoneum must consider the amount intra-abdominal pressure rises. Pneumoperitoneum will decrease respiratory system compliance through its impact on both the abdominal and rib cage components. The lungs may be impacted less since they are contained by the rib cage and abdomen (through the diaphragm), impeding lung expansion.

Respiratory System Mechanical Properties

Abdominal Pressure Change

For non-obese subjects, insufflation with 4.45 liters generates a pressure of 15 mmHg. Further insufflation of 2.3 liters increases the pressure to 30 mmHg. Abdominal compliance during distension decreases from about 218 ml/cm H_2O at 15 mmHg to 113 ml/cm H_2O at 30 mmHg.

There are no data to describe the abdominal pressure–volume characteristic of obese subjects, although their abdomen should be less compliant than in lean subjects—a similar insufflating pressure would lead to smaller volumes of insufflated gas. Opening abdominal pressure (before starting insufflation) increases with body mass index (BMI)—about $0.07\,mmHg/kg/m^2$—although there is wide variability. Intra-abdominal pressure is directly related to chest wall elastance—the higher intra-abdominal pressure, the higher the chest wall elastance (1). Insufflating the abdomen to $13.6\,mmHg$ increases intra-abdominal pressure as measured by a bladder catheter. The increase is smaller when the lungs are inflated with 10 cm H_2O positive end expiratory pressure (PEEP), suggesting that pressure-limited pneumoperitoneum competes with other activities that impact abdominal volume (2).

Functional Residual Capacity (FRC)

FRC is the volume in the lungs at end exhalation. FRC decreases with induction of general anesthesia, being higher in reverse Trendelenburg and least in the Trendelenburg position.

Pneumoperitoneum further reduces FRC. The decrease depends on body position and volume of, or pressure within, the pneumoperitoneum. The larger the pneumoperitoneum volume, the more the FRC falls (2). Normal-weight subjects have higher FRC than the obese; pneumoperitoneum may create reductions of 20%. Since FRC is largest in the reverse Trendelenburg position before insufflation, the decrease in FRC caused by pneumoperitoneum will be more pronounced in the reverse Trendelenburg position than in Trendelenburg. Compared to the supine position, the "beach chair" position (produced by 30° reverse Trendelenburg with legs lifted to the abdomen) may increase FRC (2).

Peak Inspiratory Pressure (PIP)

PIP comprises pressure generated by volumetric expansion of the lung and chest wall (compliance), and flow-rate related changes (flow-dependent or resistive properties) of the lungs. The chest wall "resistive" contribution is negligible. For a fixed tidal volume, PIP increases between 40% and 70% with pneumoperitoneum. The increase is similar for obese and non-obese subjects.

Compartment Compliances

Compliance measurements are the inverse of elastance measurements. Both types of measurements have been reported in clinical studies. In normal weight subjects, intra-abdominal insufflation to 15 and $25\,mmHg$ (3) causes:

1. Chest wall compliance to decrease almost four-fold
2. Lung compliance to decrease about two-fold
3. For pressures up to 15 mmHg, lung compliance decreases more in the Trendelenberg position than in reverse Trendelenberg. Decreases in chest wall elastance are independent of position

For a pneumoperitoneum pressure increase from 0 to 15 mmHg, subjects with higher BMI (within a range of $20–31.7\,kg/m^2$) have progressively worse pulmonary compliance but smaller changes in chest wall compliance than subjects in the lower BMI range. Pneumoperitoneum-induced compliance changes for normal-weight subjects are almost completely reversible upon termination of insufflation.

Lung elastance is about 75% higher than chest wall elastance for obese subjects. This is independent of body position or addition of 10 cm H_2O PEEP (2). Pneumoperitoneum of $13.6\,mmHg$ causes lung and chest wall elastance to become almost equal because chest wall elastance almost doubles. This is not affected by addition of 10 cm H_2O PEEP or patient position (2).

Static Respiratory System Compliance
This comprises lung and chest wall compliance but excludes flow-resistive properties. Obese subjects have about 30% lower respiratory system compliance than normal subjects. Pneumoperitoneum reduces static compliance by about 40% for both normal-weight and obese subjects (2,4).

Inspiratory Resistance
Airway resistance increases as lung volume decreases. Resistance of the lung behaves in a similar manner. Pneumoperitoneum increases inspiratory resistance, while changing body position produces relatively small resistance changes. Inspiratory resistance increases by 18% to 72% during pneumoperitoneum (2,4,5).

Dynamic Respiratory System Compliance
This is computed as the ratio of tidal volume to PIP. There is no end-inspiratory pause to allow flow-resistive pressure components to dissipate. It decreases by 20–30% during pneumoperitoneum (6).

Esophageal Pressure
Esophageal pressure is higher in supine obese subjects than in normal weight subjects (7). It increases more with 15 mmHg pneumoperitoneum in supine obese subjects than in normal weight subjects (7).

Gas Exchange Properties
Carbon Dioxide Levels
Carboperitoneum (insufflating CO_2) increases pulmonary CO_2 excretion due to gas absorption. CO_2 excretion may be higher for extraperitoneal CO_2 insufflation than for CO_2 pneumoperitoneum.

End-Tidal CO_2 (ETCO$_2$)
$ETCO_2$ may change exponentially during CO_2 pneumoperitoneum if alveolar ventilation remains constant. Subcutaneous emphysema can develop from escaped insufflating CO_2 and may contribute to extensive and prolonged rises in CO_2 excretion. $ETCO_2$ may remain elevated in the recovery room as CO_2 washout continues after evacuation of CO_2 pneumoperitoneum. Given a constant airway dead space, in order to maintain a constant $ETCO_2$ by increasing minute ventilation during CO_2 pneumoperitoneum, proportionally larger increases will be required for respiratory rate than for tidal volume.

Arterial to End-Tidal CO_2 Difference ($P_{a-ET}CO_2$)
$P_{a-ET}CO_2$ remains essentially unchanged during pneumoperitoneum for normal-weight subjects (1). In obese subjects it is increased by about 50%. Increasing tidal volume may decrease $P_{a-ET}CO_2$ in obese subjects. Interestingly, an increase in $P_{a-ET}CO_2$ with larger tidal volumes has been observed in lean subjects (8).

Dead Space to Tidal Volume Ratio (V_D/V_T)
V_D/V_T is not affected by pneumoperitoneum. It is much larger for obese than normal subjects (1).

Respiratory Quotient

It is the ratio of minute O_2 consumption to minute CO_2 excretion. As oxygen consumption remains essentially constant during pneumoperitoneum, this quotient rises from a "normal" of about 0.8 to >1.0 as CO_2 is absorbed from insufflated gas.

Arterial Shunt (Q_S/Q_T)

Studies involving pneumoperitoneum in subjects with normal BMI have shown a slight decrease in arterial shunt (9).

Alveolar to Arterial Oxygen Difference ($P_{A-a}O_2$)

$P_{A-a}O_2$ may increase or even slightly decrease for normal-weight subjects during pneumoperitoneum. A change in $P_{A-a}O_2$ during pneumoperitoneum probably depends upon whether atelectasis can be prevented, such as by maintaining alveolar nitrogen concentrations (rather than using nitrous oxide), or whether PEEP provides more alveolar recruitment than overdistension.

Arterial Oxygen Pressure (P_aO_2)

Obese subjects may increase P_aO_2 during pneumoperitoneum (2) while normal-weight subjects usually do not exhibit such improvement, despite some reports (above) of decreasing shunt (9).

Other Respiratory Issues
Mechanical Ventilation Strategies

Pressure controlled ventilation (PCV) may provide better gas exchange than volume controlled ventilation (VCV) for obese patients during laparoscopy. When both modalities are set to provide similar levels of ventilation (tidal volume, minute ventilation, plateau pressure, PEEP, and peritoneal pressure) (10):

- PCV has lower $P_{a-ET}CO_2$, $P_{A-a}O_2$, P_aCO_2 and higher P_aO_2 and P_aO_2/FiO_2 (fraction of inspired oxygen) values
- These differences were attributed to better matching of ventilation to perfusion
- There were no differences in respiratory resistance, dynamic compliance, dead space, CO_2 production, or O_2 consumption

By contrast, while maintaining a constant minute ventilation and $ETCO_2$ during abdominal insufflation (11):

- There were no meaningful differences between PCV and VCV for peak or plateau pressure, mean airway pressure, compliance, or resistance
- VCV produced higher P_aO_2, lower P_aCO_2, lower $P_{ET}CO_2$ and lower $P_{a-ET}CO_2$ values

In normal-weight patients undergoing laparoscopic radical prostatectomy, switching ventilation from VCV to PCV while maintaining identical tidal volumes resulted in (12):

- No differences in plateau pressure, respiratory system compliance, $ETCO_2$, arterial CO_2, estimated V_D/V_T, P_aO_2/FiO_2
- Smaller peak airway pressure, greater airflow rates, larger mean airway pressure, and larger dynamic respiratory system compliances with PCV versus VCV
- No change in left ventricular end systolic wall stress, the velocity-time integral for pulmonary arterial flow, or right ventricular stroke volume

Endotracheal Tube (ETT) Positioning
Pneumoperitoneum may lead to movement of the ETT tip (13). Passive ETT advances may be more common in obese subjects undergoing laparoscopy in the head-down position than in obese patients undergoing "open" surgery. ETT movement into a mainstem bronchus, even the right mainstem bronchus, did not lead to significant changes in peripheral hemoglobin saturation as measured by pulse oximetry (S_pO_2), $ETCO_2$, or PIP measurements in one study (13). However, this finding differs from the clinical observation of a decrease in S_pO_2 commonly observed with migration of the ETT into the right mainstem bronchus of obese patients undergoing laparoscopic surgery.

Atelectasis
Compared to lean patients, atelectasis (assessed by computed tomography) is more common in obese subjects. While both normal and obese subjects develop atelectasis postoperatively, when measured immediately following laparoscopic surgery, increases in the amount of atelectatic lung tissue are greater for obese subjects. Such atelectasis persists longer into the recovery period for obese subjects, while it may resolve within twenty-fours of surgery for normal weight patients.

CARDIOVASCULAR SYSTEM
Pneumoperitoneum, by affecting both the diaphragm and rib cage, will impact the heart through changes in intrathoracic pressure and cardiac orientation. In addition, abdominal insufflation changes blood volume within, and blood flow through the abdomen. The cardiovascular effects of pneumoperitoneum also result from indirect effects, such as those produced by reflexes or hormonal release.

Furthermore, the hemodynamic effects of pneumoperitoneum depend upon prior fluid hydration status and the level of insufflation pressure. Many studies do not describe preoperative fluid status when assessing changes induced by pneumoperitoneum. This chapter will describe studies where preoperative fluid replacement was assessed. Lower pressure levels (<10 mmHg) produce limited impact on inferior vena cava flow, while very high values (>20) substantially impair venous return through the vena cava. Most insufflation pressures are between about 12 and 18 mmHg.

Heart Rate
Obese subjects, similar to normal weight subjects, have small and insignificant changes in heart rate during pneumoperitoneum.

Mean Arterial Pressure (MAP)
MAP is influenced by changes in cardiac output and systemic vascular resistance. Abdominal insufflation in the supine or reverse Trendelenburg position generally increases MAP by 30% in normal weight patients (14). In normal-weight subjects, abdominal exposure produced by "gasless laparoscopy" (abdominal wall lift) results in slightly lower MAP than pneumoperitoneum. The Trendelenburg position leads to higher MAP than the supine position, while reverse Trendelenburg leads to lower MAP than the supine position for both groups (15). Obese subjects, in contrast to normal weight subjects, may have either small changes in MAP during pneumoperitoneum or increases of up to 40% (6).

Changes in arterial pressure waveform amplitude (ΔP) during mechanical ventilation may indicate volumetric status (7). Pneumoperitoneum increases ΔP for normal subjects but not for obese subjects. This might be due to the larger, initial intra-abdominal pressure in obese subjects. Combining pneumoperitoneum with the reverse Trendelenburg position increases ΔP for obese subjects, but does not create additional increases for normal subjects.

Cardiac Output or Cardiac Index

Cardiac output does not change substantially with time after onset of pneumoperitoneum. Compared to pneumoperitoneum, abdominal exposure produced by "gasless laparoscopy" (abdominal wall lift) of normal-weight subjects results in unchanged cardiac output. These changes are independent of patient position: supine, Trendelenburg, and reverse Trendelenburg. However, the power to detect a change in this study may have been insufficient (15).

Studies of patients with cardiac disease report a sustained reduction of cardiac output after pneumoperitoneum. These decreases did not achieve statistical significance and appeared to be relatively well tolerated in these small samples (16,17). Although some studies report a cardiac output increase with onset of pneumoperitoneum, in general both obese and lean subjects exhibit no change in cardiac output.

Systemic Vascular Resistance (SVR) = (MAP – CVP)/Cardiac Output

SVR rises substantially for supine, normal weight patients during abdominal insufflation. The increase is greater than that observed in the Trendelenburg position. In patients with normal BMI, SVR may decrease with time after initiation of pneumoperitoneum, but decreases are small and variable. The SVR response in obese patients during pneumoperitoneum is similar to that described for normal-weight subjects.

Pulmonary Vascular Resistance = (mPAP – PCWP)/Cardiac Output

Changes during pneumoperitoneum vary widely, both in normal and obese subjects.

Cardiac Filling Pressures (when referenced to the position of the left atrium as body position changes)

Pressure outside the pericardium (pleural pressure) increases during pneumoperitoneum—probably in proportion to the resultant decrease in FRC—although its relation to FRC change has not been studied directly. Translocation of splanchnic vascular volume to intrathoracic structures also may contribute to rises in cardiac filling pressure during pneumoperitoneum.

Central Venous Pressure (CVP)

CVP increases with pneumoperitoneum in both obese and in patients with normal BMI. In normal-weight subjects, pneumoperitoneum induces a greater proportional increase from baseline CVP in the reverse Trendelenburg compared to the supine position. The increase is least in the Trendelenburg position, due to substantial differences in baseline CVP. CVP changes, relative to changes in pneumoperitoneum pressure, may be almost independent of position.

Pulmonary Capillary Wedge Pressure (PCWP)

PCWP increases with pneumoperitoneum. Compared to CVP measurements, pneumoperitoneum induces slightly smaller increases in PCWP relative to values before insufflation. For normal-weight patients, pneumoperitoneum-induced changes of PCWP from baseline levels are greatest for those in reverse Trendelenburg and least for supine patients. Obese subjects, similar to normal weight subjects, have increases in PCWP during pneumoperitoneum.

Echocardiographic Measurements
These data should be interpreted in light of their numerous limitations.

1. Studies include either 2D or 3D echocardiograms. Since cardiac axis changes with pneumoperitoneum, multiplane transesophageal echocardiographic probes may provide more accurate evaluations (18).
2. Body position changes usually are determined in a non-randomized, predetermined order. The reader must presume there are no time-dependent changes independent of body position.
3. Studies may lack power to detect changes, while differences in factors such as anesthetic, order of change, and time allowed to detect a change, further limit applying these results to specific patient groups.
4. Small changes in end-diastolic areas and/or wall end-diastolic stresses, despite large changes in end-diastolic pressures (CVP or PCWP), may indicate that pressure measurements do not reflect changes in cardiac function (18).

Left Ventricle End-Diastolic Area (LVEDA)/Volume
Pneumoperitoneum in anesthetized, supine, normal-weight patients may either increase or produce no change in dimensions. In normal-weight patients, pneumoperitoneum produces minimal changes during shifts from supine to the Trendelenburg position. Shifts from supine to reverse Trendelenburg produce either no change or a decrease in dimensions. Compared to pneumoperitoneum, abdominal exposure produced by "gasless laparoscopy" of normal-weight subjects results in smaller LVEDA. These changes are independent of patient position (15).

Left Ventricle End-Systolic Area (LVESA)/Volume
Pneumoperitoneum produces either no change or increases dimensions for supine patients. Pneumoperitoneum for normal-weight patients produces no change when patient's position changes from supine to Trendelenburg or from supine to the reverse Trendelenburg position. Abdominal exposure produced by "gasless laparoscopy" for normal-weight subjects, results in significantly smaller LVESA compared to pneumoperitoneum. These changes are independent of patient's position.

Ejection Fraction (EF) or Fractional Area Shortening
In normal-weight, supine subjects, pneumoperitoneum is associated with a decrease or no change. In this patient population, pneumoperitoneum induces minimal changes with a shift from supine to the Trendelenburg position. A position change from supine to reverse Trendelenburg produces either no change or a decrease. Abdominal exposure produced by "gasless laparoscopy" in normal BMI subjects results in larger fractional shortening compared to pneumoperitoneum for subjects in supine or Trendelenburg positions. Fractional shortening may decrease for subjects in the reverse Trendelenburg position (15). Obese patients have small changes in EF with pneumoperitoneum.

Left Ventricle End Systolic Wall Stress (LVESWS)
LVESWS is determined by ventricular pressure, end-systolic volume and myocardial wall thickness. Short term increases result from an increase left ventricular size

or left ventricular pressure. LVESWS increases in normal-weight, supine subjects during pneumoperitoneum. In normal-weight patients, pneumoperitoneum induces minimal changes when patient position is shifted from supine to Trendelenburg, and produces no change in LVESWS for a shift from supine to the reverse Trendelenburg position. LVESWS is larger for obese subjects than for normal weight subjects. Pneumoperitoneum causes a significant increase only for obese subjects, although values increase by about 47% for both normal and obese subjects.

Electrocardiogram (19)
Changing body position alters lung volume and diaphragmatic length. As a result the heart will change its orientation relative to the chest wall electrodes. Changes in electrocardiographic parameters during pneumoperitoneum are smallest for patients in the Trendelenburg position and are greatest for patients in reverse Trendelenburg, although most changes do not reach statistical significance. Examples of effects include:

1. QRS vector magnitude duration changes (in microvolt-seconds) during pneumoperitoneum (an average of 1.6-fold) are greatest for reverse Trendelenburg, less for supine position and least for Trendelenburg position
2. QRS complex spatial area (in microvolts-squared) increases (1.5-fold on average) during pneumoperitoneum but does not change significantly with body position
3. Neither position nor pneumoperitoneum alters ST segment axis or magnitude

LIVER
Pneumoperitoneum reduces hepatic portal blood flow and alters postoperative hepatic transaminases (20–22). In normal subjects baseline portal pressure is usually <10 mmHg. Raising intra-abdominal pressure to >10 mmHg causes significant narrowing of the portal vein and significant decreases in portal blood velocity, which may lead to liver damage. The mechanisms for alteration of postoperative hepatic function include:

1. Direct operative trauma to the liver. Trauma associated with mechanical retraction of the left lobe of the liver is the primary mechanism for elevation of liver enzymes after open laparoscopic gastric bypass.
2. The use of general anesthetics. Certain hepatically metabolized anesthetic agents can be hepatotoxic and result in postoperative elevation of hepatic enzymes.
3. The reduction of portal venous flow during pneumoperitoneum. An acute increase in the intra-abdominal pressure during laparoscopy dramatically decreases portal venous flow.

During laparoscopic cholecystectomy with abdominal insufflation to 14 mmHg, there can be a 53% reduction of portal blood flow. This may lead to hepatic hypoperfusion with acute hepatocyte injury and transient elevation of liver enzymes (ALT and AST). These changes return to baseline by 72 hours postoperatively.

Few studies examine the effects of pneumoperitoneum on hepatic function in the morbidly obese. Transient elevation of hepatic transaminase levels (ALT and AST) after laparoscopic and open laparoscopic gastric bypass are reported. Transaminase levels after laparoscopic gastric bypass can increase by six-fold, peaking at 24 hours postoperatively. These levels return to baseline by the third postoperative day without long-term sequelae. Although a mild increase in hepatic enzymes is not a specific indicator of liver damage, an increase in hepatic transaminase levels exceeding three times that of baseline levels may suggest acute hepatic injury.

Overall, pneumoperitoneum in the morbidly obese is considered safe in patients with normal baseline liver function, although further studies are needed.

ENDOCRINE SYSTEM

Carbon dioxide pneumoperitoneum results in progressive and significant increases in plasma concentrations of cortisol, epinephrine, norepinephrine, and renin. Levels of prostaglandins and endothelin do not change significantly. However, there is no clear understanding of the causes and consequences of these changes, and there are no consistent studies in the obese population. We will describe catecholamine and vasopressin changes as a proxy to explain some physiological changes reported in anesthetized obese patients during pneumoperitoneum.

Catecholamine

Raising intra-abdominal pressure during CO_2 insufflation is associated with increasing plasma catecholamine concentrations. This may be due to an increase in regional spillover from the abdominal region, specifically from the portal vein. Excessive intra-abdominal pressure (20 mmHg) (independent of insufflating gas or body position) increases plasma catecholamine concentrations during pneumoperitoneum. Most clinicians use insufflation pressures ≤15 mmHg.

Vasopressin

Atrial transmural pressure gradient decreases during pneumoperitoneum. This is the presumed mechanism which triggers the excretion of antidiuretic hormone. Vasopressin plasma concentration markedly increases immediately upon abdominal insufflation. The profile of vasopressin release parallels the time course of changes in SVR.

Other Hormones

Very little data exists regarding the impact of pneumoperitoneum on other hormones such as ACTH/cortisol, TSH, T3, T4, and epinephrine.

RENAL FUNCTION

Pneumoperitoneum alters renal function (23–25) although results differ between studies.

Urine Output

Intraoperative urine output decreases during abdominal insufflation. Upon desufflation, urine output is restored, though this may be delayed for a few hours. Laboratory studies have demonstrated that the degree of intraoperative oliguria is dependent on the intra-abdominal pressure; higher intra-abdominal pressures result in a greater degree of oliguria (23,24). For critically ill patients, an acute increase in the intra-abdominal pressure to >25 mmHg results in acute renal insufficiency. Abdominal decompression leads to immediate improvement in renal function. For obese subjects, intraoperative urine output decreases immediately after initiation of pneumoperitoneum during laparoscopic gastric bypass (25). In a study by Nguyen et al. (25), urine output remained 31% to 64% less than during open gastric bypass (19 mL vs. 55 mL). Postoperative blood urea nitrogen and createnine levels remained within the normal range in both groups.

Mechanisms of Decreased Urinary Output During Laparoscopy (23–25)

1. Direct pressure effect on renal cortical blood flow: Superficial renal cortical perfusion decreases by 60% with abdominal insufflation and returns to baseline level after desufflation.
2. Direct pressure effect on the renal vasculature, resulting in reduced renal blood flow, which can decrease up to 35% below baseline during pneumoperitoneum.
3. Endocrine effect: Intraoperative release of hormones such as antidiuretic hormone (ADH), plasma renin, and serum aldosterone may diminish urine output. During pneumoperitoneum there is a surge in plasma ADH concentration, which is not observed during an open procedure. ADH facilitates water reabsorption in the distal tubules and concentrates the urine. For morbidly obese subjects, levels of ADH, aldosterone, and plasma renin activity significantly increase during laparoscopic gastric bypass (25).

Renal Tissue Damage
Despite the intraoperative oliguria, pneumoperitoneum at 15 mmHg is considered clinically safe. There are no reports showing an increase in serum creatinine after a laparoscopic procedure as compared to an open procedure. This lack of difference applies to both normal and morbidly obese subjects. Creatinine clearance measured in patients undergoing laparoscopic gastric bypass remains within the normal range on the first and second postoperative days. Laboratory studies in rats show that CO_2 pneumoperitoneum gradient and its duration affect renal function and induce apoptosis.

THERMOREGULATION
Perioperative hypothermia (usually defined as <36°C of core temperature) is common and is associated with several complications: myocardial morbidity secondary to sympathetic nervous system activation; wound infections and delayed healing; coagulopathy; more allogeneic transfusions; negative nitrogen balance; and delayed postanesthetic recovery.

Few reports address thermoregulation in the obese patients. In patients with a BMI of 40 to 60 kg/m² randomly assigned to open or laparoscopic gastric bypass, a comparison of core temperature changes revealed the following (26):

*   Core temperature decreased significantly in both groups after induction
*   Hypothermia developed in 36% of patients in the open group and 37% of patients in the laparoscopic group
*   Hypothermia progressed to comprise 46% of the open group and 41% of the laparoscopic group
*   In the recovery room, hypothermia could be measured in 6% of the patients in the open group and 8% of those in the laparoscopic group
*   Intraoperative heat loss can be minimized with the use of an upper body external warming blanket and by passive airway humidification

PAIN MANAGEMENT
In general, laparoscopic procedures are associated with both a decrease in the intensity of postoperative pulmonary dysfunction and less pain as manifested by

less opioid usage in the intraoperative and post-operative period. Laparoscopic procedures are associated with a decrease in time to mobilization, and a 50% reduction in the incidence of hypoxemia and segmental atelectasis.

REFERENCES

1. Pelosi P, Ravagnan I, Giurati G, et al. Positive end-expiratory pressure improves respiratory function in obese but not normal subjects during anesthesia and paralysis. Anesthesiology 1999; 91: 1221–3.
2. Valenza F, Vagginelli F, Tiby A, et al. Effects of the beach chair position, positive end-expiratory pressure, and pneumoperitoneum on respiratory function in morbidly obese patients during anesthesia and paralysis. Anesthesiology 2007; 107: 725–32.
3. Fahy BG, Barnas GM, Flowers JL, et al. The effects of increased abdominal pressure on lung and chest wall mechanics during laparoscopic surgery. Anesth Analg 1995; 81: 744–50.
4. Sprung J, Whalley DG, Falcone T, et al. The effects of tidal volume and respiratory rate on oxygenation and respiratory mechanics during laparoscopy in morbidly obese patients. Anesth Analg 2003; 97: 268–74.
5. Salihoglu Z, Demiroluk S, Dikmen Y. Respiratory mechanics in morbidly obese patients with chronic obstructive pulmonary disease and hypertension during pneumoperitoneum. Eur J Anaesth 2003; 20: 658–61.
6. Casati A, Comotti L, Tommasino C, et al. Effects of pneumoperitoneum and reverse Trendelenberg position on cardiopulmonary function in morbidly obese patients receiving laparoscopic gastric banding. Eur J Anaesth 2000; 17: 300–5.
7. Guenoun T, Aka EJ, Journois D, et al. Effects of laparoscopic pneumoperitoneum and changes in position on arterial pulse pressure waveform: comparison between morbidly obese and normal-weight patients. Obes Surg 2006; 16: 1075–81.
8. Sprung J, Whalley DG, Falcone T, et al. The impact of morbid obesity, pneumoperitoneum, and posture on respiratory system mechanics and oxygenation during laparoscopy. Anesth Analg 2002; 94: 1345–50.
9. Odeberg S, Solevi A. Pneumoperitoneum for laparoscopic surgery does not increase venous admixture. Eur J Anaesthesiol 1995; 12: 541–8.
10. Cadi P, Guenoun T, Journois D, et al. Pressure-controlled ventilation improves oxygenation during laparoscopic obesity surgery compared with volume-controlled ventilation. Br J Anaesth 2008; 100: 709–16.
11. DeBaerdemaeker LEC, Van der Herten C, Gillardin JM, et al. Comparison of volume-controlled and pressure-controlled ventilation during laparoscopic gastric banding in morbidly obese patients. Obes Surg 2008; 18: 680–5.
12. Balick-Weber CC, Nicolas P, et al. Respiratory and haemodynamic effects of volume-controlled vs pressure-controlled ventilation during laparoscopy: a cross-over study with echocardiographic assessment. Br J Anaesth 2007; 429–35.
13. Ezri T, Hazin V, Warters D, et al. The endotracheal tube moves more often in obese patients under laparoscopy compared with open abdominal surgery. Anesth Analg 2003; 96: 278–82.
14. Odeberg S, Ljungqvist O, Svenberg T, et al. Haemodynamic effects of pneumoperitoneum and the influence of posture during anesthesia for laparoscopic surgery. Acta Anaesth Scand 1994; 38: 276–83.
15. Larsen JF, Svendsen FM, Pedersen V. Randomized clinical trial of the effect of pneumoperitoneum on cardiac function and the haemodynamics during laparoscopic cholecystectomy. Br J Surg 2004; 91: 848–54.
16. Dhoste K, Laxoste L, Karayan J, et al. Haemodynamic and ventilatory changes during laparoscopic cholecystectomy in elderly ASA III patients. Can J Anaesth 1996; 43: 783–8.

17. Hein HAT, Joshi GP, Ramsay MAE, et al. Hemodynamic changes during laparoscopic cholecystectomy in patients with severe cardiac disease. J Clin Anesth 1997; 9: 261–5.
18. Myre K, Buanes T, Smith G, et al. Simultaneous hemodynamic and echocardiac changes during abdominal gas insufflation. Surg Laparos Endosc 1997; 7: 415–19.
19. Gannedahl P, Oderberg S, Ljungqvist O, et al. Vectorcardiographic changes during laparoscopic cholecystectomy may mimic signs of myocardial ischemia. Acta Anaesthiol Scand 1997; 41: 1187–92.
20. Spaulding L, Trainer T, Janiec D. Prevalence of non-alcoholic steatohepatitis in morbidly obese subjects undergoing gastric bypass. Obes Surg 2003; 13: 347–9.
21. Takagi S. Hepatic and portal vein blood flow during carbon dioxide pneumoperitoneum for laparoscopic hepatectomy Surg Endosc 1998 May; 12: 427–31.
22. Saranita J, Soto RG, Paoli D. Elevated liver enzymes as an operative complication of gastric bypass surgery. Obes Surg 2003; 13: 314–16.
23. Nishio S, Takeda H, Yokoyama M. Changes in urinary output during laparoscopic adrenalectomy. Br J Urol Intl 1999; 83: 944–7.
24. McDougall EM, Monk TG, Wolf JS, et al. The effect of prolonged pneumoperitoneum on renal function in an animal model. J Am Coll Surg 1996; 182: 317–28.
25. Nguyen NH, Perez RV, Fleming N, et al. Effect of prolonged pneumoperitoneum on intraoperative urine output during laparoscopic gastric bypass. J Am Coll Surg 2002; 195: 476–83.
26. Nguyen NT, Fleming NW, Singh A, et al. Evaluation of core temperature during laparoscopic and open gastric bypass. Obes Surg 2001; 11: 570–5.

13 | Intraoperative Positioning and Nerve Injury

Aalok V. Agarwala

Instructor in Anesthesia, Harvard Medical School, Assistant in Anesthesia, Department of Anesthesia and Critical Care, Massachusetts General Hospital, Boston, Massachusetts, U.S.A.

INTRODUCTION

Positioning of the obese patient for surgery has important implications for safety, both of the patient and the operating room staff. It also has physiologic implications as cardiac and pulmonary function can be further compromised. Part of the care plan of the obese surgical patient should include a discussion amongst team members (anesthesia, nursing, surgery) regarding the patient's position for the surgery. Ideally, this position would offer a balance between adequate surgical exposure and hemodynamic stability. Whenever possible, it is best for both patients and operating room staff to allow and encourage patients to move and position themselves.

PATIENT POSITIONING
Preparation and Planning
Equipment

Beds. Some severely obese patients may require special hospital beds both for transport to the operating room as well as for intraoperative use. Attention should be paid to weight limits of operating tables as limits may vary depending on the orientation of the table. In addition, standard operating tables may not be wide enough to adequately support morbidly obese patients. While wider tables are now readily available, in extreme cases, it may be necessary to place two tables side by side to accommodate the largest patients (1).

Hoists and pulleys. Several devices are commercially available to assist in the transfer of obese patients who are unable to move themselves. Some of these hoist and pulley systems may be mounted to the ceiling of the operating room, while others may be brought in and out of a given operating or procedure room. These devices can significantly reduce the risk of injury to operating room personnel.

Padding. Several different types of padding are regularly used for the protection of pressure points, including foam, gel, and air filled pads. One type has not been shown to be superior to another. Given the higher risk of nerve injury and pressure sores in the obese population, it is imperative that all pressure points be adequately padded while the patient is immobile.

Other equipment. To help minimize the risk of falls and movement after the patient is on the operating table, straps should be used for security. In addition, to prevent shifting of the patient once positioned, the use a bean bag has been recommended (2). A bean bag is a commercially available large soft pad containing small beads that may be molded to the patient's body with the assistance of wall suction. The device can be used to help hold the patient in a desired position while distributing pressure over a large area, thereby minimizing the risk of pressure sores and nerve injury.

After completion of surgery, operating room staff are at significant risk for injury as they transfer the obese patient from the operating table to the postoperative hospital bed. There are now commercially available devices that may reduce this risk of injury, such as the HoverMatt (HoverTech International, Bethlehem, PA, www.hovermatt.com). This device is an inflatable air mattress that can be placed on the operating table prior to surgery. Upon completion of the surgical procedure, the mattress is inflated using an electric pump, lifting the patient off of the operating table, and allowing personnel to slide the mattress from the operating table to the postoperative bed, all with minimal effort.

Personnel
It is critical to have adequate personnel available to assist in moving and positioning morbidly obese patients. Risk of injury to operating room staff can be significant depending both on the patient's weight as well as the patient's ability to assist in moving themselves.

Cardiopulmonary Changes with Obesity: Brief Summary
As the alterations in physiology that occur in the obese patient are covered in detail in other chapters, the discussion here will focus on the most significant of these changes in relation to positioning of the patient for surgery, specifically the effects on the cardiovascular and pulmonary systems.

Cardiovascular Changes
The increased body weight of severely obese patients results in increased strain on the cardiovascular system. All measurements of pressure are increased in the severely obese patient (3).

1. A higher cardiac output is required to support a higher metabolic demand as compared to the non-obese (4)
2. Left and right ventricular pressures increase reflecting the additional cardiac work
3. Pulmonary artery pressures are elevated, further straining a heart that is already functioning under high demand
4. Systemic pressures are also increased, evidenced by the common occurrence of arterial hypertension in these patients

All of these changes, in combination with advancing age and other risk factors, eventually lead to a significant incidence of ischemic heart disease and congestive heart failure (5–6).

Pulmonary Changes
As compared to the non-obese, obese patients demonstrate a number of important pulmonary and respiratory changes:

1. Obese patients have decreased chest wall compliance (7)
2. Obese patients have an increased work of breathing, resulting in increased O_2 consumption and increased CO_2 production (8)
3. Obese patients have increased intra-abdominal pressure, which results in decreased functional residual capacity (FRC), expiratory reserve volume (ERV), and total lung capacity (TLC) as compared to non-obese patients (9–11)

4. Obese patients also suffer from increased shunting as a result of a reduced closing capacity. There is closure of small airways during normal ventilation, thereby reducing PaO_2 as compared to non-obese patients (12)

Physiologic Changes with Various Positions
It is well known that significant changes in cardiopulmonary physiology occur with changes in position. This is true of all patients, but more significant in the obese.

Supine Position
The most commonly used position during surgery is the supine position.

Pulmonary effects. The effects on the pulmonary and gas-exchange systems are due primarily to the relatively increased intra-abdominal pressure in the supine obese patient.

As abdominal contents shift cephalad in the supine position, the result is decreased FRC, ERV, and TLC (13–14). Pelosi et al. showed that general anesthesia with muscle relaxation intensifies these changes (15). Reduced TLC in the obese results in a greater decrease in pulmonary compliance and FRC. This leads to greater ventilation/perfusion (V/Q) mismatch, a greater shunt fraction and, ultimately, relative hypoxemia as compared to non-obese patients (16–17).

The role of increased intra-abdominal pressure has been further substantiated by the demonstration that relieving it improves respiratory function by increasing pulmonary compliance and lung volumes, and improving oxygenation. This has been shown by physically lifting the panniculus (18), as well as by opening of the abdomen during laparotomy (19).

It has also been shown that the use of positive end expiratory pressure (PEEP) is useful in improving oxygenation and respiratory function in the mechanically ventilated supine obese patient (20).

Cardiovascular effects. The cardiovascular effects of the supine position in obese patients are less dramatic owing to the fact that there are no significant pressure gradients above or below the heart. There is, however, an increase in venous return to the heart as compared to the sitting or standing position. This is manifested by increased pulmonary blood flow, increased cardiac output, and increased arterial blood pressure (16).

Similar to the position used during Caesarean section, placement of a wedge under the right side of the patient, or use of a left-side down tilt of the operating table, can be helpful in reducing the impact of a large pannus on inferior vena cava compression (supine hypotension syndrome).

Trendelenburg/Head-Down Positions
The Trendelenburg, or head-down, position is routinely used to increase exposure during surgical procedures (both open and laparoscopic) involving the lower abdominal and pelvic organs. This position allows the small and large intestines to shift cephalad. Frequently, retractors and packing are also used to maximize exposure, further increasing the pressure placed on the diaphragm.

Pulmonary effects. As might be expected, the Trendelenburg position creates more perturbation in the obese patient's physiology compared to the supine position. However, the changes going from supine to Trendelenburg are not as dramatic as those seen in a change from sitting to supine position (21).

As the weight of the abdominal cavity and the panniculus is shifted towards the lungs, the pulmonary compliance, lung volumes and FRC decrease to a greater degree than they do in the supine position. It has been shown that a change in position from supine to Trendelenburg can result in a decrease in PaO_2 in obese patients (22).

It is important to note that changes in PaO_2 can also be secondary to inadvertent right mainstem intubation, as can occur with shifting of the abdominal contents and mediastinum cephalad during Trendelenburg positioning.

Cardiovascular effects. As compared to the supine position, there is a greater return of venous blood to the central circulation from the lower extremities, increasing central venous pressure and, potentially, increasing cardiac output. This may or may not be significant depending on the baseline cardiac functional status of the patient.

Other considerations. In addition to the physiologic effects, it is important to be mindful of practical aspects when placing patients in steep Trendelenburg position. Given their body habitus and weight, severely obese patients may have a tendency to shift on the operating table, especially in very steep positions. If shoulder braces are used to prevent cephalad movement, they should be well padded, and prolonged pressure should be avoided in order to prevent injury to the brachial plexus.

Reverse Trendelenburg/Head-Up Positions

The reverse Trendelenburg position displaces the abdominal contents caudally, resulting in improved ventilation and, in the awake patient, improved patient comfort.

Pulmonary effects. It has been demonstrated that during surgery in the obese patient, the reverse Trendelenburg position leads to increased tidal volume and a higher total respiratory system compliance, resulting in a significant improvement in the alveolar-arterial oxygen partial pressure gradient (23). In a study by Perilli et al., 10 cm H_2O PEEP and 30 degree reverse Trendelenburg positioning were found to be equally efficacious in increasing total pulmonary compliance and oxygenation in morbidly obese patients undergoing upper abdominal surgery (24).

Cardiovascular effects. While in theory, the head up position could result in hemodynamic compromise secondary to venous pooling in the lower extremities, at least one study showed no adverse cardiovascular effects in morbidly obese patients positioned in reverse Trendelenburg (23).

Post-operative care. It has been shown that obese patients have a greater reduction in total lung volumes after abdominal surgery as compared to non-obese patients. This can lead to a decrease in PaO_2 secondary to increased shunting (25–26). The head up position is thus recommended during extubation, patient transport, as well as during the immediate postoperative period.

Other considerations. As with the Trendelenburg position, it is important to be aware of challenges that may occur when morbidly obese patients are placed in steep positions. While in reverse Trendelenburg, the use of a footboard can be extremely helpful in preventing patients from sliding down to the caudal end of the table.

Lateral Decubitus Position

The lateral decubitus position is often used for procedures involving the kidney, aorta and other retroperitoneal structures. Changes in the pattern of ventilation and perfusion in the lateral position can lead to increased V/Q mismatching (27). Hypoxemia can ensue, especially in patients with significant pulmonary disease.

However, physiologic changes in the lateral decubitus position observed in obese patients may differ from those seen in the non-obese. For example, by allowing the weight of the obese abdomen to fall to the side, the lateral decubitus position may result in an increase in pulmonary compliance and FRC, as well as a decrease in shunting, thereby leading to improved oxygenation (28).

Prone Position

General considerations. Special attention should be paid to the face, specifically the eyes, ears and the nose, as well as breasts and genitalia. If possible, the head should be kept neutral, and the arms abducted less than 90 degrees or tucked at the patient's sides. If the patient is positioned in the kneeling position, the knees should be well padded. The endotracheal tube should be secured firmly given the potential for dislodgement with movement of the patient.

Pulmonary issues. The prone position can be helpful or harmful to the obese patient depending on whether the abdomen is allowed to hang freely. With appropriate support to the chest and pelvis, a free abdomen in the prone position decreases pressure on the diaphragm, allowing for an increase in FRC and thereby improving compliance and oxygenation (29). Portions of the lung subject to collapse due to increased intra-abdominal pressure will reopen and contribute to gas exchange. This finding holds true in patients paralyzed under general anesthesia as well (30).

Conversely, if the abdomen is not allowed to move freely, the resultant increased pressure on the diaphragm will lead to worsened pulmonary compliance (31).

Cardiovascular effects. If the abdomen is not compressed, cardiovascular status may improve, as pressure on the inferior vena cava is relieved, allowing better venous return (27).

If, however, the abdomen is restricted, the increased intra-abdominal pressure can result in compression of the inferior vena cava, mesenteric and femoral vessels, leading to engorgement of the paraverterbral venous plexus. In patients undergoing spine surgery, this can then result in increased surgical blood loss and worsened exposure (32). Furthermore, the increased intra-abdominal pressure can also decrease venous return from the lower portion of the body, leading to decreased cardiac output (33). This reduction in cardiac output may be worsened by the increased positive intra-thoracic pressure required during mechanical ventilation of patients in this position (34).

Lithotomy Position

The lithotomy position is commonly used for gynecologic and perineal surgery. This requires patients to be supine with hips and knees flexed, the feet and legs held by stirrups or leg holders. Occasionally, patients are also tilted head-down to enhance exposure of the perineum.

Cardiovascular effects. Many of the physiologic changes that occur in the Trendelenburg position also occur in the lithotomy position. With the legs elevated to a level above the heart, there is an increase in venous return from the lower portion of the body, resulting in increased central venous pressure and increased cardiac output (35). In a patient with preexisting cardiac disease, this increase in central blood volume may be poorly tolerated.

Pulmonary effects. As in the Trendelenburg position, lung volumes will decrease in the lithotomy position (27). There is a relative increase in intra-abdominal pressure, again resulting in decreased FRC and total lung volume. In order to maintain adequate ventilation and oxygenation in severely obese patients in the lithotomy position, the addition of PEEP to positive pressure ventilation may be useful.

Other considerations. A potentially devastating consequence of a prolonged period of time in the lithotomy position is a gluteal compartment syndrome. It appears that procedures lasting more than four hours place patients at additional risk for this complication, which can lead to rhabdomyolysis and renal failure. Additional padding may be helpful, as well as aggressive hydration and mannitol diuresis if creatine phosphokinase (CPK) is significantly elevated (36).

Nerve injury. It is important to pay attention to protection and padding of pressure points in the lithotomy position, as it has been found that a significant number of nerve injuries is associated with this position. These are discussed below.

NERVE INJURY

One of the most common factors in peripheral nerve injuries is inadequate attention to positioning of the patient during surgery. In fact, peripheral nerve injuries are the second most frequent cause of professional liability in the practice of anesthesia. Unfortunately, certain patients are predisposed to manifesting neuropathies despite the best care possible (37).

Obese patients may be at an increased risk of nerve injury compared to non-obese patients. Their larger size makes them more difficult to position with standard operating room equipment. They often do not fit into or onto standard equipment and their added weight increases the pressure on contact surfaces. These concerns, in addition to the prevalence of diabetes in the obese population, warrant special attention with respect to padding of pressure points.

Upper Extremity Injuries

The most commonly occurring and therefore most commonly discussed nerve injuries of the upper extremities are those involving the ulnar nerve and the brachial plexus.

Ulnar Nerve Injury

While injury to the ulnar nerve is frequently attributed to inappropriate positioning of the patient during surgery, there is a growing body of literature that supports other causes and contributing factors, including injury sustained outside of the operating room, and the predisposition of some patients to neuropathy (38). Nonetheless, it is still the responsibility of the operating room team to provide the best care possible to try to prevent such injuries. Ulnar nerve injury can result from either compression or stretch. Compression occurs with inadequate padding of the arms while stretch can occur with prolonged flexion of the elbow (39).

Obesity has been found to be an independent risk factor for developing ulnar neuropathy. Warner et al. analyzed a single institution's 35-year experience with perioperative ulnar neuropathy and found that 29% of such injuries occurred in patients with a body mass index greater than 38 kg/m². In that study, they also found that 70% of patients with injury were male (40).

In a subsequent study by the same author, it was found that ulnar neuropathies also occurred in hospitalized non-surgical patients, suggesting that patient positioning outside of the operating room also contributes to this type of injury. This could include the supine position, with elbows resting on the bed with arms on the abdomen or chest, or elbows resting on bed siderails (41).

It has been speculated that the occurrence of these injuries could be reduced or prevented by the use of wider beds to accommodate larger patients, and with increased education of caregivers (41).

Brachial Plexus
It appears that most brachial plexus injuries occur during median sternotomy. In this setting, they seem to be unrelated to positioning of the head and arms, and more likely related to stretch or compression injury during sternal separation (42–44). Brachial plexus injury can occur in other circumstances including excessive arm abduction and inadequate support of the arms.

The use of shoulder braces to prevent cephalad movement of the patient while in steep Trendelenburg position can cause either compression or stretch of the brachial plexus if care is not taken to appropriately position the braces with adequate padding (38).

Brachial plexus injuries may also occur in patients in the prone position, especially when patients are positioned with the head turned to the side and arms abducted and flexed at the elbow. This can result in stretch of the brachial plexus on the side contralateral to that on which the patient's head is turned. Though the incidence of brachial plexus injury from this mechanism is low, it might be prudent to allow the arms to be tucked by the patient's sides when possible for surgery in the prone position (45).

Lower Extremity Injuries
While injury to the nerves of the lower extremity can occur in any number of patient positions, including lateral decubitus and prone, the most common surgical position encountered when dealing with these injuries is the lithotomy position. A variety of nerves in the lower extremity are vulnerable to injury, including the common peroneal, sciatic, femoral, obturator, and lateral femoral cutaneous.

Common Peroneal Nerve Injury
In a retrospective review (46), Warner et al. found that injury to the common peroneal nerve was most commonly seen in patients undergoing procedures in the lithotomy position. This nerve is prone to injury given the superficial nature of its course, especially around the head of fibula. This area can be easily compressed while the legs are held in stirrups or leg holders. If care is not taken at the start of the surgery to carefully position the legs, inadequate padding can lead to prolonged compression of the nerve, ultimately leading to ischemia and nerve injury. This is especially true in obese patients, in whom the size of the leg holders may be inadequate to comfortably hold the legs without compression.

Injury to the common peroneal nerve can also occur distal to where it wraps around the head of the fibula (47). Proposed mechanisms for injury include compressive stockings or wraps used for deep vein thrombosis prophylaxis.

Sciatic Nerve Injury
A combination of extension of the knee and extreme flexion of the hip, as might occur in the placement of a patient in lithotomy position, can lead to sciatic nerve stretch. If this stretch is significant or prolonged, it may subsequently lead to injury. Moving patients caudally once already positioned in lithotomy with the legs secured, as is sometimes done to increase exposure of the perineum, may exacerbate the likelihood of injury.

Femoral Nerve Injury
Most femoral nerve injuries result from direct compression of either the blood supply or the nerve itself, not from poor positioning or inadequate padding. This is most frequently attributed to inappropriate abdominal wall retractor placement (48).

Obturator and Lateral Femoral Cutaneous Nerve Injury
There are currently conflicting data on the occurrence of obturator and lateral femoral cutaneous nerve injury. One prospective study found that these nerves were most commonly implicated in neuropathies associated with longer duration in lithotomy position (47). A subsequent cadaveric study found that strain on the lateral femoral cutaneous nerve did not increase with either hip flexion or mild abduction. However, abduction greater than 30 degrees without hip flexion did increase obturator nerve strain (49).

Prevention of Nerve Injury
Any exposed superficial peripheral nerves should be padded. Padding may be comprised of gel pads, foam pads, air-filled pads, blankets, or a variety of other materials. There are no studies to support the use of one type of padding over another. Areas where peripheral nerves run superficially should be protected from direct compression, from stretch, and from excessive force being placed on a small physical area. During prolonged procedures, shifting of the patient's position intermittently might reduce the risk of injury, not only to nerves, but to skin structures as well (38). This is especially true with obese patients who may not properly fit within operating room positioning devices, and who may have a greater risk of injury at pressure points due to their increased weight.

REFERENCES
1. Cooper JR, Brodsky JB. Anesthetic management of the morbidly obese patient. Semin Anesth 1987; 6: 260–70.
2. Ogunnaike BO, Jones SB, Jones DB, et al. Anesthetic considerations for bariatric surgery. Anesth Analg 2002; 95: 1793–805.
3. Whyte HM. Blood pressure and obesity. Circulation 1959; 19: 511–16.
4. Alexander JK. Obesity and cardiac performance. Am J Cardiology 1964: 14; 860–5.
5. Kannel WB, Lebauer EJ, Dawber TR, et al. Relation of body weight to development of coronary heart disease. The Framingham Study. Circulation 1967; 35: 734–44.
6. Kannel WB, D'Agostino RB, Cobb JL. Effect of weight on cardiovascular disease. Am J Clin Nutr 1996; 63(Suppl): 419S–422S.
7. Dempsey JA, Reddan W, Rankin J, et al. Alveolar-arterial gas exchange during muscular work in obesity. J Appl Physiol 1966; 21: 1807–14.
8. Luce JM. Respiratory complications of obesity. Chest 1980; 78: 626–31.
9. Biring MS, Lewis MI, Liu JI, et al. Pulmonary physiologic changes of morbid obesity. Am J Med Soc 1999; 318: 293–7.
10. Ray C, Sue D, Bray G, et al. Effects of obesity on respiratory function. Am Rev Respir Dis 1983; 128: 501–6.
11. Ladosky W, Botelho MA, Albuquerque JP Jr. Chest mechanics in morbidly obese non hypoventilated patients. Respir Med 2001; 95: 281–6.
12. Rorvik S, Bo G. Lung volumes and arterial blood gases in obesity. Scand J Respir Dis Suppl 1976; 95: 60–4.
13. Vilke GM, Chan TC, Neuman T, et al. Spirometry in normal subjects in sitting, prone, and supine positions. Respir Care 2000; 45: 407–10.
14. Rehder K. Postural changes in respiratory function. Acta Anaesthesiol Scand 1998; 113(Suppl): 13–16.
15. Pelosi P, Croci M, Ravagnan I, et al. Respiratory system mechanics in sedated, paralyzed, morbidly obese patients. J Appl Physiol 1997; 82: 811–18.
16. Paul DR, Hoyt JL, Boutrous AR. Cardiovascular and respiratory changes in response to change in posture in the very obese. Anesthesiology 1976; 45: 73–7.

17. Yap JC, Watson RA, Gilbey S, et al. Effects of posture on respiratory mechanics in obesity. J Appl Physiol 1995; 79: 1199–205.
18. Wyner J, Brodsky JB, Merrell RC. Massive obesity and arterial oxygenation. Anesth Analg 1981; 60: 691–3.
19. Aueler JO Jr, Miyoshi E, Fernandes CR, et al. The effects of abdominal opening on respiratory mechanics during general anesthesia in normal and morbidly obese patients: a comparative study. Anesth Analg 2002; 94: 741–8.
20. Pelosi P, Ravagnan I, Giurati G, et al. Positive end-expiratory pressure improves respiratory function in obese but not in normal subjects during anesthesia and paralysis. Anesthesiology 1999; 91: 1221–31.
21. Lumb AB, Nunn JF. Respiratory function and ribcage contribution to ventilation in body positions commonly used during anesthesia. Anesth Analg 1991; 73: 422–6.
22. Vaughan RW, Wise L. Intraoperative arterial oxygenation in obese patients. Ann Surg 1976; 184: 35–42.
23. Perilli, V, Sollazzi L, Bozza P, et al. The effects of reverse Trendelenburg position on respiratory mechanics and blood gases in morbidly obese patients during bariatric surgery. Anesth Analg 2000; 91: 1520–5.
24. Perilli, V, Sollazzi L, Modesti, C, et al. Comparison of positive end-expiratory pressure with reverse Trendelenburg position in morbidly obese patients undergoing bariatric surgery: effects on hemodynamics and pulmonary gas exchange. Obes Surg 2003 Aug; 13: 605–9.
25. Pelosi P, Croci M, Ravagnan I, et al. Total respiratory system, lung, and chest wall mechanics in sedated-paralyzed postoperative morbidly obese patients. Chest 1996; 109: 144–51.
26. Vaughan RW, Bauer S, Wise L. Effect of position (semirecumbent versus supine) on postoperative oxygenation in markedly obese subjects. Anesth Analg 1976; 55: 37–41.
27. Gottumukkala, V. Positioning of patients for operation. In: Longnecker DE, Brown DL, Newman MF, Zapol WM, eds. Anesthesiology. New York: McGraw-Hill, 2007: 465–75.
28. Tanskanen P, Kytta J, Randell T. The effect of patient positioning on dynamic lung compliance. Acta Anaesthesiol Scand 1997; 41: 602–6.
29. Pelosi P, Croci M, Calappi E, et al. The prone position during general anesthesia minimally affects respiratory mechanics while improving functional residual capacity and increasing oxygen tension. Anesth Analg 1995; 80: 955–60.
30. Pelosi P, Croci M, Calappi E, et al. Prone positioning improves pulmonary function in obese patients during general anesthesia. Anesth Analg 1996; 83: 578–83.
31. Palmon SC, Kirsch JR, Depper JA, et al. The effect of the prone position on pulmonary mechanics is frame-dependent. Anesth Analg 1998; 87: 1175–80.
32. McNulty SE, Weiss J, Azad SS, et al. The effect of the prone position on venous pressures and blood loss during lumbar laminectomy. J Clin Anesth 1992; 4: 220–5.
33. Lee TC, Yang LC, Chen HJ. Effect of patient position and hypotensive anesthesia on inferior vena caval pressure. Spine 1998; 23: 941–9.
34. Toyota S, Amaki Y. Hemodynamic evaluation of the prone position by transesophageal echocardiography. J Clin Anesth 1998; 10: 32–5.
35. Brodsky JB. Positioning the morbidly obese patient for anesthesia. Obes Surg 2002; 12: 751–8.
36. Bostanjian D, Anthone GJ, Hamoui N, et al. Rhabdomyolysis of gluteal muscles leading to renal failure: a potentially fatal complication of surgery in the morbidly obese. Obes Surg 2003; 13: 302–5.
37. Cheney FW, Domino KB, Caplan RA, et al. Nerve injury associated with anesthesia: a closed claims analysis. Anesthesiology 1999; 90: 1062–9.
38. Warner MA. Perioperative neuropathies. Mayo Clin Proc 1998; 73: 567–74.
39. Sawyer RJ, Richmond MN, Hickey JD, et al. Peripheral nerve injuries associated with anesthesia. Anaesthesia 2000; 55: 980–91.

40. Warner MA, Warner ME, Martin JT. Ulnar neuropathy: incidence, outcome, and risk factors in sedated or anesthetized patients. Anesthesiology 1994; 81: 1332–40.
41. Warner MA, Warner DO, Harper CM, et al. Ulnar neuropathy in medical patients. Anesthesiology 2000; 92: 613–15.
42. Hickey C, Gugino LD, Aglio LS, et al. Intraoperative somatosensory evoked potential monitoring predicts peripheral nerve injury during cardiac surgery. Anesthesiology 1993; 78: 29–35.
43. Vahl CF, Carl I, Muller-Vahl H, et al. Brachial plexus injury after cardiac surgery: the role of internal mammary artery preparation; a prospective study of 1000 consecutive patients. J Thorac Cardiovasc Surg 1991; 102: 724–9.
44. Roy RC, Stafford MA, Charlton JE. Nerve injury and musculoskeletal complaints after cardiac surgery: influence of internal mammary artery dissection and left arm position. Anesth Analg 1988; 67: 277–9.
45. Martin JT. The ventral decubitus (prone) positions. In: Martin JT, Warner MA, eds. Positioning in Anesthesia and Surgery, 3rd edn. Philadelphia: W.B. Saunders Company; 1997; 155–95.
46. Warner MA, Martin JT, Schroeder DR, et al. Lower-extremity motor neuropathy associated with surgery performed on patients in a lithotomy position. Anesthesiology 1994; 81: 6–12.
47. Warner MA, Warner DO, Harper CM, et al. Lower extremity neuropathies associated with lithotomy positions. Anesthesiology 2000; 93: 938–42.
48. Rosenblum J, Schwarz GA, Bendler E. Femoral neuropathy—a neurological complication of hysterectomy. JAMA 1966; 195: 409–14.
49. Litwiller JP, Wells RE Jr, Halliwill JP, et al. Effect of lithotomy positions on strain of the obturator and lateral femoral cutaneous nerves. Clin Anat 2004; 17: 45–9.

14 | Metabolic Surgery for the Treatment of Obesity-Related Comorbidities

Janey S. A. Pratt[1] and Fawsi S. Khayat[2]

[1]Instructor in Surgery, Harvard Medical School, Assistant Surgeon, Department of Surgery, Massachusetts General Hospital, Boston, Massachusetts, U.S.A.

[2]Minimally Invasive Surgery Fellow, Harvard Medical School, Department of Surgery, Massachusetts General Hospital, Boston, Massachusetts, U.S.A.

INTRODUCTION

Bariatric surgical procedures have traditionally been divided into two categories, malabsorptive and restrictive, based upon the mechanism by which they were thought to induce weight loss. More recent research has proposed that changes in postoperative satiety hormone level and basal metabolic rate are responsible for the majority of weight loss in bariatric procedures. Hormones such as peptide YY (PYY), glucagon-like peptide 1, oxyntomodulin, and ghrelin are thought to regulate appetite, sensations of fullness, and metabolism. The most commonly performed bariatric procedure, the gastric bypass, has been studied in this regard. This operation is characterized by immediate and prolonged loss of appetite resulting in weight loss due to decreased calorie intake rather than by restriction or malabsorption (1).

Restrictive procedures limit caloric intake by downsizing the stomach's reservoir capacity. Gastric banding and sleeve gastrectomy are restrictive procedures that limit solid food intake by restriction of stomach size. Vertical pouches, as opposed to horizontal pouches, are the current standard as they preserve the normal anatomy and prevent esophageal reflux. While restrictive procedures are simpler in comparison to malabsorptive procedures, they tend to produce more gradual weight loss. In addition to caloric restriction, these procedures may have some neuro-hormonal activity affecting weight loss through changes in PYY and perhaps other pathways (2).

Malabsorptive procedures such as the biliopancreatic diversion (BPD) in which the length of the functional small intestine is shortened, promote weight loss through decreasing the effectiveness of nutrient absorption. Profound changes in the neuro-hormonal pathways controlling appetite, metabolism, and satiety also occur. However, with increased weight loss there is a significant increase in metabolic complications, including protein calorie malnutrition, various micronutrient deficiencies, and even liver failure (3).

METABOLIC SURGICAL PROCEDURES

History

The first surgery done for the treatment of hyper-triglyceridemia and obesity was the jejeuno-ileal bypass or JIB procedure performed in 1954. This was a true mal-absorptive procedure in that the majority of the small intestine was bypassed leading to a short intestine syndrome, protein calorie malabsorption, and severe electrolyte abnormalities. Operations of this type also stimulated similar neuro-hormonal pathways leading to decreased appetite and early satiety. Unfortunately, complications of migratory polyarthralgias, calcium oxalate urinary calculi, liver failure, and severe diarrhea and flatulence caused these operations to be abandoned and replaced by stapling procedures (4).

The early gastric stapling procedures worked predominantly through restriction but also produced changes in the satiety pathways. These procedures resulted in weight loss comparable to what we see with the adjustable gastric bands done today, however, they were not durable due to staple line breakdown, pouch enlargement or diet accommodation. Many early stapling procedures were converted to Roux-en-Y gastric bypasses to provide durable results.

Choice of Procedures
Patients are referred or self-refer to a metabolic or weight loss surgery (WLS) program for the treatment of either obesity or its comorbidities. Most surgical programs and insurance companies use the NIH criteria developed by the 1991 consensus conference and updated in 1996. These state that WLS is expected to be the most effective and appropriate treatment for patients with a body mass index (BMI) > 40 or a BMI > 35 with related comorbidities (5).

The consensus conference recommendation for surgery applied only to patients between 18 and 55 years old. Today studies show that surgery in older patients leads to improved life expectancy despite increased surgical risk, with the improvement in mortality occurring at 11 months post-op as compared to 6 months in those under age 65 years (6,7). As for adolescents, there is emerging data that surgery is not only safe, but also quite effective at decreasing comorbidities as well as significantly improving quality of life (8–10).

Preoperative evaluation varies depending on the WLS program. Many patients suffering from obesity have not undergone basic medical screening such as annual pap smears or rectal exams despite the increased risk of endometrial, colon, and prostate cancer in this patient population (11). These screening tests should be included preoperatively along with screening for other often missed comorbidities such as sleep apnea, insulin resistance, diabetes, cardiovascular disease, depression, and fatty liver disease (12). At a minimum, patients are seen by a dietician, psychologist or psychiatrist, and the surgeon. Some patients are sent for evaluation by other specialists or by an obesity medicine specialist (13).

Informed consent is an important part of WLS. Patients need to be informed not only about the short term risks of blood clots, bleeding, and leaks but should also be informed about longer term issues of vitamin deficiencies, gallstones, kidney stones, ulcers, and bowel obstructions. It is extremely important that patients be apprised of the true operative mortality rate as well as the risk of weight regain or weight loss failure for the given procedure. Patients should also be educated on alternative surgical procedures. It is important to balance this information with recognition of the risks of remaining obese (13).

Most WLS programs will have both a preoperative and a postoperative education program run by a nurse, dietician, or a psychologist. These programs vary widely in their size, time commitment, and in their content. Their purpose is to educate the patients on when, what, and how to eat before, during, and after recovery from WLS. Behavior modification before surgery to provide preoperative weight loss, smoking cessation and caffeine withdrawal are included and even required by many programs. Other features include group and individual meetings with preoperative education ranging from 3 to 20 hours, and postoperative courses lasting 1 to 12 months with 3 to 40 hours of instruction. Many insurance companies require compliance with a six month preoperative weight loss program. Although there is not data to support the effectiveness of this requirement, preoperative weight loss may be beneficial (14–16).

Adjustable Gastric Banding (AGB)

For the most part, laparoscopic AGB is a restrictive procedure that compartmentalizes the stomach into two sections. The smaller section, located above the band, has a capacity of 10 to 20 ml (pouch). The larger section is below the band. The constriction created by the band is called the stoma.

The band consists of a soft, locking silicone ring connected to an infusion port placed on the anterior rectus fascia. The port may be accessed with relative ease using a Huber needle. Injection of saline into the port leads to reduction in the band diameter, resulting in an increased degree of restriction. The bands currently available are adjustable, and are placed laparoscopically. In experienced hands this procedure takes anywhere from 30 to 60 minutes.

Laparoscopic AGB is gaining significant attention among bariatric surgeons and patients primarily because of its simplicity, adjustability, and reversibility. It does not require division of the stomach or intestines. As a result, it has the lowest mortality rate (0.05–0.5%) of all bariatric procedures. The adjustability of the outlet by the band design offers a theoretical advantage of addressing various nutritional issues after surgery. Furthermore, as newer and more advanced treatments for obesity emerge, the band can be removed easily leaving the stomach anatomy intact (17).

There are two main techniques for gastric banding—the perigastric and the pars flaccida technique. Most surgeons use the pars flaccid technique where the dissection is kept outside of Morrison's pouch to prevent slipping of the band posteriorly. This procedure is well suited for patients who have a BMI < 50, are younger than 50 years old, willing to make significant changes in their daily food choices, and are motivated to come in frequently for adjustments (18). It is also a good choice for patients who require repeat endoscopic retrograde cholangiopancreatography (ERCP) or monitoring of the distal stomach (Fig. 1).

Roux-en-Y Gastric Bypass (RYGB)

RYGB was first described in 1967 by Dr. Mason, considered to be the father of bariatric surgery. He proposed the procedure based on the observation that patients who underwent partial gastrectomy experienced significant long-term weight loss. The first laparoscopic gastric bypass was performed by Wittgrove and Clark in 1993. Today, this is the most commonly performed bariatric procedure in the United States, and is considered the gold standard among bariatric procedures. Depending on the type of configuration and surgical expertise, the duration of the procedure can vary from 90 minutes to 4 hours.

The RYGB is characterized by a small (<30 ml) proximal gastric pouch divided and separated from the stomach remnant. Drainage of food to the rest of the gastrointestinal tract takes place via a stoma and a Roux-en-Y small bowel arrangement. A much larger gastric remnant becomes disconnected from the food stream, while secretion of gastric acid, pepsin, and intrinsic factor continues. It is the bypass of the duodenum which changes the neural-hormonal pathways affecting satiety and hunger. This ultimately results in decreased food intake. These same pathways affect insulin resistance and account for the immediate improvement in certain comorbidities like type II diabetes (1).

The anastomosis of the gastric pouch to the jejunum can be done by suturing, with a linear stapler, or with a circular stapler. This anastomosis was first performed

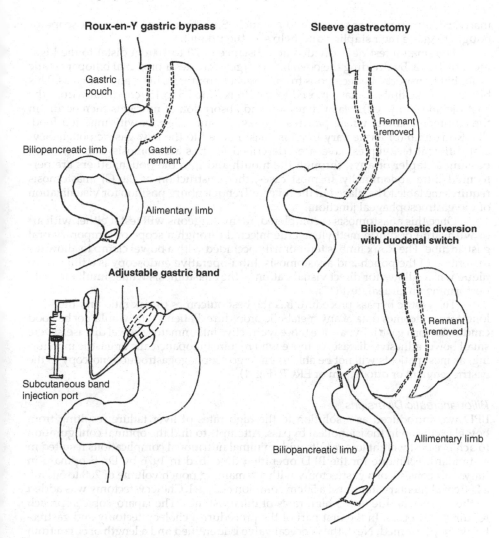

Figure 1 Four most common weight loss surgeries.

via a retrocolic passage of the jejunum, but nowadays most surgeons use an ante-colic passage. Usually in the ante-colic approach, the greater omentum has to be divided so that the Roux limb can reach the gastric pouch. The anastomosis itself is calibrated to be 1.2 to 3 cm in size.

The operation can be performed laparoscopically with five to seven trocars inserted through the upper abdominal wall, or in an open fashion through an upper midline or a left sub costal incision. Creation of the 30 ml gastric pouch is performed using mechanical staplers. It is important to ensure stapling close to the gastroesophageal junction while avoiding coming across the esophagus. Before stapling is initiated all items placed in the stomach or esophagus must be removed: nasogastric tube, esophageal stethoscope, and temperature probe. All of these have been inadvertently stapled or sewed into a pouch. Some surgeons will use a scope or bougie to guide their stapling and help size their pouch.

The small intestine is divided at a distance of 30 to 100 cm distal to the Ligament of Treitz. By dividing the bowel, the surgeon creates a proximal biliopancreatic limb that transports the secretions from the gastric remnant, liver, and pancreas. This biliopancreatic limb is anastomosed to the Roux limb 75 to 150 cm distally from the gastrojejunostomy (GJ). Major digestion and absorption of nutrients then occurs in the common channel where pancreatic enzymes and bile mix with ingested food. The Roux limb (or alimentary limb) is anastomosed to the new gastric pouch. Several different techniques have been described for this anastomosis. Some involve passing a stapler or anvil through the mouth and into the pouch; others are performed intra-abdominally. In most cases, the construction of the GJ anastomosis requires the table to be placed in the reverse Trendelenburg position for visualization of the gastroesophageal junction.

Once this anastomosis is completed, many surgeons will test it either with air or with 60 ml of dilute methylene blue injected through a scope or temporary oral gastric tube. The Roux limb is temporarily occluded with a bowel clamp to allow for distention of the pouch and anastomosis. Intra-operative endoscopy is a third technique which allows for direct visualization of the anastomosis while simultaneously performing an air leak test (17).

The gastric bypass procedure has the best outcomes to risk ratio and the most long-term outcomes data of any metabolic procedure. Patients who would not be good candidates for a gastric bypass are those with active inflammatory bowel disease, severe small bowel adhesive disease, or those who require biliopancreatic or gastric monitoring, as most patients will not be able to undergo esophagogastroduodenoscopy to the gastric remnant or duodenum or ERCP (Fig. 1).

Biliopancreatic Diversions

BPD was introduced as a solution to the high rates of liver failure resulting from bowel exclusion in the jejunoileal bypass. Attempts to find the optimal configuration to achieve best weight loss results with minimal nutritional complications resulted in a standard technique for the BPD operation described in 1976 by Dr. Scopinaro in Italy. This consists of a gastrectomy with a remaining pouch volume of 200 to 500 ml, a 200 cm alimentary limb, and a 50 cm common channel. Cholecystectomy was added to the procedure due to the high rates of biliary stones. The laparoscopic approach requires six trocars. In the first part of the procedure a cholecystectomy and gastrectomy are performed. Next, the ileocecal valve is identified and a length of 50 cm from the valve is measured and marked to be the location of the enteroenterostomy. The bowel is measured for another 200 cm and then divided to create the alimentary and biliopancreatic limbs. The Roux limb is brought retrocolic to fashion the GJ anastomosis in two layers (19).

A variant of this procedure, the biliopancreatic diversion with duodenal switch (BPD with DS) has also been described. The procedure involves a sleeve gastrectomy with preservation of the pylorus, and creation of a Roux limb with a short common channel. This procedure differs from the BPD in the portion of the stomach that is removed, as well as preservation of the pylorus. It is thought to have a lower incidence of marginal ulceration and dumping syndrome. This procedure has been advocated for patients with super-morbid obesity (BMI > 60), a group in which it has been associated with improved weight loss. It can also be performed in stages, doing the sleeve gastrectomy in one operation and the BPD as a second procedure, significantly decreasing the overall risk. Use of either of these procedures as a primary weight loss operation requires a patient willing to deal with loose bowel movements (about five times a day), as well as very high protein intake which can be difficult with the American diet (20).

Sleeve
Sleeve gastrectomy, introduced by Dr. Gagner as the first stage in the BPD with DS, is now considered a primary weight loss procedure. The procedure consists of a laparoscopic partial gastrectomy in which the majority of the greater curvature of the stomach is removed and a tubular stomach is created. Division of the greater curvature of the stomach is started 8 to 10 cm proximal to the pylorus with a 32–60 french bougie or endoscope inserted transorally. The gastrectomy is fashioned along the bougie toward the gastroesophageal junction. Patients experience approximately 51% excess weight loss in one year (21). While this operation is currently only used as a staging procedure, long term outcomes may prove the sleeve gastrectomy to be a safe and effective standalone procedure for surgical weight loss.

Future Procedures
There are several minimally invasive and natural orifice procedures which may play a significant role in the future. The directions of metabolic surgery at this point in time are twofold. There are those procedures aimed at minimizing invasiveness and complications and those aimed at specific mechanisms of obesity. An example of the first would be transoral vertical gastroplasty, a restrictive procedure involving stapling or sewing the proximal stomach from the inside to create a proximal pouch, mimicking the AGB. Another variation on an old theme is the gastric balloon. Originally filled with air, these endoscopically placed balloons, offer a mass effect in the stomach increasing early satiety (22). Today the balloons are saline filled and can be tethered to the abdominal wall similar to a gastrostomy tube (23). There are a few examples of the second category: vagal stimulation to reduce appetite (24), endoluminal sleeves that block food absorption in the duodenum (25), and/or stomach, and oral devices worn to prevent rapid eating or to monitor food intake.

Another potential future role of metabolic surgery may be in the treatment of normal weight patients who have type II diabetes or sleep apnea. There is good evidence that either standard gastric bypass or a variation thereof may be effective and appropriate in the non-obese patient with diabetes (26).

OUTCOMES
Successful surgical outcomes after WLS are most often measured by average excess body weight (EBW) lost. Unfortunately, this value represents the least important measure of success. Probably the best measures of success following WLS are resolution of comorbidities, improvement in quality of life, and increased life expectancy.

Weight Loss
Most WLS outcomes describe weight loss in the form of EBW loss as a percentage of total body weight and ideal body weight. The frequency distribution of EBW loss occurs as a bell curve in the case of gastric bypass and as a double peaked curve in the case of gastric banding (27). According to a 2005 meta-analysis by Buchwald et al., the average EBW loss with gastric bypass is 68% (77–33%) and with banding 50% (70–32%). It is more difficult to get a good idea of the actual failure rate as defined by loss of <25–30% EBW or BMI > 35. Ranges of reported

failure at 5 to 7 years varied from 36.9% after AGB (28) to 4.2% after RYGB (29). Though uncommon after RYGB, inadequate weight loss and weight regain still remain a difficult problem since there is little option for revision. Weight loss failure or regain after AGB can be treated by band removal and conversion to a RYGB or BPD either in one operation or in sequential procedures.

Resolution of Comorbidities
There are many publications looking at comorbidities, perhaps the most compelling data is on diabetes and obstructive sleep apnea. In a meta-analysis of all WLS outcomes on 22,094 patients, Buchwald et al. found diabetes to be completely resolved in 76.8% of patients, and either resolved or improved in 86.0% (combining RYGB, AGB, and BPD patients). Hyperlipidemia improved in at least 70% of patients. Hypertension either resolved or improved in 78.5%. Obstructive sleep apnea was resolved in 85.7% (17). Operation specific data is shown in Table 1.

Quality of Life
Quality of life following WLS is significantly improved (30). This is partly due to the freedom from the anti-fat bias which is pervasive in our society. Remarkable changes in health related quality of life occur in a relatively short period of time following bariatric surgery. These are related not only to physical but also to social functioning (31). In teens the effect on quality of life is perhaps most significant since obese teens suffer from significant social stigmatization which resolves with weight loss (32,33). Depression is decreased after WLS, with fewer hospital admissions and improved overall Beck Depression Index scores (34).

Mortality
Operative mortality ranges from 1.1% in BPD to 0.5% for RYGB and 0.1% for AGB (17). These rates have decreased with newer techniques, higher volume centers, and the center of excellence programs instituted in the last few years. While the initial operative risk is lowest for the AGB, the re-operative rate is significantly higher than for the other two operations. The RYGB 30 day mortality risk equals that of hip replacement and is significantly less than that for cardiac bypass.

Statistically, mortality associated with surgery in the severely obese patient remains significantly less than mortality without surgery (35). In Canada, Christou et al. looked at 1035 WLS patients and 5746 case matched controls; they showed that at five years there was a reduction in relative risk of death by 89% for those patients undergoing WLS. The mortality rate in the bariatric surgery patient was 0.68% and in the obese control group was 6.17%.

Table 1 Summary of Metabolic Surgical Outcomes of the Three Most Common Operations (17)

Metabolic procedure	Adjustable gastric band	Roux-en-Y gastric bypass	Biliopancreatic diversion
Excess weight loss	50% (70–32%)	68% (77–33%)	72% (75–62%)
Diabetes resolved	48% (29–67%)	84% (77–90%)	99% (97–100%)[a]
Hypertension resolved	43% (30–56%)	68% (58–77%)	83% (73–94%)
Obstructive sleep apnea resolved	95% (89–100%)[a]	80% (68–92%)	92% (82–100%)

[a]Comparison across studies not significant for heterogeneity.

Complications
Complications can be divided into three time periods: early, midterm, and late. Rates vary by operative type, surgeon, and hospital. As with other complex surgical procedures, the surgeon's overall experience and annual volume as well as the hospital volume affect complication rates.

Early
In a review of the Cochrane clinical data base, early peri-operative complications were more common with RYGB than with AGB (9% vs. 5%) (36). Major early complications include *anastomotic leak, thromboembolism, obstruction, urinary tract infection, bleeding, wound infection,* and *pulmonary adverse events*. The impact of many of these complications can be minimized. For example, aggressive thromboembolism prophylaxis with pre- or peri-operative injectable anticoagulants (heparin, LMWH), pneumatic compression boots and early ambulation can decrease the likelihood of postoperative thromboembolic events. Patients with obstructive sleep apnea or hypoventilation syndrome should be monitored carefully postoperatively, especially in the setting of narcotic administration. Respiratory recovery is improved by the use CPAP and BiPAP immediately postoperatively. There is no evidence that this increases nausea, vomiting, or leak rate (37).

Midterm
These complications represent the least well documented yet preventable complications. *Kidney stones, gallstones, anastomotic stenosis, internal hernias,* and *marginal ulcers* can be seen after RYGB or BPD. The rate of these complications is difficult to identify due to the mobility of our population, the often delayed onset, and the variety in techniques. For example, the rate of stenosis ranges from 1.6% to 27%. This depends greatly on the technique of anastomosis with the 21 EEA circular stapler imparting the highest risk. Endoscopic dilatation is the treatment of choice in most cases (38). The formation of gallstones due to rapid weight loss can be mitigated, and often prevented, by prescribing Ursodiol for the first six months postoperatively. Some surgeons simply opt to remove the gallbladder at the time of surgery. Both options are controversial, today most programs recommend cholecystectomy at a later date if the patient develops symptoms (39). Ulcers are most commonly seen in smokers and those using NSAIDs. Dehydration, a potentially preventable condition, probably contributes to both ulcer and kidney stone formation. Finally, internal hernias from adhesions or true mesenteric defects can be difficult to diagnose radiographically. For this reason exploratory laparoscopy is recommended in cases of severe abdominal pain following RYGB or BPD.

Complications following AGB can include gallstones, kidney stones, and internal hernias similar to the other procedures. In addition, *band slipping, erosion, infection,* and *pouch dilatation* can occur. Most of these require removal of the band. Placement of a new band or conversion to RYGB or BPD has a higher success rate than readjusting the original band both as measured by weight loss as well as by need for reoperation (40).

Late
The long-term reoperation rates are lower after RYGB than AGB (16% vs. 24%). Indications for reoperation after RYGB include: staple line breakdowns or fistulas, obstruction, gallstones, ulcers and bleeding. Re-operations after AGB are for weight loss failure, band slipping or eroding, pouch dilatation, stenosis, tubing failure, or infection.

The most common late complications of RYGB or BPD are *vitamin deficiencies* and *dumping syndrome*. In a compliant patient, vitamin levels should be checked annually. Dumping syndrome, a reaction probably mediated by incretin hormones, can generally be prevented by avoiding foods high in fats and complex carbohydrates. Late complications associated with AGB often require band removal. Similar to breast implants, the band elicits a foreign body reaction resulting in formation of a firm capsule. This capsule must be removed or ablated at the time of revision (41).

SPECIAL ANESTHETIC CONSIDERATIONS IN RE-OPERATIVE PATIENTS
The patient who has undergone WLS is likely to return to the operating room to address complications of WLS, for unrelated cancer procedures, orthopedic surgery, and plastic/reconstructive procedures. There are several considerations in these patients depending on the operation originally preformed, the operation planned, and the patients' preoperative health.

Vitamin and Mineral Deficiencies
First, it is important to remember that patients who are status post bariatric surgery are at high risk for vitamin and mineral deficiencies. These can be screened for and treated preoperatively, but may not be recognized by the patient or surgeon in many cases. The most common deficiencies include iron, B_{12}, vitamin D, and in patients with recurrent vomiting, thiamine (vitamin B_1). Patients with a RYGB or BPD are at higher risk for deficiencies than those with AGB; however, recurrent vomiting is common with banding, therefore intravenous (IV) thiamine therapy prior to administration of a dextrose infusion should be considered.

Preoperative screening and intravenous treatment of anemia should be of high priority. Vitamin B_{12} shots and IV iron infusion are sometimes required, especially in menstruating female patients. In addition, vitamins A, B_6, C, E, and folic acid deficiencies can also lead to anemia refractory to iron supplementation (41). BPD patients are at particular risk of fat soluble vitamin deficiencies (vitamin A, D, E, and K). An abnormal prothrombin time preoperatively should prompt assessment of the vitamin K level prior to surgery. Increasing evidence exists that even in patients who take vitamin supplements, deficiencies of the B vitamins, as well as vitamins A and C, zinc, selenium, and copper are not uncommon (42). These deficiencies can cause significant wound healing (C and Zinc), cardiac (selenium), and neurologic (copper) problems, and thus should be assessed in any prior WLS patient undergoing major surgery or admitted to an ICU.

Positioning and Procedures
Patients who have a Roux-en-Y gastric bypass or band are at some risk of pouch perforation with introduction of naso-gastric or oro-gastric tubes. For this reason it is recommended that these be avoided or introduced under endoscopic or fluoroscopic guidance if required. Operative table padding should be set up with attention to folds of skin present after significant weight loss. Epidural placement may be complicated by the looseness of skin, leading to more common displacement of the catheter. Securing of central venous catheters can also be difficult and requires special attention to suturing and taping. Patients who still have a large pannus may develop meralgia paresthetica, an injury of the lateral femoral cutaneous nerve leading to numbness and tingling in the upper outer thigh and groin area. This will most often resolve on its own when it occurs as a result of operative positioning (43).

Protein Malnutrition

Protein malnutrition is uncommon after AGB and RYGB; however, it may occur in as many as 10% of patients who have undergone BPD. It is important to avoid surgery in patients with this condition unless absolutely indicated. Early introduction of either enteral nutrition or IV nutrition is key. One must watch for refeeding syndrome by carefully monitoring and repleting potassium, magnesium, and phosphate levels as calories are reintroduced (44). Protein malnutrition must be distinguished from marasmus, a condition characterized by hanging dry skin and complete loss of adipose tissue. The signs of pure protein malnutrition seen after BPD are total body edema, critically low albumin and hemoglobin, vomiting, diarrhea, and Wernicke–Korsakoff encephalopathy (45).

Hypoglycemia

Hypoglycemia following oral administration of glucose after RYGB or BPD is common. In rare cases this response is exaggerated and can lead to confusion, seizures, and auto accidents. Any patient admitted to the ICU or operating room with an unexplained seizure or auto accident following WLS should have plasma glucose levels assessed, a postoperative evaluation with glucose tolerance testing, and referral to an endocrinologist for medical treatment (46).

REFERENCES

1. le Roux CW, Welbourn R, Werling M, et al. Gut hormones as mediators of appetite and weight loss after Roux-en-Y gastric bypass. Ann Surg 2007; 246: 780–5.
2. Reinehr T, Roth CL, Schernthaner GH, et al. Peptide YY and glucagon-like peptide-1 in morbidly obese patients before and after surgically induced weight loss. Obes Surg 2007; 17: 1571–7.
3. Borg CM, le Roux CW, Ghatei MA, et al. Biliopancreatic diversion in rats is associated with intestinal hypertrophy and with increased GLP-1, GLP-2 and PYY levels. Obes Surg 2007; 17: 1193–8.
4. MacDonald KG Jr. Overview of the epidemiology of obesity and the early history of procedures to remedy morbid obesity. Arch Surg 2003; 138: 357–60.
5. Brolin R. Update: NIH consensus conference. Gastrointestinal surgery for severe obesity. Nutrition 1996; 6: 403–4.
6. Perry CD, Hutter MM, Smith DB, et al. Survival and changes in comorbidities after bariatric surgery. Ann Surg 2008; 247: 21–7.
7. Flum DR, Dellinger EP. Impact of gastric bypass operation on survival: a population-based analysis. J Am Coll Surg 2004; 199: 543–51.
8. Inge TH, Zeller MH, Lawson ML, et al. A critical appraisal of evidence supporting a bariatric surgical approach to weight management for adolescents. J Pediatr 2005; 147: 10–19.
9. Ippisch HM, Inge TH, Daniels SR, et al. Reversibility of cardiac abnormalities in morbidly obese adolescents. J Am Coll Cardiol 2008; 51: 1342–8.
10. Kalra M, Inge T. Effect of bariatric surgery on obstructive sleep apnoea in adolescents. Paediatr Respir Rev 2006; 7. 260–7.
11. Cohen SS, Palmieri RT, Nyante SJ, et al. Obesity and screening for breast, cervical, and colorectal cancer in women: a review. Cancer 2008; 112: 1892–904.
12. Kelly J, Tarnoff M, Shikora S, et al. Best practice recommendations for surgical care in weight loss surgery. Obes Res 2005; 13: 227–33.
13. Commonwealth of Massachusetts Betsy Lehman Center for Patient Safety and Medical Error Reduction Expert Panel on Weight Loss Surgery: executive report. Obes Res 2005; 13: 205–26.
14. Alger-Mayer S, Polimeni JM, Malone M. Preoperative weight loss as a predictor of long-term success following Roux-en-Y gastric bypass. Obes Surg 2008; 18: 772–5.

15. Alvarado R, Alami RS, Hsu G, et al. The impact of preoperative weight loss in patients undergoing laparoscopic Roux-en-Y gastric bypass. Obes Surg 2005; 15: 1282–6.
16. Riess KP, Baker MT, Lambert PJ, et al. Effect of preoperative weight loss on laparoscopic gastric bypass outcomes. Surg Obes Relat Dis 2008.
17. Buchwald H, Avidor Y, Braunwald E, et al. Bariatric surgery: a systematic review and meta-analysis. JAMA 2004; 292: 1724–37.
18. Busetto L, Angrisani L, Basso N, et al. Safety and efficacy of laparoscopic adjustable gastric banding in the elderly. Obesity (Silver Spring) 2008; 16: 334–8.
19. Scopinaro N, Gianetta E, Adami GF, et al. Biliopancreatic diversion for obesity at eighteen years. Surgery 1996; 119: 261–8.
20. Hess DS, Hess DW. Biliopancreatic diversion with a duodenal switch. Obes Surg 1998; 8: 267–82.
21. Mognol P, Chosidow D, Marmuse JP. Laparoscopic sleeve gastrectomy (LSG): review of a new bariatric procedure and initial results. Surg Technol Int 2006; 15: 47–52.
22. Rigaud D, Trostler N, Rozen R, et al. Gastric distension, hunger and energy intake after balloon implantation in severe obesity. Int J Obes Relat Metab Disord 1995; 19: 489–95.
23. Geliebter A, Melton PM, Gage D, et al. Gastric balloon to treat obesity: a double-blind study in nondieting subjects. Am J Clin Nutr 1990; 51: 584–8.
24. Shikora SA, Storch K. Implantable gastric stimulation for the treatment of severe obesity: the American experience. Surg Obes Relat Dis 2005; 1: 334–42.
25. Tarnoff M, Shikora S, Lembo A. Acute technical feasibility of an endoscopic duodenal-jejunal bypass sleeve in a porcine model: a potentially novel treatment for obesity and type 2 diabetes. Surg Endosc 2008; 22: 772–6.
26. Depaula AL, Macedo AL, Schraibman V, et al. Hormonal evaluation following laparo-scopic treatment of type 2 diabetes mellitus patients with BMI 20-34. Surg Endosc 2008.
27. Bessler M, Daud A, DiGiorgi MF, et al. Frequency distribution of weight loss percentage after gastric bypass and adjustable gastric banding. Surg Obes Relat Dis 2008; 4: 486–91.
28. Suter M, Calmes JM, Paroz A, et al. A 10-year experience with laparoscopic gastric band-ing for morbid obesity: high long-term complication and failure rates. Obes Surg 2006; 16: 829–35.
29. Angrisani L, Lorenzo M, Borrelli V. Laparoscopic adjustable gastric banding versus Roux-en-Y gastric bypass: 5-year results of a prospective randomized trial. Surg Obes Relat Dis 2007; 3: 127–32; discussion 32–3.
30. Karlsson J, Taft C, Ryden A, et al. Ten-year trends in health-related quality of life after surgical and conventional treatment for severe obesity: the SOS intervention study. Int J Obes (Lond) 2007; 31: 1248–61.
31. Dziurowicz-Kozlowska A, Lisik W, Wierzbicki Z, et al. Health-related quality of life after the surgical treatment of obesity. J Physiol Pharmacol 2005; 56(Suppl 6): 127–34.
32. Loux TJ, Haricharan RN, Clements RH, et al. Health-related quality of life before and after bariatric surgery in adolescents. J Pediatr Surg 2008; 43: 1275–9.
33. Modi AC, Loux TJ, Bell SK, et al. Weight-specific health-related quality of life in adolescents with extreme obesity. Obesity (Silver Spring) 2008; 16: 2266–71.
34. Kosatka D, Sobow T, Strzelczyk J. [Severity and rate of depression in obese patients after surgical treatment of obesity with Roux-en-Y gastric bypass procedure]. Wiad Lek 2006; 59: 477–80.
35. Christou NV, Sampalis JS, Liberman M, et al. Surgery decreases long-term mortality, morbidity, and health care use in morbidly obese patients. Ann Surg 2004; 240: 416–23; discussion 23–4.
36. Tice JA, Karliner L, Walsh J, et al. Gastric banding or bypass? A systematic review comparing the two most popular bariatric procedures. Am J Med 2008; 121: 885–93.
37. Meng L. Postoperative nausea and vomiting with application of postoperative continuous positive airway pressure after laparoscopic gastric bypass. Obes Surg 2008.

38. Swartz DE, Gonzalez V, Felix EL. Anastomotic stenosis after Roux-en-Y gastric bypass: a rational approach to treatment. Surg Obes Relat Dis 2006; 2: 632–6; discussion 7.
39. Caruana JA, McCabe MN, Smith AD, et al. Incidence of symptomatic gallstones after gastric bypass: is prophylactic treatment really necessary? Surg Obes Relat Dis 2005; 1: 564–7; discussion 7–8.
40. Muller MK, Attigah N, Wildi S, et al. High secondary failure rate of rebanding after failed gastric banding. Surg Endosc 2008; 22: 448–53.
41. Fishman SM, Christian P, West KP. The role of vitamins in the prevention and control of anaemia. Public Health Nutr 2000; 3: 125–50.
42. Gasteyger C, Suter M, Gaillard RC, et al. Nutritional deficiencies after Roux-en-Y gastric bypass for morbid obesity often cannot be prevented by standard multivitamin supplementation. Am J Clin Nutr 2008; 87: 1128–33.
43. Grossman MG, Ducey SA, Nadler SS, et al. Meralgia paresthetica: diagnosis and treatment. J Am Acad Orthop Surg 2001; 9: 336–44.
44. Gariballa S. Refeeding syndrome: a potentially fatal condition but remains underdiagnosed and undertreated. Nutrition 2008; 24: 604–6.
45. Gracia JA, Martinez M, Elia M, et al. Obesity surgery results depending on technique performed: long-term outcome. Obes Surg 2008.
46. Goldfine AB, Mun EC, Devine E, et al. Patients with neuroglycopenia after gastric bypass surgery have exaggerated incretin and insulin secretory responses to a mixed meal. J Clin Endocrinol Metab 2007; 92: 4678–85.

15 | Regional Anesthesia in the Obese Patient

Shubha V. Y. Raju[1] and Tim Canty[2]

[1]Clinical Fellow in Anesthesia, Harvard Medical School, Resident, Department of Anesthesia and Critical Care, Massachusetts General Hospital, Boston, Massachusetts, U.S.A.

[2]Instructor in Anesthesia, Harvard Medical School, Assistant in Anesthesia, Department of Anesthesia and Critical Care, Massachusetts General Hospital, Boston, Massachusetts, U.S.A.

INTRODUCTION

The increasing prevalence of obesity has led to an increase in the number of anesthetics performed in overweight and obese patients. There are numerous physiologic considerations associated with the administration of general anesthesia to patients with increased BMI. Some areas of concerns include:

Airway

A recent meta-analysis revealed a two to three times higher rate of difficult laryngoscopy in the obese compared to the lean patient. This despite optimal positioning (1).

Cardiovascular

Obesity is associated with increased cardiac output (2,3), hypertension (4), and left ventricular hypertrophy which may progress to diastolic dysfunction (5,6). The metabolic syndrome associated with obesity increases the risk of myocardial infarction (7) and cerebro-vascular accident in affected patients. Chronic hypoxia resulting from sleep apnea can cause pulmonary hypertension, which may progress to right ventricular hypertrophy and congestive cardiac failure (8). Hemodynamic changes associated with induction of general anesthesia and emergence may exacerbate these pre-existing conditions.

Pulmonary

Increased weight of the thoracic and abdominal components of the chest wall results in marked reduction of total respiratory compliance, functional residual capacity, expiratory reserve volume, and total lung capacity (9–11). The reduction in lung volumes and increase in ventilation/perfusion mismatching are responsible for an increased risk of hypoxemia during and after surgery. Obese patients often suffer from obstructive sleep apnea (10). This, coupled with an increased sensitivity to opiates, may predispose them to respiratory depression.

Gastrointestinal

Diabetic gastroparesis in conjunction with an increased incidence of gastro-esophageal reflux disease (12,13) increases the propensity of aspiration pneumonitis. Given these and other potential complications of general anesthesia, it may be prudent to consider regional anesthesia as an alternative for procedures in which it is a viable option.

ADVANTAGES OF REGIONAL ANESTHESIA

A regional anesthetic technique is less likely than general anesthesia to cause or exacerbate preexisting cardio-pulmonary depression. When regional anesthesia is used either as the sole anesthetic or as an adjunct to general anesthesia, there may be a lower requirement for post-operative opiates. Use of high dose narcotics is associated with post-operative respiratory depression and hypoxemia in the obese. Consequently, lowering its use can diminish the likelihood of respiratory complications (7). In the obese and non-obese patient populations, lowering the total parenteral perioperative opioid requirement decreases the degree and frequency of opioid related side effects, particularly, respiratory depression (14). By avoiding airway manipulation, there can be a decrease in potential risk for aspiration pneumonitis. Regional techniques have been shown to decrease post-operative nausea and vomiting (PONV), and to lower length of stay both in the post-anesthetic care unit (PACU) and in the hospital (15,16).

DIFFICULTIES WITH REGIONAL ANESTHETIC TECHNIQUES

While a regional anesthetic technique offers significant benefits to the obese patient compared to a general anesthetic, it is not devoid of challenges such as:

1. Proper patient positioning prior to and upon completion of the block (15)
2. Successful identification of appropriate anatomic landmarks (15)
3. Inadequate equipment such as block needles of insufficient length
4. Higher rates of complications from misplaced needles
5. Higher incidence of failed blocks which may result in delayed start of cases or conversion to general anesthesia under less than optimal conditions (15,17)
6. Multiple attempts may be required before a successful block is achieved. Additionally, it may be necessary to supplement blocks with local or general anesthesia (17)

SPECIAL CONSIDERATIONS FOR DIFFERENT REGIONAL ANESTHETIC TECHNIQUES
Neuraxial Blocks
Epidural
The distance from the skin to the epidural space differs significantly among patients, increasing in patients with high BMI. It also varies with the position of the patient (18). The distance from the skin to the epidural space is least in the sitting flexed position, which makes it the preferred patient position for epidural catheter placement. This distance increases as the obese patient sits upright or lies in the lateral decubitus position. As patients change position, from sitting to the lateral decubitus position for example, an epidural catheter already secured to the skin can migrate out of the epidural space (19,20). Thus, it has been suggested that in order to reduce the risk of catheter dislodgement, the obese patient should assume either the sitting upright or lateral decubitus position before the catheter is secured to the skin (20).

In the obese obstetric population, lower doses and volume of local anesthetic are required to obtain a similar surgical level of epidural anesthesia compared to non-obese parturients (21–23). An important factor in this difference is a smaller epidural space in the obese, presumably resulting from abundance of epidural fat as well as engorged epidural veins caused by the increased intraabdominal pressure and higher blood volume. The success of catheter placement in the obese population increases with ultrasound (USG) (24,25) or fluoroscopic assistance (26).

Spinal

Studies have clearly shown a decreased requirement for intrathecal local anesthetic doses in the obese population secondary to smaller cerebrospinal fluid (CSF) volumes. For a given dose of local anesthetic, higher sensory levels have been demonstrated in the obese population (27–30). A potential complication of spinal anesthesia, post dural puncture headache (PDPH) is seen less frequently in the obese population. This may be secondary to lowering of the pressure gradient between the subarachnoid and epidural spaces by the abdominal panniculus functioning much like an abdominal binder. With elevated intra-abdominal pressures, there is a decrease in the degree of spinal fluid leakage through the dural puncture site (31).

There is an increased risk of transient neurologic symptoms (TNS) following spinal anesthesia with lidocaine in patients with obesity (32). Use of either USG or fluoroscopic (26) assistance improves the success rate of spinal anesthesia. However, time and cost benefit of using these techniques in the operating room setting have yet to be demonstrated.

Peripheral Nerve Blocks

In one small study of supraclavicular blocks in obese patients, there was only a slightly decreased rate of block success with no difference in complication rate (33). A large review of prospectively gathered data on 7160 patients showed that obesity incrementally increases the difficulty and decreases the success rate of several single shot blocks and peripheral catheters. Some of the blocks studied include interscalene, supraclavicular, axillary, lumbar plexus, femoral, ankle, sciatic, paravertebral, and spinal. All blocks in this study were performed with nerve stimulator localization, not ultrasound guidance (34).

Interscalene blocks are frequently associated with phrenic nerve blockade, which may result in clinically significant hypoxia and respiratory distress in the obese patient. In our experience, avoidance of phrenic nerve blockade can be achieved through the use of lower volumes of local anesthetics or injection posteriorly, deeper, or more distal along the plexus, if appropriate for the surgery (35).

Despite the paucity of data, it is possible to conclude that peripheral regional anesthetic techniques can be applied safely to the obese patient with minimal difference in complication rates, albeit with a slightly greater need for block supplementation or conversion to general anesthesia. Obese patients should not be excluded from having the option of regional anesthesia.

The use of ultrasound guidance in obese patients has been shown to decrease block performance time. The high quality images generated allow for better visualization of landmarks, reducing the number of needle passes, shortening the block onset time, and allowing the block to be performed using lower local anesthetic doses (36,37). In general, the use of USG in peripheral nerve blocks helps in the direct visualization of nerves, minimizing the risk of intraneural injection; decreases block latency; is a dynamic and safe teaching tool; and allows for visualization of anatomical variations. Consequently, the risks of intravascular injection, pleural puncture and complications from local anesthetic toxicity are reduced, resulting in an overall better quality of the blockade (37).

IMAGING GUIDANCE FOR NEURAXIAL BLOCKS
Ultrasound (USG)
Advantages
One of the main advantages of USG is accurate identification of anatomy, specifically:

1. The exact spinal level and insertion point at which the procedure will be performed (38)
2. The ideal level as defined by the clearest sonoanatomy (38)
3. The depth of the epidural space from the skin (38)
4. Anatomical abnormalities (e.g., scoliosis) (38)
5. It serves as a valuable teaching tool and has been shown to improve learning curves (39)
6. It increases efficacy as well as patient satisfaction (40)
7. It has been shown to increase patient safety by decreasing the number of attempts (40) and subsequent tissue trauma. As it allows for identification of abnormal sonoanatomy of the ligamentum flavum, the number of accidental dural punctures can be reduced as well (38)
8. May help identify potentially difficult epidurals (38)
9. May help convert what was previously considered to be difficult epidurals into easy epidurals (38)
10. By accurately identifying the depth of the epidural and subarachnoid spaces, it helps the clinician in choosing the best equipment for the spinal/epidural, e.g., length of needle (38)

Methods
Extensive description of the methods is beyond the scope of this chapter. Please refer to the review by Carvalho (38) for further details.

Transverse mid-line approach. The probe is placed horizontally and the midline of the spine, corresponding to the hyperechoic spinous process, is identified. From this point the probe is moved cephalad or caudad to identify the optimal interspace. Ligamentum flavum and dura mater can be seen and the depth measured to gauge needle placement.

Longitudinal paramedian approach. The probe is placed vertically, parallel to the long axis of the spine, slightly off the midline just lateral to the spinous processes. In this view, ligamentum flavum and dura can be visualized in the spaces between the hyperechoic lamina. With the aid of this view, the needle can be advanced while avoiding contact with lamina or spinous processes.

Special Considerations
The quality of USG imaging depends on the amount of fat tissue that exists between the surface of the skin and the tip of the spinous process as well as the depth of the ligamentum flavum. As both these factors are increased in the obese patient, the sharpness of the image may be compromised, although appropriate visualization is still possible (38). In the obese population, it is important to realize that the depth of the epidural space from the skin may be underestimated if the subcutaneous tissues are compressed by the USG probe. For an accurate estimation, it is recommended that the pressure on the skin be relieved prior to obtaining the measurement of depth (38).

It has been estimated that in most obese patients use of an extra-long epidural or spinal needle is unnecessary as the epidural space is located at a maximum of 8 cm from the skin, provided the puncture is done at the optimal insertion point

(38). Based on the amount of sub-cutaneous tissue in the paraspinous groove, the estimation of depth may vary by a few millimeters depending on the method chosen (i.e., the midline approach or the paramedian approach) (38). The use of dynamic USG helps in identifying ideal patient positioning as small changes in patient position can dramatically open up interspinous spaces while ensuring minimal spinal rotation or lateral flexion (38).

Limitations
1. Lack of technical prowess
2. Increased costs
3. Increased time

Fluoroscopy
Advantages
1. Accurate identification of anatomic landmarks
2. Determination of distance to the intrathecal space
3. Advancement of needle in real-time thereby confirming proper positioning
4. It is the standard for many types of injections in the specialty of pain management
5. Decreased frequency of traumatic taps

Methods
A detailed discussion of the trans-foraminal and inter-laminar approaches can be found in reference 37.

Special Considerations
While evaluating the use of fluoroscopy for placement of a difficult spinal, Nomura et al. found that the prone position resulted in significant improvement in the clarity of the fluoroscopic image compared with the sitting position. They hypothesized that there was probably less attenuation of the radiographic beam as it passed through the tissues compressed by a massive abdomen in the prone position. Additionally, it was felt that this position may alter the curvature of the spinal cord, causing the angle of the fluoroscopic beam to be more perpendicular in relation to the spinal axis (26).

Limitations
On of the main limitations is that of increased cost—fluoroscopic guidance may not be feasible for routine needle placements. However, the cost benefit may be appropriate in certain circumstances such as when caring for a patient with a history of multiple failed attempts, or when there is an absolute necessity of confirmation of needle placement (i.e., intrathecal chemotherapy). Radiation exposure may be an additional concern in the obese parturient.

CONCLUSION
The paucity of data evaluating the safety and risks of regional anesthesia in the obese population underscores the need for studies in these areas. Available literature reveals that regional anesthesia can be performed safely with a high degree of patient satisfaction. During performance of a neuraxial block in an obese patient it is important to consider their decreased requirement for local anesthetic doses compared to a lean patient, as well as the greater likelihood of a high sensory block. The

need for patient monitoring and availability of resuscitation equipment cannot be overemphasized.

Emerging technologies such as ultrasound guidance may facilitate and improve success rates of regional anesthesia techniques in this difficult patient population. Additionally, peripheral regional anesthesia can be applied safely to the obese patient with no difference in complication rates, albeit with a slightly greater need for block supplementation or conversion to general anesthesia compared to patients with normal BMI. Thus, obese patients should not be excluded from having the option of regional anesthesia, which in certain cases may be a suitable alternative to general anesthesia.

REFERENCES

1. Shiga T, Wajima Z, Inoue T, et al. Predicting difficult intubation in apparently normal patients: a meta-analysis of bedside screening test performance. Anesthesiology 2005; 103: 429–37.
2. Backman L, Freyschuss V, Hallberg D, et al. Cardiovascular function in extreme obesity. Acta Med Scand 1973; 193: 437–46.
3. Palmieri V, de Simone G, Arnett DK, et al. Relation of various degrees of body mass index in patients with systemic hypertension to left ventricular mass, cardiac output, and peripheral resistance (The Hypertension Genetic Epidemiology Network Study). Am J Cardiol 2001; 88: 1163–8.
4. Diaz ME. Hypertension and obesity. J Hum Hypertens 2002; 16(Suppl 1): 18–22.
5. Alpert MA, Lambert CR, Panayiotou H, et al. Relation of duration of morbid obesity to left ventricular mass, systolic function, and diastolic filling, and effect of weight loss. Am J Cardiol 1995; 75: 1194–7.
6. Alpert MA, Lambert CR, Terry BE, et al. Interrelationship of left ventricular mass, systolic function and diastolic filling in normotensive morbidly obese patients. Int J Obes Relat Metab Disord 1995; 19: 550–7.
7. Casati A, Putzu M. Anesthesia in the obese patient: pharmacokinetic considerations. J Clin Anesth 2005; 17: 134–45.
8. Alpert MA. Obesity cardiomyopathy: pathophysiology and evolution of the clinical syndrome. Am J Med Sci 2001; 321: 225–36.
9. Ray C, Sue D, Bray G, et al. Effects of obesity on respiratory function. Am Rev Respir Dis 1983; 128: 501–6.
10. Biring MS, Lewis MI, Liu JI, et al. Pulmonary physiologic changes of morbid obesity. Am J Med Sci 1999; 318: 293–7.
11. Pelosi P, Croci M, Ravagnan I, et al. Total respiratory system, lung, and chest wall mechanics in sedated paralyzed postoperative morbidly obese patients. Chest 1996; 109: 144–51.
12. Geiss LS, Pan L, Cadwell B, Gregg EW, et al. Changes in incidence of diabetes in U.S. adults, 1997–2003. Am J Prev Med 2006; 30: 371–7.
13. Hampel H, Abraham NS, El-Serag HB. Meta-analysis: obesity and the risk for gastroesophageal reflux disease and its complications. Ann Intern Med 2005; 143: 199–211.
14. Michaloudis D, Fraidakis O, Petrou A, et al. Continuous spinal anesthesia/analgesia for perioperative management of morbidly obese patients undergoing laparotomy for gastroplastic surgery. Obes Surg 2000; 10: 220–9.
15. Brodsky JB, Lemmens HJ. Regional anesthesia and obesity. Obes Surg 2007; 17: 1146–9.
16. Wong J, Marshall S, Chung F, et al. Spinal anesthesia improves the early recovery profile of patients undergoing ambulatory knee arthroscopy. Can J Anaesth 2001; 48: 369–74.
17. Nielsen KC, Guller U, Steele SM, et al. Influence of obesity on surgical regional anesthesia in the ambulatory setting: an analysis of 9,038 blocks. Anesthesiology 2005; 102: 181–7.
18. Clinkscales CP, Greenfield ML, Vanarase M, et al. An observational study of the relationship between lumbar epidural space depth and body mass index in Michigan parturients. Int J Obstet Anesth 2007; 16: 323–7.

19. Hamza J, Smida M, Benhamou D, et al. Parturient's posture during epidural puncture affects the distance from skin to epidural space. J Clin Anaesth 1995; 7: 1–4.

20. Hamilton CL, Riley ET, Cohen SE. Changes in the position of epidural catheters associated with patient movement. Anesthesiology 1997; 86: 778–84.

21. Panni MK, Columb MO. Obese parturients have lower epidural local anaesthetic requirements for analgesia in labour. Br J Anaesth 2006; 96: 106–10.

22. McCulloch WJ, Littlewood DG. Influence of obesity on spinal analgesia with isobaric 0.5% bupivacaine. Br J Anaesth 1986; 58: 610–14.

23. Taivainen T, Tuominen M, Rosenberg PH. Spinal anaesthesia with hypobaric 0.19% or plain 0.5% bupivacaine. Br J Anaesth 1991; 66: 272–3.

24. Nomura JT, Leech SJ, Shenbagamurthi S, et al. A randomized controlled trial of ultrasound-assisted lumbar puncture. J Ultrasound Med 2007; 26: 1341–8.

25. Wallace DH, Currie JM, Gilstrap LC, et al. Indirect sonographic guidance for epidural anesthesia in obese pregnant patients. Reg Anesth 1992; 17: 233–6.

26. Eidelman A, Shulman MS, Novak GM. Fluoroscopic imaging for technically difficult spinal anesthesia. J Clin Anesth 2005; 17: 69–71.

27. McCulloch WJ, Littlewood DG. Influence of obesity on spinal analgesia with isobaric 0.5% bupivacaine. Br J Anaesth 1986; 58: 610–14.

28. Hogan QH, Prost R, Kulier A, et al. Magnetic resonance imaging of cerebrospinal fluid volume and the influence of body habitus and abdominal pressure. Anesthesiology 1996; 84: 1341–9.

29. Pitkanen MT. Body mass and spread of spinal anesthesia with bupivacaine. Anesth Analg 1987; 66: 127–31.

30. Reyes M, Pan P. Very low-dose spinal anesthesia for cesarean section in a morbidly obese preeclamptic patient and its potential implications. Int J Obstet Anesth 2004; 13: 99–102.

31. Jones N, Peck M, Gowrie S, et al. Post dural puncture headache in morbidly obese patients. Can J Anaesth 2006; 53: 26343.

32. Freedman JM, Li D-K, Drasner K, et al. Transient neurologic symptoms after spinal anesthesia: an epidemiologic study of 1,863 patients. Anesthesiology 1998; 89: 633–41.

33. Franco CD, Gloss FJ, Voronov G, et al. Supraclavicular block in the obese population: an analysis of 2020 blocks. Anesth Analg 2006; 102: 1252–4.

34. Cotter JT, Nielsen KC, Guller U, et al. Increased body mass index and ASA physical status IV are risk factors for block failure in ambulatory surgery—an analysis of 9,342 blocks. Can J Anaesth 2004; 51: 810–16.

35. Rau RH, Chan YL, Chuand HI, et al. Dyspnea resulting from phrenic nerve paralysis after interscalene brachial plexus block in an obese male—a case report. Acta Anaesthesiol Sin 1997; 35: 113–18.

36. Nelson T. Ultrasound guided femoral nerve block in an obese patient with a patellar tendon tear and severe obstructive sleep apnea. The Internet Journal of Anesthesiology 2007; 12.

37. Escovedo Helayel P, Brüggemann da Conceição D, Rodrigues de Oliveira Filho G. Ultrasound-guided nerve blocks. Rev Bras Anestesiol 2007; 57: 106–23.

38. Carvalho JC. Ultrasound-facilitated epidurals and spinals in obstetrics. Anesthesiol Clin 2008; 26: 145–58, vii–viii.

39. Grau T, Bartusseck E, Conradi R, et al. Ultrasound imaging improves learning curves in obsteric epidural anesthesia: a preliminary study. Can J Anaesth 2003; 50: 1047–50.

40. Grau T, Leipold RW, Conradi R, et al. Efficacy of ultrasound imaging in obstetric epidural anesthesia. J Clin Anesth 2002; 14: 169–75.

16 | Postanesthesia Care of the Obese Patient

Nicholas C. Watson[1] and Edward A. Bittner[2]

[1]Fellow in Critical Care Anesthesiology, Harvard Medical School, Department of Anesthesia and Critical Care, Massachusetts General Hospital, Boston, Massachusetts, U.S.A.

[2]Instructor in Anesthesia, Harvard Medical School, Assistant in Anesthesia and Intensivist, Department of Anesthesia and Critical Care, Massachusetts General Hospital, Boston, Massachusetts, U.S.A.

INTRODUCTION

Postoperative complications are common in the obese surgical patient (Table 1). Obesity is a risk factor for postoperative morbidity and morbid obesity is a risk factor for mortality (1–3). In a large study of postoperative complications in patients who underwent a variety of elective and emergency noncardiac surgical procedures, obese patients had a higher prevalence of myocardial infarction, peripheral nerve injury, wound infection, and urinary tract infection (1). Morbidly obese patients had a higher prevalence of tracheal reintubation, cardiac arrest, and death. Thus, obese patients require close observation during their recovery room/postanesthesia care unit (PACU) stay. An understanding of the pathophysiological changes that occur with obesity and the postoperative complications unique to this group of patients should result in improved outcome.

PULMONARY CONSIDERATIONS AND MANAGEMENT

Morbid obesity has a significant effect on pulmonary function including a reduction in respiratory compliance, increased work of breathing, reduced lung volume, and increased airway resistance (4). Morbidly obese patients expend a disproportionately greater percentage of total oxygen consumption on breathing, resulting in decreased ventilatory reserve and predisposition to respiratory failure in the setting of mild pulmonary or systemic insults (5). These physiologic alterations are worsened by sedation and the supine position, particularly in patients who have undergone abdominal or thoracic procedures (5).

Desaturation

Hypoventilation frequently occurs among hospitalized patients with morbid obesity (6). Irrespective of the presence of sleep apnea, morbidly obese patients experience frequent episodes of oxygen desaturation despite supplemental oxygen administration (7).

Atelectasis is common in the postoperative period due to the effects of retraction during laparatomy or pneumoperitoneum during laparoscopy. In the morbidly obese, atelectasis persists for 24 hours after the surgical procedure whereas it resolves within hours in nonobese patients (8).

Intrapulmonary shunt is significantly increased in obese patients compared to lean individuals (9).

Obstructive Sleep Apnea and Obesity Hypoventilation Syndrome

Obstructive sleep apnea (OSA) is characterized by repetitive episodes of either partial or complete airway obstruction resulting in desaturation and sleep fragmentation.

Table 1 Postoperative Complications of Special Interest in Obesity

System	Complication
Neurologic	Peripheral nerve injury, ?delayed awakening from anesthesia
Pulmonary	Airway obstruction, hypoxemia, hypercarbia, atelectasis, pneumonia, tracheal reintubation
Cardiovascular	Hypovolemia, myocardial infarction/ischemia, cardiac arrest, atrial fibrillation
Renal	UTI
Gastrointestinal	Anastomotic leak, abdominal compartment syndrome, ?PONV
Hematologic	VTE
Endocrine	Hyperglycemia
Musculoskeletal	Pressure induced rhabdomyolysis
Integumentary	Wound infection, wound dehiscence

? indicates possible association with obesity.
The complications listed are either associated with or exacerbated by obesity.
Abbreviations: PONV, postoperative nausea/vomiting; UTI, urinary tract infection; VTE, venous thromboembolism.

Patients with OSA, a frequently undiagnosed condition, are at increased risk for postoperative respiratory depression. Risk factors for respiratory depression include systemic and neuraxial administration of opioids, use of sedatives, site and invasiveness of surgical procedure, and the underlying severity of sleep apnea (10–12). Exacerbation of respiratory depression may occur on the third or fourth postoperative day as sleep patterns are reestablished and "REM rebound" occurs (13). The American Society of Anesthesiologists has published practice guidelines for the perioperative management of patients with OSA (14). Postoperative concerns in the management of these patients include: analgesia, oxygenation, patient positioning, and monitoring.

Obesity-hypoventilation syndrome is manifested by hypoventilation, a diminished response to CO_2 and hypoxia, and hypercapnia not related to obstructive pulmonary disease (15). It appears to have significant overlap with OSA syndrome. At the most extreme, obesity hypoventilation syndrome culminates in Pickwickian syndrome which is characterized by hypoxia, hypercapnia with resulting pulmonary hypertension, and right ventricular failure (4).

Postoperative Pulmonary Management
Management strategies to prevent postoperative pulmonary complications include proper monitoring, avoidance of recumbent position, adequate pain control to permit cough and deep breathing, incentive spirometry, pulmonary toilet, and continuous positive airway pressure (CPAP). A major therapeutic goal of these interventions is maintenance or restoration of functional residual capacity (16).

Supplemental oxygen and *continuous monitoring with pulse oximetry* should be administered to all morbidly obese patients in the postoperative period. Given the increased risk of respiratory failure and emergent airway management, the PACU must be equipped with a *difficult airway cart* and trained personnel. Postoperative pulmonary dysfunction is accentuated by pain. *Pain control* strategies associated with minimal respiratory depression are discussed below. Given the high risk of postoperative *atelectasis* (8), deep breathing and coughing exercises as well as the use of incentive spirometry should be aggressively practiced postoperatively. The patient's upper body should be elevated 30 to 45° (17). If an abdominal binder is used after abdominal surgery, it should be evaluated to ensure that it does not cause overconstriction fostering splinting and atelectasis.

Unless contraindicated by the surgical procedure, *CPAP* or *bi-level positive airway pressure* (BiPAP) should be administered postoperatively to patients with sleep apnea who were receiving it preoperatively. It may also be beneficial in patients who were not previously treated with these modalities. Compliance can be improved if the patients use their own equipment. BiPAP is associated with improved pulmonary function in the first 12 to 24 hours following gastric bypass surgery in the morbidly obese. Longer-term postoperative benefits remain unproven (18). CPAP has been shown to improve hemodynamics during sleep in patients with OSA and congestive heart failure (19).

CARDIOVASCULAR CONSIDERATIONS AND MANAGEMENT
Hypertension, congestive heart failure, ischemic heart disease, cardiomyopathy, cardiac arrhythmias, and sudden cardiac death contribute to increased mortality and morbidity in the obese (20).

Hypertension
Mild to moderate hypertension is present in 50% to 60% of patients with obesity and severe hypertension in 10% (20). Patients with preexisting hypertensive disease are more likely to develop *postoperative hypertension*. Sympathetic nervous system activation resulting from noxious stimuli such as pain, anxiety, fluid overload, hypoxemia, hypercarbia, and bladder distension are common precipitants.

Complications of severe postoperative hypertension include myocardial ischemia, congestive heart failure, stroke, and increased surgical bleeding. The decision to *treat postoperative hypertension* should take into consideration the patient's baseline blood pressure, coexisting diseases, and perceived risk of complications.

Ischemic Heart Disease and Congestive Heart Failure
Increased circulating blood volume associated with obesity results in increased preload, stroke volume, cardiac output, and myocardial work. Elevated circulating concentrations of catecholamines, mineralocorticoids, renin, and aldosterone increase afterload. Myocardial hypertrophy, diastolic dysfunction, and ventricular failure can ensue.

Postoperative stressors such as pain, hypoxemia, hypercapnia, anemia, large fluid replacement, shivering, etc. can alter the balance between myocardial oxygen supply and demand further exacerbating the cardiovascular changes of obesity resulting in myocardial ischemia and congestive heart failure.

Management of *perioperative myocardial ischemia* involves decreasing myocardial oxygen demand and increasing oxygen supply with supplemental oxygen, aggressive pain control, beta-blockade, aspirin, and nitrates.

For acute decompensated *congestive heart failure* management strategies differ according to whether or not the patient has significant systolic versus diastolic dysfunction. Some of the initial therapies are similar in systolic and diastolic congestive heart failure, including supplemental oxygen and assisted ventilation (if necessary), diuresis, morphine, and vasodilator therapy. Among patients with acute systolic dysfunction, medications that either impair contractility (e.g., beta-blockers) or result in hypotension should be avoided or used with caution. For patients with primarily diastolic dysfunction, treatment of hypertension and tachycardia is particularly important. Preferred antihypertensive agents include beta-blockers, calcium channel blockers, and angiotensin receptor blockers (21).

Postoperative Arrhythmias

In this patient population, postoperative arrhythmias may be precipitated by a number of factors including hypoxia, hypercapnia, electrolyte abnormalities, increased catecholamine levels, OSA, and fatty infiltration of the conduction system. The risk of *atrial fibrillation* increases 50% in the obese population (22). Beta-blockade should be used with caution in morbidly obese patients because of impaired contractility due to decreased B-adrenergic receptors (23).

ECG abnormalities frequently encountered in the morbidly obese patient include low QRS voltage, leftward shift of the P wave, QRS wave, T wave axes, criteria for LVH, left atrial abnormalities, and T wave flattening in the inferior and lateral leads (24).

Management of a postoperative arrhythmia is focused on stabilizing hemodynamics and treating the underlying problem. Specific antiarrhythmic therapy will generally not be effective unless the precipitants are identified and treated.

RECOVERY OF CONSCIOUSNESS

Since obese patients are at risk for critical respiratory events in the PACU, a predictably prompt and complete recovery of consciousness from anesthesia is desirable (25). A paucity of primary literature exists comparing emergence times and techniques for obese and non-obese patients, thus the idea that obesity is related to prolonged emergence from anesthesia remains controversial.

Emergence from General Anesthesia

In morbidly obese patients, time to emergence and extubation in the operating room and time to numerous postoperative recovery metrics are more rapid after desflurane than after propofol, isoflurane, or sevoflurane anesthesia (26,27). General anesthesia with desflurane is associated with enhanced postoperative patient mobility and a reduced incidence of postoperative desaturation (27).

Delayed Awakening

The major causes of delayed awakening after general anesthesia apply to the obese and nonobese alike. These causes can be divided into three major groups: prolonged pharmacologic effects (volatile anesthetic, sedative, opioid, neuromuscular blockers), metabolic abnormalities (hypoxemia, hypercarbia, hepatic, renal, or endocrine dysfunction, and glucose and electrolyte abnormalities) and neurologic injury. Given the elevated risk for respiratory depression associated with the use of sedatives and opioids, hypoxemia and hypercarbia should be high on the differential diagnosis for delayed awakening in the obese patient.

POSITIONING AND MOBILIZATION
Positioning

Proper positioning of morbidly obese patients in the postoperative period has a number of benefits. First, arterial oxygenation is superior with the head of the bed elevated at 30 to 45° when compared to the supine position (28,29). Also, in comparison to the supine position, obese patients in the sitting position demonstrate favorable respiratory mechanics (30). In the event of emergent airway management the *reverse Trendelenburg* position provides the longest time of apneic normoxia when compared to supine and back-up Fowler positions (31). Furthermore, head elevation combined with neck flexion has been shown to improve view of the glottic opening during direct laryngoscopy (32).

Mobilization
Mobilization helps to prevent respiratory infections, deconditioning, venous thrombosis, and skin breakdown. The postoperative obese patient should be mobilized as soon as possible; complete bedrest is best avoided.

Explaining to the patient what to expect ahead of time and providing reassurance before and throughout the procedure can reduce fear of mobilization and improve cooperation. Physical therapists can design a program of passive and active exercise that is safe and effective for the morbidly obese patient.

Specialized equipment and mobilization techniques to prevent injury and ensure dignity should be employed. Extra large gowns are important to promote patient comfort and modesty during mobilization.

POSTOPERATIVE PAIN MANAGEMENT
Unrelieved pain can have adverse physiologic, behavioral, and psychological effects which can hinder recovery. Only a limited number of studies have been published which focus on postoperative pain management in the obese patient. A major challenge in this area involves determining the appropriate doses of analgesics which result in a balance between pain relief and minimal sedation/respiratory depression (33).

Rationale for Pain Control
Postoperative pain can contribute to pulmonary insufficiency and delay ambulation (16). Optimal analgesia permits coughing and movement without pain or discomfort as well as control of pain at rest. Given the high risk for pulmonary complications and immobility in postoperative obese patients, adequate analgesia is of paramount importance.

Assessment of Pain
Pain should be assessed, documented, and treated expeditiously. The intervals for pain assessment should be based on the intensity of the pain and the potential for analgesia-related complications. Self reports are the most reliable indicators of pain intensity (34).

Approaches to Pain Control
Strategies allowing for normal respiratory function and a timely return to ambulation must be evaluated while considering the associated risks (35). A multimodal drug regimen with minimal opioid is perhaps the best method of treating postoperative pain in the obese patient. The rationale is adequate analgesia resulting from the additive or synergic effects of the different analgesics combined with the reduction of dose related side effects (36).

Use of *opioids* in morbidly obese patients, particularly continuous infusions of long duration and high dose, may be limited by the drug's accumulation in fatty tissue. Redistribution could result in variable, prolonged or increased adverse effects such as sedation, respiratory depression, nausea/vomiting, etc. As dosing by actual body weight may overestimate an obese patient's opioid requirement, it has been suggested that initial doses be based on ideal body weight and titrated subsequently (37).

Nonopioid analgesics have been used successfully in the management of acute postoperative pain. These include: non-steroidal anti-inflammatory drugs (NSAIDs), $\alpha 2$ receptor agonists, NMDA receptor antagonists, and local anesthetics. In the absence of contraindications, supplementation with oral acetaminophen or NSAIDs is recommended. In a recent meta-analysis, Marret et al. found a 30% to 50% morphine sparing effect and reductions in nausea, vomiting, and sedation when a variety of NSAIDs were combined with morphine patient controlled analgesia (PCA) (38).

Clonidine and dexmedetomidine are α2 receptor agonists with sedative, sympatholytic, and analgesic properties. They have been used successfully for the postoperative pain management of obese patients (39–41). Administration of small doses of ketamine postoperatively can result in minimal side effects while achieving a significant reduction in pain intensity and morphine usage. Increased wakefulness, improved oxygenation, and decrease in postoperative nausea and vomiting (PONV) compared with morphine alone have been reported by Weinbrum (42).

Route of Pain Medication

The *oral* route for postoperative analgesic administration is the route of choice in surgeries with low nociceptive impact and in the ambulatory setting. Oral absorption of drugs is essentially unchanged in the obese patient (43). The most commonly administered oral drugs are NSAIDs and opioids.

The *intramuscular* route of administration is not recommended for postoperative pain management due to unpredictable effects and demonstrated poorer analgesia compared with other routes. *Intravenous* bolus injection of opioids is a common method of postoperative pain control; however, the altered pharmacologic effects in the obese patient should be taken into account.

PCA can be effective for acute postoperative pain although respiratory depression has been reported (44). Dosing should be based on ideal body weight and close monitoring of respiratory rate, sedation level, and pulse oximetry is essential.

Epidural or *spinal* analgesia may provide the safest and most effective postoperative analgesic management. The epidural route for opioid administration may be preferred over other routes because it results in less sedation, respiratory depression, and nausea, as well as earlier return of bowel function and mobilization (45–47). Nevertheless, the advantages of postoperative regional analgesia techniques must be weighed against the potential disadvantages when selecting a pain control regimen for the obese patient.

PCA intravenous morphine is comparable to epidural analgesia by several standard metrics in post gastric-bypass surgery; however, epidural analgesia was associated with increased wound infection rate when compared to PCA in one study (48). Respiratory depression following epidural morphine administration is a concern for up to 24 hours following the dosing (49–51). The combination of epidural opioids with systemic sedatives poses a risk of respiratory compromise in patients with OSA syndrome (12). Although not a consistent recommendation in the literature, epidural dosing for obese patients may need to be decreased by as much as 20% compared to lean individuals (34,52–56). Even after successful placement, inadequate epidural function requiring replacement is more common in obese than nonobese patients (57).

POSTOPERATIVE NAUSEA AND VOMITING
Obesity May Be a Risk Factor for PONV

Historically obesity has been cited as a risk factor for PONV for the following reasons (58):

1. Large *residual gastric volume* and higher incidence of *gastro-esophageal reflux*
2. Increased risk of *gastric inflation* due to difficulty with mask ventilation

3. Adipose tissue functions as a reservoir for *fat-soluble anesthetics*, releasing these into the blood and potentially promoting prolonged PONV after the cessation of anesthetic administration

However, a 2001 systematic review on the subject concluded that increased BMI is not a risk factor for PONV (59). Neither the Society for Ambulatory Anesthesia nor the American Society of Perianesthesia Nursing identifies obesity as a risk factor for PONV (60,61). There is no recommendation for PONV prophylaxis or treatment on the basis of obesity alone.

WOUND INFECTION
Obesity is a risk factor for nosocomial and surgical site infection (62).

Etiologies
Etiologies of wound infection in the obese include decreased oxygen tension, immune impairment, and secondary ischemia along suture lines (63). The higher incidence of diabetes mellitus in the obese population may be a contributing factor. In patients undergoing gastric bypass, epidural analgesia has been associated with an increased wound infection rate when compared to PCA (48).

Prevention
Wound and tissue hypoxia are common in obese patients in the perioperative period. Risk of wound infection is inversely related to tissue oxygen partial pressure. During the postoperative period, wound and tissue hypoxia are commonly seen in obese patients. Although supplemental oxygen administration only slightly increases tissue oxygenation, postoperative administration may be beneficial (64). Other strategies to minimize wound infection include prevention of hypothermia and treatment of hyperglycemia (65).

VENOUS THROMBOEMBOLISM
Obesity is an independent risk factor for venous thromboembolism (VTE) and is reported to be the most common cause of mortality after bariatric surgery (66,67). One to two of every three deaths after bariatric surgery are attributed to pulmonary embolism (68). VTE is reviewed in a separate chapter within this work.

COMPLICATIONS ASSOCIATED WITH BARIATRIC SURGERY
Bariatric surgery carries unique risks and complications in addition to the general, obesity-related complications discussed throughout this chapter (69,70).

Early Complications
Early complications of bariatric surgery deserve consideration in the deteriorating gastric bypass patient during the hours and days following the procedure (70). Meticulous communication of intraoperative events and data from the surgical and anesthetic teams to the postoperative team is essential to the rapid recognition and diagnosis of early postoperative complications.

Hypovolemia is often the result of inadequate fluid resuscitation in the operating room. Other causes are hemorrhage and, less commonly, anastomotic leak. Urine output should be calculated based on adjusted body weight (IBW + 40% of excess body weight), with the typical 0.5 to 1.0 ml/kg/hr as a minimum accepted value. Treatment is intravenous fluid administration and continued observation.

Bleeding, which may be intraluminal (causing gastrointestinal bleeding) or intra-peritoneal (causing bloody drainage output), is typically self-limited. Supportive management of hemorrhage should be initiated while work-up of coagulopathy and serial hematocrit measurements are performed. Unstable or continuously bleeding patients should undergo abdominal exploration.

Intestinal or anastomotic leak is the most serious of the early complications. Anastomotic leak carries a risk of abscess, fistula, peritonitis, sepsis, multisystem organ failure, and death. Diagnosis of anastomotic leak can be difficult due to patient's habitus and atypical presentation of peritonitis. Respiratory distress and severe tachycardia (HR > 120 bpm) are the most sensitive indicators of leak following laparoscopic RYGB (71). Additionally, fever, worsening abdominal pain, hiccups, and isolated left pleural effusion on x-ray should raise suspicion of intra-abdominal pathology and should be aggressively investigated. Workup of suspected leak may involve upper gastrointestinal series, abdominal CT, and/or evaluation by laparotomy or laparoscopy. Exploratory laparotomy should strongly be considered even if radiologic studies are inconclusive. In rapidly deteriorating patients an exploratory laparotomy should be performed without radiologic investigation (68).

Late Complications

Late complications of bariatric surgery can involve any organ system. The most common of these are prolonged nausea/vomiting, VTE, anastomotic stricture, anemia, electrolyte derangement, and nutritional deficiencies (69).

OTHER OBESITY ASSOCIATED COMPLICATIONS
Wound Dehiscence

Wound dehiscence has been ascribed to decreased perfusion combined with tension at the fascial edges (72).

1. Compromised vascularity may predispose to wound infection, necrosis, and dehiscence
2. The formation of hematoma or seroma may increase tension on the sutured incision and thus contribute to dehiscence
3. Reducing pressure on the wound with the use of elastic binders may help reduce tension resulting from coughing or transfers etc.

Pressure Induced Rhabdomyolysis

Pressure induced rhabdomyolysis is a rare but well described postoperative complication resulting from prolonged pressure on muscle during surgery. Obesity, prolonged surgery, and diabetes mellitus are risk factors. Muscles of the lower limbs, gluteal or lumbar regions are most commonly affected. Rhabdomyolysis from ischemia of the gluteal muscles leading to renal failure has been reported in morbidly obese patients (73).

Patients generally present in the postoperative period with numbness and muscular pain, symptoms which can be masked by epidural anesthesia. Muscle breakdown leads to *myoglobinuria*, which is suspected by the presence of brown urine and confirmed by the presence of hemoglobin on a urine dipstick in the absence of erythrocytes. Treatment consists of aggressive hydration, alkalinization of the urine, and maintenance of urine output with mannitol. Complications of severe rhabdomyolysis include *acute renal failure* as well as *compartment syndrome* of the involved body part.

Nerve Injury
Peripheral nerve injuries are more common in morbidly obese patients (74). Stretch injuries of the brachial plexus from excessive arm abduction and/or inadequate support of outstretched arms during surgery may contribute. Ulnar neuropathies also occur in hospitalized nonsurgical patients suggesting a multifactorial etiology (75). Consequently patient positioning should be given extra attention. This includes use of wider beds which will accommodate the arms, preventing them from resting on side rails.

Abdominal Compartment Syndrome
Morbid obesity is associated with increased intra-abdominal pressure (76). This intra-abdominal pressure is a function of central obesity and is associated with increased morbidity (76,77).

Superimposed factors such as multiple trauma, massive hemorrhage, and volume resuscitation can lead to abdominal compartment syndrome, which is associated with increased central venous pressure, pulmonary capillary wedge pressure, systemic vascular resistance, peak airway pressure, and renal vein pressure. It is also marked by decreased venous return, cardiac output, visceral and renal blood flow, and abdominal wall compliance (78). Treatment involves reduction of the intra-abdominal pressure through decompression of the abdomen.

TRIAGE
Guidelines for triaging postoperative morbidly obese patients should take into account the operative procedure, patient's coexisting diseases, and the institution's resources.

Postanesthesia Care Unit
Most morbidly obese patients who undergo surgical procedures are triaged to the surgical ward after a PACU recovery. Patients should not be discharged from the recovery area to an unmonitored setting until they are no longer at risk for postoperative respiratory depression. Adequacy of postoperative respiratory function may be documented by observing patients in an unstimulated state, preferably while they are asleep, to establish that they are able to maintain their baseline oxygen saturation while breathing room air.

ICU
Patients who are at high risk because of comorbid diseases, intraoperative complications, or failed postoperative extubation may require admission to the ICU or an intermediate level care unit (79). Approximately 20% to 24% of patients who undergo gastric bypass have been reported to require admission to the ICU (80,81). Risk factors for ICU admission after bariatric surgery include: male gender, age > 50 years, BMI > 60 kg/m^2, diabetes mellitus, cardiovascular disease, OSA, venous stasis, and intraoperative complications (82).

REFERENCES

1. Bamgbade OA, Rutter TW, Nafiu OO, et al. Postoperative complications in obese and nonobese patients. World J Surg 2007; 31: 556–60.
2. Besnoit S, Panis Y, Alves A, et al. Impact of obesity on surgical outcomes after colorectal resection. Am J Surg 2000; 179: 275–81.
3. Pasulka PS, Bistrian BR, Benotti PN, et al. The risks of surgery in obese patients. Ann Intern Med 1986; 104: 540–6.
4. Adams JP, Murphy PG. Obesity in anaesthesia and intensive care. Br J Anaesth 2000; 85: 91–108.
5. Gibson GJ. Obesity, respiratory function, breathlessness. Thorax 2000; 55: S41–S44.
6. Nowbar S, Burkart KM, Gonzales R, et al. Obesity-associated hypoventilation in hospitalized patients: prevalence, effects, and outcome. Am J Med 2004; 116: 1–7.
7. Ahmad S, Nagle A, McCarthy RJ, et al. Postoperative hypoxemia in morbidly obese patients with and without obstructive sleep apnea undergoing bariatric surgery. Anesth Analg 2008; 107: 138–43.
8. Eichenberger AS, Proietti S, Wickey S, et al. Morbid obesity and postoperative pulmonary atelectasis: an underestimated problem. Anesth Analg 2002; 95: 1788–92.
9. Ray C, Sue D, Bray G et al. Effect of obesity on respiratory function. Am Rev Respir Dis 1983; 128: 501–6.
10. Dhonneur G, Combes X, Leroux B, et al. Postoperative obstructive apnea. Anesth Analg 1999; 89: 762–7.
11. Boushra NN. Anaesthetic management of patients with sleep apnoea syndrome. Can J Anaesth 1996; 43: 599–616.
12. Ostermeier AM, Roizen MF, Hautkappe M, et al. Three sudden postoperative respiratory arrests associated with epidural opioids in patients with sleep apnea. Anesth Analg 1997; 85: 452–60.
13. Bell RL, Rosenbaum SH. Postoperative considerations for patients with obesity and sleep apnea. Anesthesiol Clin N Am 2005; 23: 493–500.
14. Practice guidelines for the perioperative management of patients with obstructive sleep apnea. A report by the American Society of Anesthesiologists Task Force on the Perioperative Management of Patients with Obstructive Sleep Apnea. Anesthesiology 2006; 104: 1081–93.
15. Kessler R, Chaouat A, Schinkewitch P, et al. The obesity-hypoventilation syndrome revisited: a prospective study of 34 consecutive cases. Chest 2001; 120: 369–76.
16. Craig DB. Postoperative recovery of pulmonary function. Anesth Analg 1981; 60: 46–52.
17. Flores JC. Post-anesthetic care unit management. In: Alvarez AO, ed. Morbid Obesity: Perioperative Management. Cambridge, UK: Cambridge University Press, 2004: 340–51.
18. Ebeo CT, Benotti PN, Byrd RP, et al. The effect of bi-level positive airway pressure on postoperative pulmonary function following gastric surgery for obesity. Respir Med 2002; 96: 672–6.
19. Tkacova R, Rankin F, Fitzgerald FS, et al. Effects of continuous positive airway pressure on obstructive sleep apnea and left ventricular afterload in patients with heart failure. Circulation 1998; 98: 2269–75.
20. Cheah MH and Kam PAC. Obesity: basic science and medical aspects relevant to anaesthetists. Anaesthesia 2005; 60: 1009–21.
21. Chinnaiyan KM, Alexander D, McCullough PA. Role of angiotensin II in the evolution of diastolic heart failure. J Clin Hypertens 2005; 7: 740–7.
22. Wang TJ, Parise H, Levy D, et al. Obesity and the risk of new-onset atrial fibrillation. JAMA 2004; 292: 2471–7.
23. Pieracci FM, Barie PS, Pomp A. Critical care of the bariatric patient. Crit Care Med 2006; 34: 1796–804.

24. Alpert MA, Terry BE, Cohen MV, et al. The electrocardiogram in morbid obesity. Am J Cardiol 2000; 85: 908–10.
25. Rose DK, Cohen MM, Wigglesworth DF, et al. Critical respiratory events in the postanesthesia care unit. Patient, surgical, and anesthetic factors. Anesthesiology 1994; 81: 410–18.
26. La Colla L, Albertin A, La Colla G, et al. Faster wash-out and recovery for desflurance vs sevoflurane in morbidly obese patients when no premedication is used. Br J Anaesth 2007; 99: 353–8.
27. Juvin P, Vadam C, Malek L, et al. Postoperative recovery after desflurane, propofol, or isoflurane anesthesia among morbidly obese patients: a prospective, randomized study. Anesthesia and analgesia 2000; 91: 714–19.
28. Vaughan RW, Bauer S, Wise L. Effect of position (semirecumbent versus supine) on postoperative oxygenation in markedly obese subjects. Anesth Analg 1976; 55: 37–41.
29. Vaughan RW, Wise L. Postoperative arterial blood gas measurement in obese patients: effect of position on gas exchange. Ann Surg 1975; 182: 705–9.
30. Yap JC, Watson RA, Gilbey S, et al. Effects of posture on respiratory mechanics in obesity. J Appl Physiol 1995; 79: 1199–205.
31. Boyce J, Ness T, Castroman P, et al. A Preliminary study of the optimal anesthesia positioning for the morbidly obese patient. Obes Surg 2003; 13: 4–9.
32. Levitan R, Mechem C, Ochroch A, et al. Head-elevated laryngoscopy position: improving laryngeal exposure during laryngoscopy by increasing head elevation. Ann Emerg Med 2003; 41: 322–30.
33. Choi YK, Brolin RE, Wagner BKJ, et al. Efficacy and safety of patient controlled analgesia for morbidly obese patients following gastric bypass surgery. Obes Surg 2000; 10: 154–9.
34. Haidbauer A. Post-operative analgesia. In: Alvarez AO, ed. Morbid Obesity: Perioperative Management. Cambridge, UK: Cambridge University Press, 2004: 381–95.
35. Kehlet H, Dahl JB. The value of "multimodal" or "balanced analgesia" in postoperative pain treatment. Anesth Analg 1993; 77: 1048–56.
36. Michaloudis D, Fraidakis O, Petrou A, et al. Continuous spinal anesthesia/analgesia for perioperative management of morbidly obese patients undergoing laparotomy for gastroplastic surgery. Obes Surg 2000; 10: 220–9.
37. Bouillon T, Shafer SL. Does size matter? Anesthesiology 1998; 89: 557–60.
38. Marret E, Kurdi O, Zufferey P, et al. Effects of nonsteroidal anti-inflammatory drugs on patient controlled analgesia morphine side effects. Anesthesiology 2005; 102: 1249–60.
39. Marinangeli F, Ciccozzi A, Donatelli F, et al. Clonidine for the treatment of postoperative pain: a dose finding study. Eur J Pain 2002; 6: 35–42.
40. Hofer RE, Sprung J, Sarr MG, et al. Anesthesia for a patient with morbid obesity using dexmedetomidine without narcotics. Can J Anaesth 2005; 52: 176–80.
41. Jeffs SA, Hall JE, Morris S. Comparison of morphine alone with morphine plus clonidine for postoperative patient-controlled analgesia. Br J Anaesth 2002; 89: 424–7.
42. Weinbrum AA. A single small dose of postoperative ketamine provides rapid and sustained improvement in morphine analgesia in the presence of morphine resistant pain. Anesth Analg 2003; 96: 789–95.
43. Cheymol G. Clinical pharmacokinetics of drugs in obesity: an update. Clin Pharmacokinet 1993; 25: 103–14.
44. Choi YK, Brolin RE, Wagner BK, et al. Efficacy and safety of patient-controlled analgesia for morbidly obese patients following gastric bypass surgery. Obes Surg 2000; 10: 154–9.
45. Brodsky JB, Merel RC. Epidural administration of morphine postoperatively for morbidly obese patients. West J Med 1984; 140: 750–3.
46. Fox GS, Whalley DG, Bevan OR. Anesthesia for the morbidly obese: experience with 110 patients. Br J Anaesth 1981; 53: 811–16.

47. Rawal N, Sjostrand U, Christofferson E, et al. Influence on postoperative ambulation and pulmonary function. Anesth Analg 1984; 63: 583–92.
48. Charghi R, Backman S, Christou N, et al. Patient controlled i.v. analgesia is an acceptable pain management strategy in morbidly obese patients undergoing gastric bypass surgery. A retrospective comparison with epidural analgesia. Can J Anaesth 2003; 50: 672–8.
49. Kafer ER, Brown JT, Scott D, et al. Biphasic depression of ventilatory responses to CO2 following epidural morphine. Anesthesiology 1983; 58: 418–27.
50. Stenseth R, Sellevold O, Breivik H. Epidural morphine for postoperative pain: experience with 1085 patients. Acta Anaesthesiol Scand 1985; 29: 148–56.
51. Gustafsson LL, Schildt B, Jacobsen K. Adverse effects of extradural and intrathecal opiates: report of a nationwide survey in Sweden, 1982. Br J Anaesth 1998; 81: 86–93.
52. Usubiaga JE, Wikinski JA, Usubiaga LE. Epidural pressure and its relation to spread of anesthetic solutions in epidural space. Anesth Analg 1967; 46: 440–6.
53. Duggan J, Bowler GM, McClure JH, et al. Extradural block with bupivacaine: influence of dose, volume, concentration and patient characteristics. Br J Anaesth 1988; 61: 324–31.
54. Curatolo M, Orlando A, Zbinden AM, et al. A multifactorial analysis of the spread of epidural analgesia. Acta Anaesthesiol Scand 1994; 38: 646–52.
55. Higuchi H, Adachi Y, Kazama T. Factors affecting the spread and duration of epidural anesthesia with ropivacaine. Anesthesiology 2004; 101: 451–60.
56. Visser WA, Lee RA, Gielen MJ. Factors affecting the distribution of neural blockade by local anesthetics in epidural anesthesia and a comparison of lumbar versus thoracic epidural anesthesia. Anesth Analg 2008; 107: 708–21.
57. Schumann R, Shikora S, Weiss JM, et al. A comparison of multimodal perioperative analgesia to epidural pain management after gastric bypass surgery. Anesth Analg 2003; 96: 469–74.
58. Watcha M, White P. Postoperative nausea and vomiting: its etiology, treatment, and prevention. Anesthesiology 1992; 77: 162–84.
59. Kranke P, et al. An increased body mass index is no risk factor for postoperative nausea and vomiting. A systematic review and the results of original data. Acta Anaesthesiol Scand 2001; 45: 160–6.
60. Gan TJ, Meyer TA, Apfel CC, et al. Society for Ambulatory Anesthesia. Society for Ambulatory Anesthesia guidelines for the management of postoperative nausea and vomiting. Anesth Analg 2007; 105: 1615–28.
61. American Society of PeriAnesthesia Nurses PONV/PDNV Strategic Work Team. ASPAN's evidence-based clinical practice guideline for the prevention and/or management of PONV/PDNV. J Perianesth Nurs 2006; 21: 230–50.
62. Cantürk Z, Cantürk NZ, Cetinarslan B, et al. Nosocomial infections and obesity in surgical patients. Obes Res 2003; 11: 769–75.
63. DeMaria EJ and Carmody BJ. Perioperative management of special populations: obesity. Surg Clin N Am 2005; 85: 1283–9.
64. Kabon B, Nagele A, Reddy A, et al. Obesity decreases perioperative tissue oxygenation. Anesthesiology 2004; 100: 274–80.
65. Mauermann WJ, Nemergut EC. The anesthesiologist's role in the prevention of surgical site infections. Anesthesiology 2006; 105: 413–21.
66. Pieracci F, Barie P, Pomp A. Critical care of the bariatric patient. Crit Care Med 2006; 34: 1796–804.
67. Podnos YD, Jimenez JC, Wilson SE, et al. Complications after laparoscopic gastric bypass: a review of 3464 cases. Arch Surg 2003; 138: 957–61.
68. Levi D, Goodman ER, Patel M, et al. Critical care of the obese and bariatric surgical patient. Crit Care Clin 2003; 19: 11–32.
69. Schauer PR, Ikramuddin S, Gourash W, et al. Outcomes after laparoscopic Roux-en-Y gastric bypass for morbid obesity. Ann Surg 2000; 232: 515–29.

70. Hess D, Forse R. Immediate postoperative complications. In: Farraye F, Armour R, eds. Bariatric Surgery: A Primer for Your Medical Practice, 1st edn. Thorofare, NJ: Slack Incorporated, 2006.

71. Hamilton E, Sims T, Hamilton T, et al. Clinical predictors of leak after laparoscopic Roux-en-Y gastric bypass for morbid obesity. Surg Endosc 2003; 17: 679–84.

72. Hahler B. Surgical wound dehiscence. MEDSURG Nursing 2006; 15: 296–300.

73. Bostanjian D, Anthone GJ, Hamoui N, et al. Rhabdomyolysis of gluteal muscles leading to renal failure: a potentially fatal complication of surgery in the morbidly obese. Obes Surg 2003; 13: 302–5.

74. McGlinch BP, Que FG, Nelson JL, et al. Perioperative care of patients undergoing bariatric surgery. Mayo Clin Proc 2006; 81: S25–S34.

75. Warner MA, Warner DO, Harper CM, et al. Ulnar neuropathy in medical patients. Anesthesiology 2000; 92: 613–15.

76. Sugerman H. Effects of increased intra-abdominal pressure in severe obesity. Surg Clin North Am 2001 Oct; 81: 1063–75.

77. Lambert DM, Marceau S, Forse RA. Intra-abdominal pressure in the morbidly obese. Obes Surg 2005; 15: 1225–32.

78. Schein M, Wittman DH, Aprahamian CC, et al. The abdominal compartment syndrome: the physiological and clinical consequences of elevated intraabdominal pressure. J Am Coll Surg 1995; 180: 745–53.

79. Davidson JE, Callery C. Care of the obesity surgery patient requiring immediate-level or intensive care. Obesity Surgery 2001; 11: 93–7.

80. Levi D, Goodman ER, Patel M, et al. Critical care of the obese and bariatric surgical patient. Crit Care Clin 2003; 19: 11–32.

81. Helling TS, Willoughby TL, Maxfield DM, et al. Determinants of the need for intensive care and prolonged mechanical ventilation in patients undergoing bariatric surgery. Obes Surg 2004; 14: 1031–41.

82. Pieracci FM, Barie PS, Pomp A. Critical care of the bariatric patient. Crit Care Med 2006; 34: 1796–804.

17 | Critical Care of the Obese Patient

Nicholas C. Watson[1] and Edward A. Bittner[2]

[1]Fellow in Critical Care Anesthesiology, Harvard Medical School, Department of Anesthesia and Critical Care, Massachusetts General Hospital, Boston, Massachusetts, U.S.A.

[2]Instructor in Anesthesia, Harvard Medical School, Assistant in Anesthesia and Intensivist, Department of Anesthesia and Critical Care, Massachusetts General Hospital, Boston, Massachusetts, U.S.A.

INTRODUCTION

Obesity results in pathophysiologic changes in most organ systems. Inflammation, hypercoagulability and insulin resistance characterize obesity as a process that mimics critical illness. Increased BMI requires increased cardiovascular, respiratory, and metabolic demand resulting in a markedly diminished physiologic reserve (1). Care of the critically ill obese patient requires knowledge of these changes and specific intensive care unit-related issues (Table 1) in order to anticipate common complications and provide timely and effective treatment.

The prevalence of obese patients in the ICU varies with the subgroup studied, ranging from 5.4% of blunt trauma patients and 17% of postoperative patients in cardiac surgical ICUs to 25% of general medical/surgical ICU patients (2). A significant percentage of patients undergoing bariatric surgery (7.6% laparoscopic, 21% open) require ICU care after surgery (3).

This chapter describes some of the most common and challenging aspects of the critical care of obese patients including airway and ventilator management, vascular access, hemodynamic monitoring and management, pharmacology, nutrition, positioning, skin care, and psychological issues.

IMPACT OF OBESITY ON OUTCOME
The Relationship of Obesity to Outcome Is Unclear

Although obesity would seem to have a negative impact on the outcome of critically ill patients, this is not a universal finding. In the medical/surgical ICU, morbidly obese patients have been reported to suffer from increased mortality, have greater length of stay and longer duration of mechanical ventilation (4–6). In contrast, other studies have reported no differences in mortality, length of stay, or cost (7–9). A recent meta-analysis found that mild and moderate obesity may be protective during critical illness and morbid obesity did not have an adverse effect on outcome (10).

Obesity as a Predictive Factor

Morbid obesity was not included as a comorbid variable in the development of commonly used (APACHE II, III, SAPS II, or MPM II) prognostic scoring indices (5). Consequently, assessment of severity of illness by general scoring systems may not accurately predict mortality in obese critically ill patients. El-Solh et al. found that multiorgan failure, PaO_2/FiO_2 <200 for >48 hours, and LVEF <40% are independent predictors of mortality in morbidly obese ICU patients (5).

Table 1 Important Critical Care Considerations in Obesity

System	Critical care implications
Pulmonary	Difficult intubation, need for close post-extubation observation, difficult mask ventilation, rapid desaturation, atelectasis, hypercarbia, technically difficult tracheostomy, calculation of Vt based on IBW (not TBW)
Cardiovascular	Ventricular dysfunction, risk for heart failure, poor tolerance of fluid loading, baseline hypertension
Gastrointestinal	Increased risk of GERD and aspiration
Renal	Extended duration of renally excreted drugs
Immunologic	Obesity as a pro-inflammatory state, increased risk of infection and sepsis
Hematologic	Hypercoagulability, elevated VTE risk
Endocrine, nutrition	Insulin resistance, hyperglycemia, protein malnutrition
Integument and body habitus	Difficult PIV and CVC placement, inaccurate NIBP measurements, poor quality radiographic imaging, special equipment needs

Abbreviations: CVC, central venous catheter; GERD, gastroesophageal reflux disease; IBW, ideal body weight; NIBP, non-invasive blood pressure; PIV, peripheral intravenous access; TBW, total body weight; Vt, tidal volume; VTE, venous thromboembolism.
Source: Adapted from Ref. 1.

AIRWAY MANAGEMENT

Airway management in the critically ill obese patient may be challenging due to the physiologic derangements of obesity.

Endotracheal Intubation

Endotracheal intubation may be more difficult in obese patients; however, this assertion remains controversial. One reason for this discrepancy is the lack of a consensus definition of difficult intubation (11). A large neck circumference appears to be one of the best predictors of a difficult intubation (12). Gonzalez et al. found that a neck circumference of >43 cm had 92% sensitivity and 84% specificity for predicting difficult intubation (11).

Proper positioning is essential to a successful intubation. In addition to the reverse Trendelenburg or back-up position, blankets placed under the patient's shoulders and occiput are often helpful in achieving the sniffing position. Head elevation combined with neck flexion has also been shown to improve view of the glottic opening during direct laryngoscopy (13).

Obese patients desaturate more rapidly than nonobese patients (14). Effective *preoxygenation* is vitally important because the morbidly obese patient has a reduced FRC, often falling below the closing capacity of the airways. This leads to atelectasis, increased intrapulmonary shunting, and impaired oxygenation (15–17). Preoxygenation in the obese is more effective in the head-up position compared to supine (18). Similarly, the reverse Trendelenburg position provides a longer period of apneic normoxia during intubation when compared to the supine position (19).

Noninvasive positive pressure ventilation has been shown to enhance preoxygenation in morbidly obese patients in the operating room and may also be useful for rapid preoxygenation prior to urgent intubation in the ICU (20). *Mask ventilation* in the obese may be more difficult due to reduced pulmonary compliance, abnormal diaphragmatic position, and increased upper airway obstruction. Langeron et al. found an almost threefold increase in difficult ventilation in patients with BMI >26 kg/m² (21). If mask ventilation is required, higher than normal airway pressures may be needed. Adding PEEP to the ambu bag may be helpful.

It is commonly believed that the risk of aspiration is greater in obese patients due to larger volumes of gastric fluid, increased intra-abdominal pressure, and a higher incidence of GERD (22). However, there is conflicting data on gastric pH, gastric volume, gastric emptying, and barrier pressure in morbidly obese patients (23,24). Despite the conflicting evidence, it is sensible to take precautions against aspiration. Prophylaxis against acid aspiration has been recommended in morbidly obese patients even in the absence of symptoms of reflux (25).

Tracheostomy
If prolonged ventilation is anticipated then early tracheostomy may facilitate weaning. Tracheostomy is common in obese patients due to the likelihood of increased duration of mechanical ventilation and as a means to minimize complications related to sleep apnea (26). Compared to endotracheal intubation, tracheostomy is more comfortable for the patient, improves pulmonary toilet, and allows communication with the addition of a speaking valve. In obese patients, speaking valves may have the added advantage of preserving FRC, making trials of spontaneous breathing more successful (26).

Anatomical distortions and increased thickness of subcutaneous tissues make tracheostomy technically more difficult in the obese. Locating the trachea deep in fatty tissue and selecting a tube of appropriate size are surgical challenges. Standard tracheotomy tubes may not be appropriate for the morbidly obese patient. Custom fit or adjustable tubes may be needed to accommodate the increased neck girth (27). Once in place, these tubes may be more likely to be dislodged or occluded (28). An endotracheal tube advanced through the incision may serve a temporary measure to resecure the airway if dislodgement occurs. As the tracheostomy wound is often extensive, care must focus on preventing infection. In a potentially deep wound, protection of the skin surrounding the tube from excessive pressure and prevention of the trachea tube from eroding the trachea or surrounding vessels (by tube immobilization), are important aspects of the respiratory care.

Percutaneous tracheostomy has conventionally been considered a poor choice for morbidly obese patients due to their large and thick necks. Byhahn et al. reported a 2.7 fold increased risk of complications in obese patients with an overall complication rate of 43.8% in those who underwent percutaneous tracheostomy (29). However, other reports have suggested that it can be successfully performed with a low complication rate (30,31).

PULMONARY MANAGEMENT
Non-invasive Positive Pressure Ventilation (NIPPV)
Continuous positive airway pressure (CPAP) or bi-level positive airway pressure (BiPAP) acts to displace the tongue and pharyngeal soft tissue, preventing airway obstruction. NIPPV has been demonstrated to be effective for support of patients with acute postoperative respiratory failure (32). NIPPV is delivered via nasal or face mask. Alert and cooperative patients are the best candidates for NIPPV. NIPPV is typically initiated at low pressure and increased gradually as tolerated. BiPAP allows independent adjustment of inspiratory positive airway pressure (IPAP) and expiratory positive airway pressure (EPAP). The lower EPAP reduces resistance during exhalation, improving patient tolerance as well as reducing the risk of barotrauma.

Mechanical Ventilation

Calculating tidal volume based on ideal body weight rather than total body weight will avoid high airway pressures and potential barotrauma. Because of reduced compliance of the respiratory system in obese patients, inflation pressures should be interpreted with caution. Limiting transpulmonary pressures to 35 cm H_2O has been suggested (28).

PEEP helps to prevent airway closure and reduces the development of atelectasis. In the postoperative period, morbidly obese patients who are sedated and pharmacologically paralyzed have worse oxygenation compared to their baseline (33). In this situation, addition of 10 cm H_2O of PEEP has been shown to improve respiratory function (34). PEEP should be cautiously applied as excessive pressure can overdistend alveoli, impair venous return, and redistribute pulmonary blood flow leading to ventilation-perfusion mismatch and worsening oxygenation (34).

Weaning obese patients from mechanical ventilation may be difficult due to high oxygen requirements, increased work of breathing, reduced lung volumes, and ventilation-perfusion mismatching. In addition, the shift from fat to carbohydrate metabolism increases the respiratory quotient and may cause hypercarbia, which can impair weaning from the ventilator (1).

The reverse Trendelenburg position, rather than 90° head-up, results in larger tidal volumes and lower respiratory rate and may be of use during weaning (35). *Extubation* in the obese patient is a critical event requiring optimal conditions. The airway should be extubated when the patient is fully awake. Supplemental oxygen should be administered immediately and chest physical therapy initiated as soon as possible. Some patients may benefit from extubation directly to CPAP or BiPAP. Use of BiPAP has been shown to improve pulmonary function after open gastric bypass and may be useful as an adjunct (28,36). Clinicians should always be prepared for the possibility of emergency reintubation. Extubation should be planned when adequate personnel and resources are available, especially if the initial intubation was difficult. An ICU should have immediate access to a difficult airway cart at all times.

Failure to wean or sudden respiratory decompensation should alert the clinician to the possibility of pulmonary embolism or anastomotic leak. A high degree of suspicion and prompt investigation are essential (37).

CARDIOVASCULAR CONSIDERATIONS
Cardiac Output

Variations in BMI translate into predictable yet modest differences in CO and SV even at the extremes of body size. Each 1 kg/m^2 increase in BMI is associated with a 0.08 L/min increase in CO (1.35 ml increase in SV) (38). Compared to lean patients, heart rate is largely unchanged in morbidly obese non-hypertensive patients (39). Obesity is marked by a reduction in total blood flow relative to body weight despite an increased circulating blood volume and elevated resting oxygen consumption. In obese subjects splanchnic blood flow is slightly increased and renal blood flow slightly reduced; otherwise, cardiac output is similarly distributed to organs as in the nonobese (2).

Impaired Ventricular Performance

Morbidly obese patients have greater left ventricular mass and decreased left ventricular systolic and diastolic function. The extent of ventricular performance impairment is influenced both by the magnitude and duration of obesity. Increased hemodynamic load, neurohumeral activation, and oxidative stress contribute to ventricular dysfunction (40). Obesity is an independent risk factor for heart failure (41). Obese patients have elevated cardiac filling pressures which may increase further when the patient is in the supine position (42,43). As a consequence of cardiovascular impairment, the morbidly obese patient is likely to tolerate fluid loading poorly. This is potentially exacerbated in critical illness.

VENOUS THROMBOEMBOLISM
Risk Factors for VTE
Although obesity is a well known risk factor for development of venous thromboembolism (VTE), the incidence in critically ill morbidly obese patients is unknown. A higher prevalence of VTE is associated with a BMI > 50 kg/m^2, truncal obesity, venous stasis disease or history of VTE (1). Critically ill obese patients are at risk for VTE due to the prevalence of *Virchow's triad*: venous stasis, hypercoagulability from prothrombotic abnormalities, and endothelial injury from a chronic proinflammatory state. The prothrombotic abnormalities in morbidly obese include increased levels of fibrinogen, plasminogen activator inhibitor (PAI-1), antithrombin III deficiency, and decreased fibrinolysis (1).

Prevention of VTE
Prevention of VTE is the key to reducing morbidity and mortality. Limited data exist regarding prophylactic regimens in the morbidly obese patients. Accepted *prophylactic strategies* include low dose unfractionated heparin (5000 U subcutaneously every eight hours) with or without sequential compression devices. Data extrapolated from morbidly obese patients undergoing bariatric surgery suggest that enoxaparin 40 mg administered every 12 hours was superior to 30 mg every 12 hours in preventing postoperative deep venous thrombosis (44).

Low molecular weight heparin must be adjusted in renal insufficiency. Dosing adjustment may be accomplished by monitoring anti-Xa levels. *Sequential compression devices* have not been well studied in the obese population and achieving an adequate fit can be problematic. Early, aggressive mobilization of the critically ill obese patient is likely to reduce the risk for venous thrombosis, although specific data supporting this notion is lacking. Patients with pulmonary hypertension have limited cardiopulmonary reserve and may be at high risk of death even with mild or moderate pulmonary embolism. *Prophylactic IVC filter* placement may be of benefit in this subgroup (37).

VASCULAR ACCESS
Vascular access can be technically challenging in obese patients. Obesity can obscure anatomic landmarks, increase the depth of insertion, and potentially interfere with the angle of insertion.

Peripheral Venous Access
Peripheral veins are the first choice in gaining vascular access. However, peripheral venous line insertion is more difficult in obese than in lean patients (45).

Central Venous Access
Standard central venous catheters may not be long enough in some obese patients (46). In morbidly obese patients catheter position can change with movement so

position should be reconfirmed periodically (47). Because of respiratory difficulties, most severely obese patients will not tolerate the Trendelenberg position for central line placement. Abduction of the arm, rather than adduction, and retraction of the chest tissue away from the clavicle can reduce excess tissue at the subclavian insertion site (48).

Femoral vein cannulation may be difficult due do the presence of a large panniculus or contraindicated due to the presence of intertrigo. Studies support the use of ultrasound guidance for central venous cannulation, with fewer insertion attempts and reduced complications, especially in obese patients (49). Central venous access poses an infectious risk. In the ICU central line use in the obese is increased and lines remain in place for a longer duration relative to nonobese patients (5). Consequently, line infection rates may be higher resulting in a greater risk of line sepsis and death. Vigilant line care and monitoring are essential to prevent infection. The need for maintaining central venous access should be reassessed on a daily basis. Removal should occur expeditiously when no longer needed.

Peripherally Inserted Central Catheters (PICC)
PICC lines are a potential alternative to centrally placed catheters for routine infusion needs and as a means for blood sampling. They are relatively safer to place and allow greater mobility of the patient without risk of dislodgment (26).

MONITORING
Monitoring of hemodynamic and respiratory parameters can be challenging in the obese critically ill patient.

Arterial Blood Pressure Monitoring
Use of standard *non-invasive blood pressure cuffs* can result in inaccurate blood pressure readings (50–52). The blood pressure cuff used may be improperly sized and, due to the shape of the arm in obese patients, often does not fit properly. The length of the cuff bladder should be at least 80% of the measured arm circumference and the width should be at least 40% of the measured arm circumferece at the midpoint of the upper arm (53). Following the trend in blood pressure rather than the absolute number or obtaining the reading using a standard cuff applied to the forearm are alternate management strategies (54). The ankle or wrist may also be used as sites for measuring blood pressure (55).

Intra-arterial monitoring should be used for severely obese individuals, patients with significant cardiopulmonary disease, and in cases where noninvasive blood pressure monitoring is unreliable. The radial artery is typically the first site selected for placement of an arterial catheter. The axillary artery has been suggested as an alternative (56).

Monitoring Central Pressures and Cardiac Performance
Invasive measurement of cardiac filling pressures and function may be helpful. Obese patients have higher resting cardiac filling pressures. These may increase further when the patient is supine, exceeding pressures necessary for the development of pulmonary edema. Physical exam findings of congestive heart failure may be difficult to assess due to body habitus (2). Indexing hemodynamic measurements to body surface area attenuates the effects of BMI. Obesity should not complicate the interpretation of hemodynamic data (38).

Pulse Oximetry
Pulse oximetry can be unreliable secondary to increased finger tissue thickness and poorly transmitted light waves. The earlobe presents an alternative site to the finger as its skin is thinner, well perfused, and holds the probe more readily (48).

Capnography
End-tidal capnography is a poor indicator of the adequacy of ventilation in morbidly obese patients due to a large alveolar to arterial difference (17). Serial arterial blood gas analysis should be used to assess adequacy of ventilation.

INFECTION AND SEPSIS
There is increasing evidence that obesity is a chronic inflammatory state. This may play a role in the higher incidence of infectious complications and sepsis in the obese (57). Multiple mechanisms including secretion of proinflammatory adipokines, increased secretion of various cytokines, activation of leukocytes, and oxidative stress act together to produce an environment that leads to inflammation and endothelial dysfunction in obesity (58,59).

    The chronic inflammatory state of obesity together with accompanying hyperglycemia/insulin resistance create an environment in which an additional inflammatory stimulus, such as sepsis, results in a "second hit" and leads to an exaggerated inflammatory response (60).

METABOLIC, NUTRITIONAL, AND ENDOCRINE CONSIDERATIONS
Metabolic Syndrome
The metabolic abnormalities associated with obesity (termed "Metabolic Syndrome") are characterized by insulin resistance, hyperinsulinemia, hyperglycemia, CAD, HTN, and hyperlipidemia (61). Substrate overload leads to baseline resistance to insulin and pancreatic polypeptides which leads to glucotoxicity and lipotoxicity (37).

Nutritional Management
Operative stress, trauma, and critical illness cause marked metabolic changes resulting in *protein catabolism* and *negative nitrogen balance*. A hypermetabolic response results in increased energy expenditure, myocardial oxygen demand, and pulmonary work which exacerbate these preexisting metabolic derangements of obesity.

    Despite excess fat stores, morbidly obese patients are prone to develop *protein malnutrition* during metabolic stress. Elevated basal insulin levels suppress lipid mobilization from body stores resulting in breakdown of protein to support gluconeogenesis and rapid loss of lean body mass. Nutrition should not be withheld during critical illness in the mistaken belief that weight reduction is beneficial. Caloric intake of 20 to 30 Kcal/kg obesity adjusted body weight per day, and 1.5 to 2 g/kg ideal body weight (IBW) per day of protein to ensure nitrogen balance has been recommended (62). Obesity adjusted body weight is calculated as IBW + (ABW – IBW) × 0.25 where ABW is the actual body weight. The reader is referred to Table 2 for calculation of IBW.

    In morbidly obese patients *indirect calorimetry* is the method of choice to determine energy expenditure and nutritional requirements (63). Standard energy expenditure equations are unreliable in critically ill obese patients (62,64). Expert advice on nutritional requirements of the critically ill obese patient should be obtained from consultation with a dietician.

Table 2   Medication Dosing Guidelines for Morbidly Obese Patients in the ICU

Medication	Loading dose	Maintenance dose
Analgesics		
Fentanyl	ABW	0.8 × IBW
Morphine	IBW	IBW
Remifentanyl	IBW	IBW
Antiarrythymics		
Amiodarone	IBW	IBW
Lidocaine	ABW	IBW
Procainamide	IBW	IBW
Antibiotics		
Beta-lactams	–	IBW + 0.3(ABW – IBW)
Aminoglycosides	–	IBW + 0.4(ABW – IBW)
Vancomycin	–	ABW
Sulfonamides	–	IBW
Quinolones	–	IBW + 0.45(ABW – IBW)
Macrolides	–	IBW
Anticoagulants		
Heparin	IBW + 0.4(ABW – IBW)	IBW + 0.4(ABW – IBW)
Enoxaparin	Standard dose	Standard dose
Drotrecogin alfa	–	ABW
Anticonvulsants		
Carbamezepine	–	IBW
Phenytoin	IBW + 1.33(ABW – IBW)	IBW
Valproic acid	–	IBW
Antifungals		
Amphotericin	–	ABW
Fluconazole	–	6 mg/kg/day
Beta blockers		
Metoprolol	IBW	IBW
Esmolol	IBW	IBW
Propanolol	IBW	IBW
Labetalol	IBW	IBW
Calcium channel blockers		
Diltiazem IV	ABW	Titration
Verapamil	ABW	IBW
Catecholamines		
Dobutamine	–	IBW + 0.4(ABW – IBW)
Corticosteroids		
Methylprednisolone	IBW	IBW
GI prophylaxis		
H-2-blocker	–	Standard dosing

(Continued)

Table 2 Medication Dosing Guidelines for Morbidly Obese Patients in the ICU *(Continued)*

Neuromuscular blockers		
Succinylcholine	ABW	–
Rocuronium	ABW	ABW
Vecuronium	IBW	IBW
Cisatracurium	–	–
Medication	Loading dose	Maintenance dose
Other cardiac medications		
Adenosine	IBW	IBW
Digoxin	IBW	IBW
Sedatives/anesthetics		
Benzodiazepine	ABW	IBW
Propofol	ABW	IBW + titration
Thiopental	ABW	IBW
Ketamine	IBW	IBW
Etomidate	ABW	–

IBW for men = 48.2 kg + 2.7 kg per 2.54 cm of height >1.54 m.
IBW for women = 45.4 kg + 2.3 kg per 2.54 cm of height >1.54 m.
Abbreviations: ABW, actual body weight; IBW, ideal body weight.
Source: Adapted from Refs. 1,48,68.

Nutritional support with a hypocaloric, high protein diet has also been suggested as beneficial in critically ill morbidly obese patients. Small trials in critically ill obese patients demonstrated that hypocaloric enteral nutrition support is as least as effective as eucaloric feeding (65,66). It has been postulated that if obligatory glucose requirements are satisfied and adequate protein is provided, endogenous fat stores will be used for energy. Other potential benefits include reduced incidence of hyperglycemia, decreased CO_2 production, and improved protein anabolism, wound healing and immune function. Although data addressing the critically ill morbidly obese patient are lacking, total parenteral nutrition (TPN) has not been shown to decrease major postoperative complication rates or mortality in critically ill postoperative patients (67).

Insulin Resistance
Obesity is a risk factor in the development of insulin resistance and Type 2 diabetes mellitus. The adipocyte actively regulates the complex hormonal and neuronal signals responsible for energy balance. In insulin resistance, signaling in the adipocyte is impaired and this results in decreased cellular uptake and metabolism (40). Hyperglycemia from gluconeogenesis and glycogenolysis is common after surgery. Persistence of hyperglycemia for more than 72 hours is suggestive of insulin resistance that is caused by sepsis (37). The importance of normalizing blood glucose is based on the association of hyperglycemia with increased infections, delayed wound healing, fluid and electrolyte imbalance, and impaired nutrient utilization. Tight glucose control has been advocated to improve ICU outcomes; however guidelines for morbidly obese patients are not available at this time. Insulin infusions are commonly needed in obese patients due to unpredictable effects of subcutaneous administration.

PHARMACOLOGIC CONSIDERATIONS
Of the very few published studies on medication dosing for morbidly obese patients, none is specific to the ICU setting. Therefore the clinician must extrapolate drug dosing regimens from the limited studies conducted in nonobese patients (68). Pharmacologic alterations in morbid obesity are the result of changes in several parameters including: volume of distribution, hepatic metabolism, protein binding, and renal clearance (69). Critical illness, particularly shock states, alter regional blood flow resulting in further impairment of renal function and altering plasma protein levels responsible for drug binding.

Dose Selection
Drug dosing in obese patients can be based on ideal body weight, total body weight or an intermediate amount (IBW plus some percentage of TBW). The suggested doses for medications commonly used in the intensive care unit are listed in Table 2.

Dosing weight = IBW + 0.3 (TBW–IBW) is sometimes used for hydrophilic drugs. This is based on the fact that the water content of adipose tissue is approximately 30% of that in other tissue (48). For maintenance dosing, IBW should be used when weight based dosing is desired and once a weight has been chosen, the same weight should be used to maintain consistency with subsequent adjustments. Monitoring of clinical endpoints, signs of toxicity, clinical response, and drug levels (when available) is essential.

Dosing of highly lipophilic drugs in obese patients is generally best approximated using the actual body weight rather than the ideal body weight (70). Volume of distribution (Vd) of drugs is generally related to lipophilicity (i.e., drugs that have a high affinity for adipose tissue) have an increased Vd whereas those with lower affinity have a lower Vd. Accumulation of lipophilic drugs in adipose tissue not only increases the dose necessary to gain clinical effect but also prolongs the elimination (1). The volume of distribution of hydrophilic drugs in general relates to the lean body mass and is better approximated by ideal body weight. Dosing of hydrophilic drugs based on actual body weight in obese patients may grossly overestimate dosages leading to toxicity. The volume of distribution of hydrophilic drugs is altered by the excessive fluid gains that follow intraoperative or postoperative resuscitation. This state may be exacerbated by renal failure. Oral absorption of drugs is relatively unchanged in the morbidly obese patient (71).

Hepatic Metabolism
Obesity has differing effects on hepatic metabolism. In general, clearance of drugs that undergo biotransformation as the primary route of elimination are not significantly altered (72,73). Obesity is commonly associated with liver and gallbladder pathology which may affect the metabolism and clearance of various drugs (37). Protein binding of drugs bound to albumin is not altered in obesity, although liver disease resulting in diminished albumin levels would be expected to alter the total amount of drug that can be protein bound (74).

Renal Clearance
The glomerular filtration rate (GFR) and creatinine clearance are increased in morbidly obese patients with normal renal function. In morbidly obese patients with impaired renal function, creatinine clearance estimates using standard weight based formulae correlate poorly with measured creatinine clearance (75). Therefore dosing should be calculated on measured creatinine clearance.

RADIOLOGIC PROCEDURES
Radiologic imaging of the morbidly obese patient can be challenging.

Body Habitus Limits Quality of Radiographic Images
Standard films are often underpenetrated. Portable x-ray equipment which is generally easier to use is of lower quality. Use of grids can increase the quality of x-ray imaging in obese patients (76).

   Ultrasound imaging is difficult with poor visualization of target organs resulting in an indeterminate exam.

Body Habitus Limits Fit of Radiographic Devices
Standard radiographs may be unable to fit the entire body part being imaged necessitating multiple images. *CT* and *MRI* are limited by the weight and girth restrictions of the scanners, approximately 300 to 350 lbs. Veterinary hospitals and zoos may have CT scanners that can accommodate a greater weight. This may be an option for morbidly obese patients who exceed the weight limits of standard scanners.

INTRA-HOSPITAL TRANSFER
Intra-hospital transfer is usually best accomplished on the patient's own hospital bed. Before transporting to diagnostic or procedural areas it is essential to ensure that the equipment to be used at the site can accommodate the patient safely. When transferring the obese patient extra attention must be paid to ensure that artificial airways, vascular catheters, and other tubes and drains are guarded to prevent accidental removal. To ensure availability of appropriate support for transfer and positioning, "road trips" should be scheduled for normal business hours whenever possible.

NURSING CARE CONSIDERATIONS
Skin and Wound Care
Pressure from the weight of overlying tissue in combination with moisture and friction predisposes the obese patient to skin breakdown. Fatty tissues are poorly perfused resulting in delayed wound healing. Periodic episodes of hypotension, hyperglycemia and tissue hypoxemia predispose to compromised skin integrity and infection. Critically ill patients who cannot participate in active turning are at increased risk of pressure ulcers. Patients should be turned every two hours at a minimum (77). Use of bariatric beds with pressure relief features may help to reduce pressure related injuries in morbidly obese patients with prolonged bedrest (28).

   The extremities and head are areas of particular concern. The arms deserve special attention as they may rub against the side rails of the bed when a patient fills the bed side to side. The occiput and the heels of the feet are areas of high risk and should be examined for breakdown regularly. Patients should be turned and all skin folds inspected immediately upon stabilization in the ICU. Inspection requires lifting, cleansing, and drying all skin folds. The panniculus should be lifted and retracted to allow examination of the skin of the lower abdomen and perineum. Additional personnel may be needed to assist with visualization. Care must be taken when using "lift" or "turn" sheets for positioning or transferring to avoid shearing or abrading the skin. Drainage tubes can become trapped, or hidden in skin folds resulting in skin erosion. In addition they can become kinked or dislodged resulting in impaired drainage and/or decreased measured output. The moist environment of skin folds of obese patients encourages microbial growth, especially fungal infections. Efforts to reduce skin friction and absorb moisture, such as non-medicated powders, may be helpful. An absorbent gauze placed between skin folds can absorb moisture and reduce friction. Antifungal powders can be used to treat actual infection but should not be used prophylactically (78).

Positioning and Mobilization
Not all positions may be well tolerated in the obese patient. Many patients experience a decrease in oxygenation when turning, with oxygen desaturation persisting for some time following turns.

Supine, Trendelenburg, lithotomy and prone positions may result in significant hemodynamic and respiratory changes. The *lateral decubitus position* displaces weight from the chest wall and may allow greater diaphragmatic excursion. *The reverse Trendelenburg position* may result in larger tidal volumes and lower respiratory rates (35).

Simple patient care activities like turning, bathing, changing linens, or urinary catheter insertion require planning and coordination. Creating a patient focused plan for patient turns is essential. Once the plan has been tested it should be treated as a protocol and adhered to consistently. The plan should be refined during the patient's ICU stay, with changes being guided by the severity of illness (56).

Positioning and mobilization of morbidly obese patients pose increased risk of back injury to the health care worker (26). Education of hospital personnel on patient care routines which emphasize back safety is recommended. Specialized equipment and mobilization techniques promote patient comfort and dignity and prevent injury to the patient and health care team.

Elimination
Managing the elimination needs of the morbidly obese patient can be challenging. Undetected incontinence of urine or stool can rapidly lead to skin breakdown. It is therefore essential to keep the perineum clean and dry. Urinary catheters and rectal bags are useful to keep the skin protected from exposure to waste products as well as monitoring of output. Diarrhea can be managed with a rectal tube and collection bag. Generally a urinary catheter remains in place until a patient can cooperate with elimination. Urinary catheters should be removed as soon as possible to decrease the risk of urinary tract infection.

Psychological Considerations
The obese population is acutely aware of body size and, if conscious, may be easily embarrassed by plans to manage the patient with either special equipment and/or expanded staff. Bedside or doorway conversations should be discrete so as to minimize embarrassment and maintain patient dignity. Families are also quite sensitive to discussions regarding size and weight (56).

Healthcare providers also often hold negative attitudes toward morbidly obese patients and this probably contributes to the decreased quality of health care that obese patients receive (1). It is essential that obese patients be treated with compassion and respect. Health care providers need to be educated regarding the prejudice that occurs with obesity and how this may negatively impact patient outcome.

REFERENCES
1. Pieracci FM, Barie PS, Pomp A. Critical care of the bariatric patient. Crit Care Med 2006; 34: 1796–804.
2. Joffe A, Wood K. Obesity in critical care. Curr Opin Anaesthesiol 2007; 20: 113–18.
3. Nguyen NT, Goldman C, Rosenquist J, et al. Laparoscopic versus open gastric bypass: randomized study of outcomes, quality of life and costs. Ann Surg 2001; 234: 279–91.
4. Bercault N, Boulain T, Kuteifan K, et al. Obesity-related excess mortality rate in an adult intensive care unit: a risk-adjusted matched cohort study. Crit Care Med 2004; 32: 998–1003.
5. El-Solh AA, Sikka P, Bozkanat E, et al. Morbid obesity in the medical ICU. Chest 2001; 120: 1989–97.
6. Goulenok C, Monchi M, Chiche JD, et al. Influence of overweight on ICU mortality: a prospective study. Chest 2004; 125: 1441–5.
7. Ray DE, Matchett SC, Baker K, et al. The effect of body mass index on patient outcomes in a medical ICU. Chest 2005; 127: 2125–31.
8. O'Brien JM, Welch CH, Fish RH, et al. Excess body weight is not independently associated with outcome in mechanically ventilated patients with acute lung injury. Ann Intern Med 2004; 140: 338–45.
9. Peake SL, Moran JL, Ghelani DR, et al. The effect of obesity on 12-month survival following admission to intensive care: a prospective study. Crit Care Med 2006; 34: 2929–39.
10. Akinnusi ME, Pineda LA, El Solh AA. Effect of obesity on intensive care morbidity and mortality: a meta-analysis. Crit Care Med 2008; 36: 151–8.
11. Gonzalez H, Minville V, Delanoue K, et al. The importance of increased neck circumference to intubation difficulties in obese patients. Anesth Analg 2008; 106: 1132–6.
12. Brodsky JB, Lemmens HJ, Brock-Utne JG, et al. Morbid obesity and tracheal intubation. Anesth Analg 2002; 94: 732–6.
13. Levitan R, Mechem C, Ochroch A, et al. Head-elevated laryngoscopy position: improving laryngeal exposure during laryngoscopy by increasing head elevation. Ann Emerg Med 2003; 41: 322–30.
14. Jense HG, Dubin SA, Silverstein PI, et al. Effect of obesity on safe duration of apnea in anesthetized humans. Anesth Analg 1991; 72: 89–93.
15. Yap JC, Watson RA, Gilbey S, et al. Effects of posture on respiratory mechanics in obesity. J Appl Physiol 1995; 79: 1199–205.
16. Biring M, Lewis M, Liu J, et al. Pulmonary physiologic changes of morbid obesity. Am J Med Sci 1999; 318: 293–7.
17. Adams J, Murphy P. Obesity in anaesthesia and intensive care. Brit J Anaesth 2000; 85: 91–108.
18. Dixon B, Dixon J, Carden, et al. Preoxygenation is more effective in the 25 degrees head-up position than in the supine position in severely obese patients: a randomized controlled study. Anesthesiology 2005; 102: 1110–15.
19. Boyce J, Ness T, Castroman P, et al. A preliminary study of the optimal anesthesia positioning for the morbidly obese patient. Obes Surg 2003; 13: 4–9.
20. Delay J, Sebbane M, Nocca D, et al. The effectiveness of noninvasive positive pressure ventilation to enhance preoxygenation in morbidly obese patients: a randomized controlled study. Anesth Analg 2008; 107: 1707–12.
21. Langeron O, Masso E, Huraux C, et al. Prediction of difficult mask ventilation. Anesthesiology 2000; 92: 1229–36.
22. Suter M, Dortr G, Giusti V, et al. Gastro-esophageal reflux and esophageal motility disorders in morbidly obese patients. Obes Surg 2004; 14: 959–66.
23. Zacchi P, Mearin F, Humbert P, et al. Effect of obesity on gastroesophageal resistance to flow in man. Dig Dis Sci 1991; 36: 1473–80.
24. Gallagher TK, Geoghegan JG, Baird AW, et al. Implications of altered gastrointestinal motility in obesity. Obes Surg 2007; 17: 1399–407.

25. Vila P, Valles J, Canet J, et al. Acid aspiration prophylaxis in morbidly obese patients: famotidine vs ranitidine. Anaesthesia 1991; 46: 967–9.
26. Burns SM, Charlebois D, Deivert M, et al. Nursing management. In: Alvarez AO, ed. Morbid Obesity: Perioperative Management. Cambridge, UK: Cambridge University Press, 2004: 371–9.
27. Ghorayeb BY. Tracheotomy in the morbidly obese patient. Arch Otolaryngol 1987; 113: 556–8.
28. El-Solh AA. Clinical Approach to the critically ill, morbidly obese patient. Am J Respir Crit Care Med 2004; 169: 557–61.
29. Byhahn C, Lischke V, Meninger D, et al. Perioperative complications during percutaneous tracheostomy in obese patients. Anaesthesia 2005; 60: 12–15.
30. Mansharamani NG, Koziel H, Garland R, et al. Safety of bedside percutaneous dilational tracheostomy in obese patients in the ICU. Chest 2000; 117: 1426–9.
31. Aldawood AS, Arabi YM, Hadda S. Safety of percutaneous tracheostomy in obese critically ill patients: a prospective cohort study. Anaesth Intensive Care 2008; 36: 69–73.
32. Garpestad E, Brennan J, Hill NS. Noninvasive ventilation for critical care. Chest 2007; 132: 711–20.
33. Pelosi P, Croci M, Ravagnan I, et al. Total respiratory system, lung and chest wall mechanics in sedated-paralyzed postoperative morbidly obese patients. Chest 1996; 109: 144–51.
34. Pelosi P, Ravagnan I, Giurati G, et al. Positive end-expiratory pressure improves respiratory function in the obese patients but not the normal patients during anesthesia and paralysis. Anesthesiology 1999; 91: 1221–31.
35. Burns SM, Egloff MB, Ryan B. Effect of body position on spontaneous respiratory rate and tidal volume in patients with obesity, abdominal distension and ascites. Am J Crit Care 1994; 3: 102–6.
36. Joris JL, Sottiaux TM, Chiche JD, et al. Effect of bi-level positive airway pressure (Bipap) nasal ventilation on the postoperative pulmonary restrictive syndrome in obese patients undergoing gastroplsty. Chest 1997; 111: 665–70.
37. Levi D, Goodman ER, Patel M, et al. Critical care of the obese and bariatric surgical patient. Crit Care Clin 2003; 19: 11–32.
38. Stelfox HT, Ahmed SB, Ribeiro RA, et al. Hemodynamic monitoring in obese patients: the impact of body mass index on cardiac output and stroke volume. Crit Care Med 2006; 34: 1243–6.
39. Alpert MA, Lambert CR, Terry BE, et al. Influence of left ventricular mass on left ventricular diastolic filling in normotensive morbid obesity. Am Heart J 1995; 130: 1068–73.
40. Cheah MH, Kam PAC. Obesity: basic science and medical aspects relevant to anaesthetists. Anaesthesia 2005; 60: 1009–21.
41. Kenchaiah S, Evans JC, Levy D, et al. Obesity and the risk of heart failure. N Eng J Med 2002; 347: 305–13.
42. De Divitiis O, Fazio S, Petitto M, et al. Obesity and cardiac function. Circulation 1981; 64: 477–82.
43. Paul DR, Hoyt JL, Boutros AR. Cardiovascular and respiratory changes in response to change in posture in the very obese. Anesthesiology 1976; 45: 73–8.
44. Scholten DJ, Hoedema RM, Scholten SE. A comparison of two different prophylactic dose regimens of low molecular weight heparin in bariatric surgery. Obes Surg 2002; 12: 1924.
45. Juvin P, Blarel A, Bruno F, et al. Is peripheral line placement more difficult in obese than in lean patients? Anesth Analg 2003; 96: 1218.
46. Ottestad E, Schmiessing C, Brock-Utne JG, et al. Central venous access in obese patients: a potential complication. Anesth Analg 2006; 102: 1293–4.
47. Thompson EC, Wilkins HE, Fox VJ, et al. Insufficient length of pulmonary artery introducer in an obese patient. Arch Surg 2004; 139: 794–6.
48. Brunette DD. Resuscitation of the morbidly obese patient. Am J Emerg Med 2004; 22: 40–7.

49. Joffe A, Wood K. Obesity in critical care. Curr Opin Anaesthesiol 2007; 20: 113–18.
50. Maxwell MH, Waks AU, Schroth PC, et al. Error in blood pressure measurement due to incorrect cuff size in obese patients. Lancet 1982; 2: 33–6.
51. Bur A, Herkner H, Vicek M, et al. Factors influencing the accuracy of occillometric blood pressure monitoring in critically ill patients. Crit Care Med 2003; 31: 793–9.
52. Bur A, HirschL MM, Herkner H, et al. Accuracy of occillometric blood pressure measurement according to the relation between cuff size and upper arm circumference in critically ill patients. Crit Care Med 2000; 28: 371–6.
53. Perloff D, Grim C, Flack J, et al. Human blood pressure determination by sphygmomanometry. Circulation 1993; 88: 2460–70.
54. Nasraway SA, Hudson-Jinks TM, Kelleher RM. Multidisciplinary care of the obese patient with chronic critical illness after surgery. Crit Care Clin 2002; 18: 643–57.
55. DeMaria EJ, Carmody BJ. Perioperative management of special populations: obesity. Surg Clin N Am 2005; 85: 1283–9.
56. Nasraway SA, Hudson-Jinks TM, Kelleher RM. Multidisciplinary care of the obese patient with chronic critical illness after surgery. Crit Care Clin 2002; 18: 643–57.
57. Vachharajani V, Vital S. Obesity and sepsis. J Intensive Care Med 2006; 21: 287–95.
58. Wisse BE. The inflammatory syndrome: the role of adipose tissue cytokines in metabolic disorders linked to obesity. J Am Soc Nephrol 2004; 15: 2792–800.
59. Olusi SO. Obesity is an independent risk factor for plasma lipid peroxidation and depletion of erythrocyte cytoprotective enzymes in humans. Int J Obes Relat Metab Disord 2002; 26: 1159–64.
60. Vachharajani V. Influence of obesity on sepsis. Pathophysiology 2008; 15: 123–34.
61. Bray GA. Pathophysiology of Obesity. Am J Clin Nutr 1992; 55: 488S–494S.
62. Cutts ME, Dowdy RP, Ellersieck MR, et al. Predicting energy needs in ventilator-dependent critically ill patients: effect of adjusting weight for edema or adiposity. Am J Clin Nutr 1997; 66: 1250–6.
63. Breen HB, Ireton-Jones CS. Predicting energy needs in obese patients. Nutr Clin Pract 2004; 19: 284–9.
64. Glynn CC, Greene GW, Winkler MF, et al. Predictive versus measured energy expenditure using limits-of-agreement analysis in hospitalized, obese patients. J Parenter Enteral Nutr 1999; 23: 147–54.
65. Dickerson RN, Boschert KJ, Kudsk KA, et al. Hypocaloric enteral feeding in critically ill obese patients. Nutrition 2002; 18: 241–6.
66. Choban PS, Dickerson RN. Morbid obesity and nutrition support: is bigger different? Nutrition Clin Pract 2005; 20: 480–7.
67. Heyland DK, MacDonald S, Keefe L, et al. Total parenteral nutrition in the critically ill patient. JAMA 1998; 280: 2013–19.
68. Erstad BL. Dosing of medications in morbidly obese patients in the intensive care unit setting. Intensive Care Med 2004; 30: 18–32.
69. Cheymol G. Effects of obesity on pharmacokinetics implications for drug therapy. Clin Pharmacokinet 2000; 39: 215–31.
70. Morgan DJ, Bray KM. Lean body mass as a predictor of drug dosage: implications for drug therapy. Clin Pharmacokinet 1994; 26: 292–307.
71. Cheymol G. Clinical pharmacokinetics of drugs in obesity: an update. Clin Pharmacokinet 1993; 25: 103–14.
72. Varon J, Marik P. Management of the obese crtically ill patient. Crit Care Clin 2001; 17: 187–200.
73. Abernathy DR, Greenblatt DJ. Pharmacokinetics of drugs in obesity. Clin Pharmacokinet 1982; 7: 108–24.
74. Girardin E, Bruguerolle B. Pharmacokinetic changes in obesity. Therapie 1993; 48: 397–402.

75. Snider RD, Kruse JA, Bander JJ, et al. Accuracy of estimated creatinine clearance in obese patients with stable renal function in the intensive care unit. Pharmacotherapy 1995; 15: 747–53.
76. Uppot RN, Sahani DV, Hahn PF, et al. Impact of obesity on medical imaging and image-guided intervention. Am J Roentgenol 2007; 188: 433–40.
77. Gallagher S. Tailoring care for obese patients. RN 1999; 62: 43–50.
78. Hidalgo G. Dermatological complications in obesity. Am J Clin Dermatol 2002; 3: 497–506.
79. Hebl MR, Xu J. Weighing the care: physicians reactions to the size of a patient. Int J Obes Relat Metab Disord 2001; 25: 1246–52.

18 | The Obese Parturient

Heather A. Panaro[1] and Vilma E. Ortiz[2]

[1]Clinical Fellow in Anesthesia, Harvard Medical School, Resident, Department of Anesthesia and Critical Care, Massachusetts General Hospital, Boston, Massachusetts, U.S.A.

[2]Assistant Professor in Anesthesia, Harvard Medical School, Department of Anesthesia and Critical Care, Associate Anesthetist, Massachusetts General Hospital, Boston, Massachusetts, U.S.A.

INTRODUCTION

The incidence of overweight and obesity in women of childbearing age has reached epidemic proportions. High maternal body mass index (BMI) is associated with an increase in peripartum complications for both mother and baby. To appropriately prepare for the needs and challenges of this patient population, anesthetic care should begin in the prenatal period with an antepartum consultation.

PHYSIOLOGIC CHANGES IN THE OBESE PARTURIENT
Pulmonary

Decreased lung volume results from reduced chest wall compliance secondary to deposition of excess adipose tissue (1). Cephalad displacement of the diaphragm by the gravid uterus contributes to a decreased functional residual capacity (FRC) (2). In the supine and Trendelenburg positions, FRC may fall below closing capacity leading to small airway collapse, worsening atelectasis, and desaturation (1).

Increased metabolic requirements from both obesity and pregnancy result in a higher rate of O_2 utilization and increased CO_2 production (3). Sleep disordered breathing (SDB) is not uncommon in obese pregnant patients (4). Paradoxically, the physical and hormonal changes with pregnancy may both diminish and worsen the risk of development of SDB. Factors such as the respiratory stimulating effect of progesterone, the preference for the lateral position during sleep as well as the reduction in REM sleep during late pregnancy seem to have a protective effect. Factors which may predispose pregnant women to SDB include excess weight gain, nasal congestion, reduced upper airway caliber, increased stage 1 sleep and sleep fragmentation (5).

Cardiovascular

Both obesity and pregnancy are associated with increased circulating blood volume, stroke volume, and cardiac output. The incidence of pregnancy induced hypertension and preeclampsia is higher in obese women, and rates positively correlate with increasing BMI (6). Increased cardiac output and hypertension, both essential and pregnancy induced, increase left ventricular demands beyond what is normally seen during pregnancy.

Aortocaval compression (supine hypotension syndrome) results in reduction of uteroplacental blood flow when the parturient lies flat. This can be exacerbated in obese patients as excess adipose tissue increases abdominal mass and inferior vena cava compression; hence, the importance of left uterine displacement in preventing significant cardiovascular compromise cannot be overemphasized (7).

Long-standing obesity can lead to dilated cardiomyopathy with systolic dysfunction, which can worsen during pregnancy. In addition, sleep apnea may lead to pulmonary hypertension and deterioration of right heart function. An ECG should be obtained in patients with suspected cardiac disease, and cardiology consultation should be sought if the patient's condition warrants it.

Gastrointestinal
Approximately two-thirds of pregnant women develop heartburn. This is mainly the result of decreased lower esophageal sphincter tone due to elevated progesterone levels as well as gastric compression from the enlarged uterus. Other contributing factors include a decrease in the physiologic function of the lower esophageal sphincter as well as changes in esophageal peristalsis (8). In the laboring patient, gastroesophageal reflux is compounded by the recumbent position and the slowing of gastric emptying by pain and parenteral opioids. These changes contribute to an increase in the risk of aspiration during induction of general anesthesia.

Gastric motility is not delayed throughout pregnancy, but has been shown to decrease during active labor (9). In accordance with the ASA Practice Guidelines for Obstetric Anesthesia, pregnant patients scheduled for elective surgery should abstain from solids for six to eight hours prior to induction. Clear liquids may be taken up to two hours prior (10).

Hepatic
Non-alcoholic steatohepatitis leading to elevated liver function tests can be seen in obese parturients, making the diagnosis of severe preeclampsia more difficult (11). It may be beneficial to obtain baseline values on obese patients to help prevent misdiagnosis later in pregnancy.

Hematologic
Thromboembolism is one of the leading causes of maternal death, and its risk is increased in obese patients (12,13). Consensus guidelines do not exist regarding thromboprophylaxis for this patient population, but consideration should be given to providing either mechanical and/or chemical prophylaxis to this high risk group (14).

Endocrine
Gestational diabetes is more prevalent in women with an elevated pregravid BMI (15). Both gestational and pre-existing type II diabetes can lead to increased morbidity for mother and baby. Consideration should be given to testing for glucose intolerance before the standard 24 to 28 weeks (11).

INTRAPARTUM CONCERNS
Maternal
An increased BMI has been shown to lead to an increase in the following:

1. *Induction of labor* (16–18)
2. *Labor augmentation with oxytocin*: This may be the result of abnormal myometrial activity. In vitro studies of uterine contractility have demonstrated a marked

decline with increasing patient weight (16). Additionally, enhanced uterine contractility from oxytocin may be inhibited by higher levels of leptin present in obese patients. This, in turn, may contribute to the increased Cesarean section (C-section) rate in this patient population (19). It is also theorized that larger doses of oxytocin are required in order to obtain similar tissue levels due to an increase in body mass compared with lean patients

3. *C-section rates*: The risk of C-section (primary and repeat) increases with BMI and is thought to be due to several factors including increased fetal weight, difficulty with abdominal and vaginal examination, failure to progress and difficulty in fetal monitoring (20–22)
4. Increasing BMI has been directly associated with higher rates of *failed trial of labor after C-section* as well as an increased incidence of uterine rupture and dehiscence (18)
5. Although conflicting data exists, operative vaginal delivery with forceps or vacuum may be increased in obese and severely obese patients (6,22,23). However, *failed operative vaginal delivery* rates do increase with higher BMI (24)
6. Maternal obesity has been linked to increased *peripartum morbidity and mortality*. Severely obese women are exposed to longer durations of hospital stay regardless of the mode of delivery, higher rate of infectious complications (such as endometriosis) and higher health care cost (14,25). Duration of C-section, intraoperative blood loss, wound infection rates and risk of postpartum hemorrhage are also higher in the obese (26)

Neonatal
Prenatal complications include a higher rate of spontaneous abortion and neonatal death (22). Pregnancies resulting from assisted reproduction also have higher rates of miscarriage (22). *Congenital malformations* such as neural tube defects, omphalocele, and cardiac anomalies are more common in infants of obese mothers (27). These defects can be more difficult to diagnose in utero due to the technical challenge of obtaining and adequately interpreting ultrasound images in obese patients. The risk of fetal macrosomia is increased in both overweight and obese women (25,28), which may contribute to the increased rates of operative deliveries as well as birth trauma.

Infants of obese mothers have an almost six-fold increase in the risk of *neonatal mortality* over those born to normal weight women. A contributing factor is the increased risk of preterm delivery secondary to preterm premature rupture of membranes (29). Macrosomic babies born to obese women are more likely to have lower Apgar scores and to be admitted to the special care nursery (29,30). Excessive gestational weight gain has also been shown to increase a term infant's risk of meconium aspiration syndrome, respiratory distress, infection, hypoglycemia, and increased hospital stay (31).

The morbidity for children born to obese mothers is not isolated to the prenatal and neonatal period. Children born to obese women are more likely to become overweight themselves (32), and obese women who are diabetic during pregnancy have children who are more likely to develop insulin resistance (33).

Pregnancy After Bariatric Surgery
With an estimated one-third of U.S. women being obese and >200,000 bariatric surgical procedures performed each year, the incidence of pregnant patients who have undergone gastric bypass or bariatric surgery is rising. Traditionally considered

very high risk, pregnancies in women after gastric bypass have increasingly been shown to have similar perinatal outcomes, assuming patients receive appropriate prenatal medical care (34,35).

Despite a paucity of data, it is recommended that pregnancy be delayed for at least 12 to 18 months after bariatric surgery (36). This time period is marked by rapid weight loss and is a highly catabolic state. However, small retrospective studies comparing women who became pregnant within one year of their gastric bypass surgery with those who waited more than one year have demonstrated similar fetal outcomes and rates of pregnancy related complications (37).

Nutritional deficiencies (e.g. thiamine, calcium, vitamin B_{12} and iron deficiency leading to anemia) can be seen after bariatric surgery, especially malabsorptive procedures (38). Perhaps of greatest concern is a depletion of folic acid, which may lead to an increase in neural tube defects in post bypass patients who are not provided with appropriate supplementation (39).

A high index of suspicion must be maintained throughout pregnancy for catastrophic intra-abdominal processes that can complicate patients who are post gastric bypass. Fatal outcomes for both mother and fetus have been reported due to internal intestinal herniation; therefore, a low threshold should be maintained to perform appropriate imaging, including CT scan if indicated to appropriately evaluate these patients (40).

ANESTHETIC CONCERNS
Labor Analgesia
Epidural
Adequate epidural analgesia offers several benefits to the laboring obese parturient including:

1. Pain relief with minimal motor weakness
2. Minimal effects on respiratory and cardiovascular status with careful titration of drugs
3. Ability to transition to a surgical anesthetic in the event of a C-section or instrumented vaginal delivery
4. Option to use for postpartum pain management

Catheter placement can be challenging despite optimal patient positioning and ultrasound assistance (7). Obese patients are likely to have distorted anatomic landmarks, and misidentification of spinal anatomy is frequent. This has been associated with higher rates of inadvertent dural puncture (41). Epidural catheters in obese patients are also more likely to become dislodged and to be placed intravascularly. In one study, severely obese patients had an initial catheter failure rate of >40% (25). For this reason, early catheter placement is recommended along with frequent assessment of proper catheter function. To minimize its movement out of the epidural space, it has been suggested that the catheter be secured to the patient's back once she is sitting upright or in the lateral position (42).

Compared to lean patients, laboring obese parturients have been shown to have lower local anesthetic requirements in order to achieve similar levels of sensory block (43,44). Beginning in the first trimester and continuing throughout gestation, the increased intra-abdominal pressure, with its attendant increase in collateral circulation, contributes to engorgement of epidural veins. The resulting reduction in the size of the epidural space may allow for enhanced spread of local anesthetics (45).

Combined Spinal Epidural
This technique can be utilized in the laboring parturient who is at an advanced stage of labor in order to achieve rapid analgesia. A theoretical disadvantage of this technique is that the epidural catheter is untested.

Continuous Spinal
Spinal catheters can provide profound analgesia throughout labor and, like epidurals, can be incrementally dosed to an appropriate sensory level if surgical anesthesia is needed. Vigilance and attention to vital signs are extremely important given the risk of an inadvertent high sensory and motor block. Should this occur, equipment must be in place to provide respiratory and cardiovascular support. One of the most frequent complications after spinal catheter placement, post dural puncture headache, is seen less frequently in the obese population. It is possible that the dural defect is more readily occluded by epidural fat (7). In addition, the increase in contents of the epidural space may decrease the pressure gradient between the subarachnoid and epidural space. An intrathecal catheter should be removed as soon as possible to minimize the risk of meningitis.

Anesthesia for C-section
General Considerations
The obese parturient presenting for an operative delivery poses a challenge not only for the anesthesiologist but also for all members of the labor and delivery team. From equipment such as operating room tables, retractors, patient-transferring devices, sphygmomanometer cuffs, short handle laryngoscopes to individuals trained in the care of the obese patient, the operating room needs to be fully equipped to accommodate patients of large body mass. Whether the C-section is elective, urgent or emergent, a careful assessment of the patient's history, comorbidities and physical exam (particularly the airway exam) is imperative for the development of a cogent anesthetic plan.

The physiologic changes associated with pregnancy are superimposed on those accompanying obesity. The potential for increased operative time and blood loss means that the patient should be positioned in a manner that facilitates safe induction of a general anesthetic at any moment. In addition to left uterine displacement, this position includes either elevation of the head of the bed, blankets under the upper torso and occiput (ramped) or the reverse Trendelenburg position with use of a footboard to support the patient. The goal is to improve lung mechanics and patient comfort while allowing the patient to maintain adequate ventilation. All pressure points should be padded to protect against nerve injury.

As it is current practice, the obese parturient coming to the operating room should be given an oral non-particulate antacid (i.e., sodium citrate) and intravenous antibiotic prophylaxis. Sodium citrate immediately works to raise the pH of gastric contents thereby decreasing the severity of pneumonitis should aspiration occurs. Prophylaxis with H_2 blockers has been shown to be more efficacious than a proton pump inhibitor in raising the pH and decreasing gastric volume when administered several hours prior to induction (46). Unless indicated by the patient's underlying condition, standard non-invasive monitors should be applied. Once in the operating room, supplemental oxygen should be provided.

Epidural
A continuous epidural catheter allows for incremental dosing of local anesthetics to achieve a surgical level with minimal hemodynamic changes. A well functioning catheter can provide prolonged surgical anesthesia, which may be necessary, as operative times have been shown to be longer in obese patients. Additionally, the catheter may be left in place to provide post-operative analgesia in patients who are not candidates for systemic or neuraxial narcotics or in patients who may be at risk for reoperation. The sacral sparing associated with intraoperative patient discomfort is a potential drawback of this technique.

Combined Spinal Epidural
This technique provides a rapid, dense block from the spinal and allows for prolongation of anesthesia through dosing of the epidural catheter should the surgical time exceed the duration of the spinal. However, there is a risk that the untested epidural will not function appropriately once dosing is initiated and resolution of the spinal block occurs (7). In order to ensure proper catheter placement, some practitioners will use lower doses of spinal anesthetic or maintain the seated position until the block has begun to set and then raise the level to a full surgical plane using the epidural (1).

Spinal
Spinal anesthesia provides a fast onset, dense, highly reliable block with limited duration of action. A block extending to the high thoracic dermatomes has been shown to decrease spirometric parameters including vital capacity, FVC, FEV_1, peak expiratory flow rate, and mid-expiratory flow (47). The decrease in vital capacity is more significant in obese patients than in normal weight parturients. This decrease has been shown to extend even after resolution of the block (47). Consideration must be given to the changes in the obese parturient, which may place her at an increased risk of a higher cephalad spread compared with parturients of normal BMI (48).

Anatomic changes. In the later stages of pregnancy, the normally seen lumbar lordosis becomes flattened, the thoracic kyphosis reduced (49), and engorged epidural veins compress the subarachnoid space (50). Once the patient is placed supine, these changes can contribute to a higher spread of a hyperbaric spinal anesthetic solution injected in the lumbar region.

Cerebrospinal fluid (CSF) changes. Obese and pregnant patients have been shown by MRI to have decreased CSF volume, presumably resulting from increased abdominal pressure. This is likely from CSF displacement as soft tissue moves into the intervertebral foramen (51).

Hormonal changes. Hormonal changes associated with pregnancy, including increased levels of progesterone, have also been postulated to increase the pregnant patient's sensitivity to local anesthetic agents (52).

General Anesthesia

General anesthesia has been traditionally considered to be higher risk in the obstetric population, largely due to an increased incidence of difficulty in airway management (53). The incidence of failed intubation in the parturient has been estimated between 0.1% and 0.6%, occurring mostly during emergency situations and involving individuals with lesser training and expertise in airway management (48,53,54). Two recent publications examining anesthesia-related maternal deaths have underscored obesity as a significant contributing factor in maternal deaths, especially during emergence from a general anesthetic and in the recovery period (55,56).

Airway exam. Preparation for a general anesthetic should start with a thorough assessment of the patient's airway. This should include not only the Mallampati score, but also evaluation of the thyromental distance, dentition, neck mobility, size of the tongue, and ability to protrude the lower teeth beyond the upper teeth (57). Factors contributing to a decreased upper airway caliber in the third trimester of pregnancy include: fat deposition infiltrating pharyngeal muscle tissue, soft tissue deposition in the neck, nasal mucosal engorgement, and increased neck circumference during pregnancy (5). If the airway evaluation reveals that a difficult intubation is a possibility, all members of the care team, including the patient, should be informed that an awake intubation would be necessary should a general anesthetic be required. A dedicated difficult airway cart, equipped with a fiberoptic bronchoscope, as well as personnel skilled in the management of the difficult airway should be part of every obstetric operating room.

Positioning. Studies in non-pregnant severely obese patients have revealed that the 25° head-up position is associated with higher preinduction oxygen tensions and longer time to desaturation than the supine position (58). When compared to the horizontal and to the 30° back up positions during induction, the reverse Trendelenburg position was associated with the longest safe apnea period (59). Reverse Trendelenburg allows for gravitational displacement of the breasts, pannus and abdominal contents away from the diaphragm, thus improving patient comfort, FRC, and oxygenation. In addition to allowing better access to the airway and neck, bag-mask ventilation is facilitated, as less pressure would be required to move the diaphragm caudad. To our knowledge no comparable studies exist in the obese parturient. A potential drawback of this position is the possibility of hypotension due to a decrease in venous return.

Preoxygenation. Preoxygenation is essential in the obese pregnant patient prior to the induction of a general anesthetic. The decrease in FRC coupled with the increased metabolic demands seen in late pregnancy account for rapid desaturation during apnea. Parturients should be preoxygenated for three to five minutes of tidal volume breathing, as this has been shown to maximize PaO_2 and the safe apnea period compared to several vital capacity breaths (46,60–62).

Intubation. For patients in whom a difficult airway is not expected, intubation should follow a rapid sequence induction once the abdomen is prepped and draped and the surgical team is ready to start upon confirmation of tracheal intubation. A difficult airway algorithm must be in place and ready to be implemented should airway difficulties be encountered.

Extubation. After a general anesthetic, the obese parturient should be extubated when fully awake and after full recovery of neuromuscular function. She should be maintained in the semi recumbent position, provided with supplemental oxygen and closely monitored during the recovery phase. For those with sleep apnea, continuous positive airway pressure or bilevel positive airway pressure may be necessary to prevent airway obstruction. Depending on the level of respiratory compromise, these patients may need to be observed in an intensive care setting.

Post-operative Pain Management
Optimal pain relief facilitates improved pulmonary function, early ambulation and prompt return to baseline functional status. Options available include continuous epidural analgesia, neuraxial opioids, patient controlled analgesia, and parenteral opioids. If no contraindications, adjuvant use of non-opioid analgesics such as NSAIDs is recommended to decrease the total dose of opioids required for pain relief. Narcotic use is associated with respiratory depression in severely obese patients and those with sleep apnea, thus these patients may need to be monitored more closely before discharge to the postpartum floor.

ACKNOWLEDGMENT
The authors would like to thank to Dr. Robert R. Gaiser (Professor of Anesthesiology and Critical Care at the Hospital of the University of Pennsylvania) for his invaluable assistance editing this chapter.

REFERENCES
1. Mhyre JM. Anesthetic management for the morbidly obese pregnant woman. Int Anesthesiol Clin 2007; 45: 51–70.
2. Kapoor R, Min JC, Leffert L. Anesthesia for obstetrics and gynecology. In: Dunn PF, Alston TA, Baker KH, et al., eds. Clinical Anesthesia Procedures of the Massachusetts General Hospital, 7th edn. Philadelphia: Lippincott Williams & Wilkins, 2007.
3. Sullivan JT, Wong CA. Anesthetic management for the obese parturient. In: Alvarez A, Brodsky J, Albert M, et al., eds. Morbid Obesity: Perioperative Management. Cambridge, UK: Cambridge University Press, 2005.
4. Saravanakumar K, Rao SG, Cooper GM. Obesity and obstetric anaesthesia. Anaesthesia 2006; 61: 36–48.
5. Izci B, Vennelle M, Liston WA, et al. Sleep-disordered breathing and upper airway size in pregnancy and post-partum. Eur Respir J 2006; 27: 321–7.
6. Weiss JL, Malone FD, Emig D, et al. Obesity, obstetric complications and cesarean delivery rate—a population-based screening study. Am J Obstet Gynecol 2004; 190: 1091–7.
7. Vallejo MC. Anesthetic management of the morbidly obese parturient. Curr Opin Anaesthesiol 2007; 20: 175–80.
8. Richter JE. Gastroesophageal reflux disease during pregnancy. Gastroenterol Clin North Am 2003; 32: 235–61.
9. Carp H, Jayaram A, Stoll M. Ultrasound examination of the stomach contents of parturients. Anesth Analg 1992; 74: 683–7.
10. American Society of Anesthesiologists Task Force on Obstetric Anesthesia. Practice guidelines for obstetric anesthesia: an updated report by the American Society of Anesthesiologists Task Force on Obstetric Anesthesia. Anesthesiology 2007; 106: 843–63.
11. Catalano PM. Management of obesity in pregnancy. Obstet Gynecol 2007; 109(2 Pt 1): 419–33.
12. de Swiet M. Maternal mortality: confidential enquiries into maternal deaths in the United Kingdom. Am J Obstet Gynecol 2000; 182: 760–6.
13. Berg CJ, Chang J, Callaghan WM, et al. Pregnancy-related mortality in the United States, 1991–1997. Obstet Gynecol 2003; 101: 289–96.

14. Duhl AJ, Paidas MJ, Ural SH, et al. Antithrombotic therapy and pregnancy: consensus report and recommendations for prevention and treatment of venous thromboembolism and adverse pregnancy outcomes. Am J Obstet Gynecol 2007; 197: 457. e1–21.
15. Cheng YW, Caughey AB. Gestational diabetes: diagnosis and management. J Perinatol 2008 Jul 17.
16. Zhang J, Bricker L, Wray S, et al. Poor uterine contractility in obese women. BJOG 2007; 114: 343–8.
17. Ray A, Hildreth A, Esen UI. Morbid obesity and intra-partum care. J Obstet Gynaecol 2008; 28: 301–4.
18. Hibbard JU, Gilbert S, Landon MB, et al. Trial of labor or repeat cesarean delivery in women with morbid obesity and previous cesarean delivery. Obstet Gynecol 2006; 108: 125–33.
19. Moynihan AT, Hehir MP, Glavey SV, et al. Inhibitory effect of leptin on human uterine contractility in vitro. Am J Obstet Gynecol 2006; 195: 504–9.
20. Bergholt T, Lim LK, Jorgensen JS, et al. Maternal body mass index in the first trimester and risk of cesarean delivery in nulliparous women in spontaneous labor. Am J Obstet Gynecol 2007; 196: 163.e1,163.e5.
21. Lynch CM, Sexton DJ, Hession M, et al. Obesity and mode of delivery in primigravid and multigravid women. Am J Perinatol 2008; 25: 163–7.
22. Yu CK, Teoh TG, Robinson S. Obesity in pregnancy. BJOG 2006; 113: 1117–25.
23. Steinfeld JD, Valentine S, Lerer T, et al. Obesity-related complications of pregnancy vary by race. J Matern Fetal Med 2000; 9: 238–41.
24. Gopalani S, Bennett K, Critchlow C. Factors predictive of failed operative vaginal delivery. Am J Obstet Gynecol 2004; 191: 896–902.
25. Hood DD, Dewan DM. Anesthetic and obstetric outcome in morbidly obese parturients. Anesthesiology 1993; 79: 1210–18.
26. Wali A, Suresh MS. Maternal morbidity, mortality, and risk assessment. Anesthesiol Clin 2008; 26: 197, 230, ix.
27. Cedergren MI, Kallen BA. Maternal obesity and infant heart defects. Obes Res 2003; 11: 1065–71.
28. Driul L, Cacciaguerra G, Citossi A, et al. Prepregnancy body mass index and adverse pregnancy outcomes. Arch Gynecol Obstet 2008; 278: 23–6.
29. Nohr EA, Vaeth M, Bech BH, et al. Maternal obesity and neonatal mortality according to subtypes of preterm birth. Obstet Gynecol 2007; 110: 1083–90.
30. Jolly MC, Sebire NJ, Harris JP, et al. Risk factors for macrosomia and its clinical consequences: a study of 350,311 pregnancies. Eur J Obstet Gynecol Reprod Biol 2003; 10: 111: 9–14.
31. Stotland NE, Cheng YW, Hopkins LM, et al. Gestational weight gain and adverse neonatal outcome among term infants. Obstet Gynecol 2006; 108(3 Pt 1): 635–43.
32. Salsberry PJ, Reagan PB. Dynamics of early childhood overweight. Pediatrics 2005; 116: 1329–38.
33. Nathanielsz PW, Poston L, Taylor PD. In utero exposure to maternal obesity and diabetes: animal models that identify and characterize implications for future health. Obstet Gynecol Clin North Am 2007; 34: 201–12, vii–viii.
34. Beard JH, Bell RL, Duffy AJ. Reproductive considerations and pregnancy after bariatric surgery: current evidence and recommendations. Obes Surg 2008; 18: 1023–7.
35. Wax JR, Cartin A, Wolff R, et al. Pregnancy following gastric bypass surgery for morbid obesity: maternal and neonatal outcomes. Obes Surg 2008; 18: 540–4.
36. Miller RJ, Xanthakos SA, Hillard PJ, et al. Bariatric surgery and adolescent gynecology. Curr Opin Obstet Gynecol 2007; 19: 427–33.

37. Dao T, Kuhn J, Ehmer D, et al. Pregnancy outcomes after gastric-bypass surgery. Am J Surg 2006; 192: 762–6.
38. Malinowski SS. Nutritional and metabolic complications of bariatric surgery. Am J Med Sci 2006; 331: 219–25.
39. Moliterno JA, DiLuna ML, Sood S, et al. Gastric bypass: a risk factor for neural tube defects? Case report. J Neurosurg Pediatrics 2008; 1: 406–9.
40. Moore KA, Ouyang DW, Whang EE. Maternal and fetal deaths after gastric bypass surgery for morbid obesity. N Engl J Med 2004; 351: 721–2.
41. Jones N, Peck M, Gowrie S, et al. Postdural puncture headache in morbidly obese patients. Can J Anesth 2006; 53: 26343.
42. Hamilton CL, Riley ET, Cohen SE. Changes in the position of epidural catheters associated with patient movement. Anesthesiology 1997; 86: 778–84; discussion 29A.
43. Panni MK, Columb MO. Obese parturients have lower epidural local anaesthetic requirements for analgesia in labour. Br J Anaesth 2006; 96: 106–10.
44. Visser WA, Lee RA, Gielen MJ. Factors affecting the distribution of neural blockade by local anesthetics in epidural anesthesia and a comparison of lumbar versus thoracic epidural anesthesia. Anesth Analg 2008; 107: 708–21.
45. Igarashi T, Hirabayashi Y, Shimizu R, et al. The fiberscopic findings of the epidural space in pregnant women. Anesthesiology 2000; 92: 1631–6.
46. Russell GN, Smith CL, Snowdon SL, et al. Preoxygenation techniques. Anesth Analg 1987; 66: 1341–2.
47. von Ungern-Sternberg BS, Regli A, Bucher E, et al. Impact of spinal anaesthesia and obesity on maternal respiratory function during elective caesarean section. Anaesthesia 2004; 59: 743–9.
48. Barnardo PD, Jenkins JG. Failed tracheal intubation in obstetrics: a 6-year review in a UK region. Anaesthesia 2000; 55: 690–4.
49. Hirabayashi Y, Shimizu R, Fukuda H, et al. Anatomical configuration of the spinal column in the supine position. II. Comparison of pregnant and non-pregnant women. Br J Anaesth 1995; 75: 6–8.
50. Takiguchi T, Yamaguchi S, Tezuka M, et al. Compression of the subarachnoid space by the engorged epidural venous plexus in pregnant women. Anesthesiology 2006; 105: 848–51.
51. Hogan QH, Prost R, Kulier A, et al. Magnetic resonance imaging of cerebrospinal fluid volume and the influence of body habitus and abdominal pressure. Anesthesiology 1996; 84: 1341–9.
52. Datta S, Hurley RJ, Naulty JS, et al. Plasma and cerebrospinal fluid progesterone concentrations in pregnant and nonpregnant women. Anesth Analg 1986; 65: 950–4.
53. Hawkins JL, Koonin LM, Palmer SK, et al. Anesthesia-related deaths during obstetric delivery in the United States, 1979–1990. Anesthesiology 1997; 86: 277–84.
54. Goldszmidt E. Principles and practices of obstetric airway management. Anesthesiol Clin 2008; 26: 109–25, vii.
55. Mhyre JM, Riesner MN, Polley LS, et al. A series of anesthesia-related maternal deaths in Michigan, 1985–2003. Anesthesiology 2007; 106: 1096–104.
56. Cooper GM, McClure JH. Anaesthesia chapter from saving mothers' lives; reviewing maternal deaths to make pregnancy safer. Br J Anaesth 2008; 100: 17–22.
57. American Society of Anesthesiologists Task Force on Management of the Difficult Airway. Practice guidelines for management of the difficult airway: an updated report by the American Society of Anesthesiologists Task Force on Management of the Difficult Airway. Anesthesiology 2003; 98: 1269–77.
58. Dixon BJ, Dixon JB, Carden JR, et al. Preoxygenation is more effective in the 25 degrees head-up position than in the supine position in severely obese patients: a randomized controlled study. Anesthesiology 2005; 102: 1110–15; discussion 5A.

59. Boyce JR, Ness T, Castroman P, et al. A preliminary study of the optimal anesthesia positioning for the morbidly obese patient. Obes Surg 2003; 13: 4–9.
60. Chin EY, Chan SY, Yip YY, et al. Preoxygenation in parturients: a comparison of 4, 6 and 8 vital capacity breaths to 5 minutes of tidal volume breathing. Singapore Med J 1990; 31: 138–41.
61. Gold MI. Preoxygenation. Br J Anaesth 1989; 62: 241–2.
62. Gambee AM, Hertzka RE, Fisher DM. Preoxygenation techniques: comparison of three minutes and four breaths. Anesth Analg 1987; 66: 468–70.

19 | The Obese Pediatric Patient

Roland Brusseau

Instructor, Harvard Medical School, Assistant in Anesthesia, Department of Anesthesiology, Perioperative and Pain Medicine, Children's Hospital Boston, Boston, Massachusetts, U.S.A.

INTRODUCTION

Overweight and obesity are increasingly prevalent in the pediatric population, paralleling the adult epidemic, both in the United States and worldwide. Pediatric anesthesiologists see many of these children in the operating room and are now dealing with many perioperative issues formerly reserved for their adult counterparts.

Definition
BMI

Adult obesity is defined as a body mass index (BMI) of 30 or higher, with overweight considered to be a BMI greater than 25 (1). [BMI = weight in kg divided by the square of the height in meters, or (kg/m²)].

Age-adjusted BMI

As BMI varies with age and gender in children, the definition of pediatric obesity is based on a percentile of age-adjusted BMI, represented on standard growth charts, rather than a specific BMI. Pediatric obesity has been defined as a BMI greater than the 95th percentile for age and gender on sex-specific BMI growth charts. Overweight is considered to be greater than the 85th percentile on such charts (2) (Figs. 1 and 2).

Prevalence

The Centers for Disease Control and Prevention and other United States government agencies have found that approximately one-third of U.S. children were overweight or obese in 2006 (3). This is a dramatic increase from roughly 5% of adolescents and 6.5% of children classified as overweight or obese in 1976 (4). Weight appears to increase with advancing age:

Overweight or Obese (BMI ≥ 85 Percentile)
- 24% of preschool children (2–5 years)
- 33% of school age children (6–11 years)
- 34% of adolescents (12–19 years)

Obese (BMI ≥ 95 Percentile)
- 12.4% of preschool children
- 17.0% of school age children
- 17.6% of adolescents

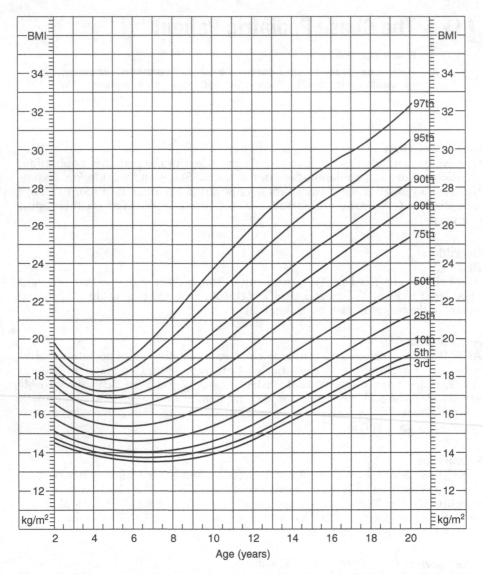

Figure 1 Body mass index-for-age percentiles, boys, 2 to 20 years, CDC growth charts: United States. Developed by the National Center for Health Statistics in collaboration with the National Center for Chronic Disease Prevention and Health Promotion (2000).

Severely Obese (BMI ≥ 97 Percentile)
- 8.5% of preschool children
- 11.4% of school age children
- 12.6% of adolescents

NHANES data suggest variations between ethnic and gender populations of the pediatric overweight. Mexican-American children are more likely to be overweight

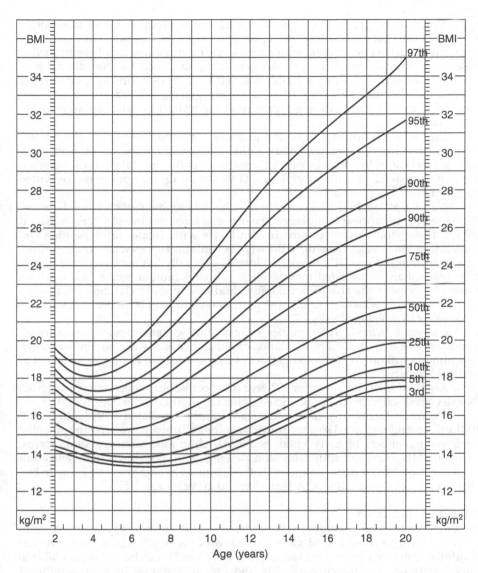

Figure 2 Body mass index-for-age percentiles, girls, 2 to 20 years, CDC growth charts: United States. Developed by the National Center for Health Statistics in collaboration with the National Center for Chronic Disease Prevention and Health Promotion (2000).

(23%) than non-Hispanic black or white children (21% and 14%, respectively). Amongst males, 27.5% of Mexican-American males are overweight or obese and amongst girls, non-Hispanic black girls have the greatest prevalence at 26.6%.

Etiology
The causes of obesity are many and often interrelated.

Ninety-five percent of pediatric obesity has *no apparent identifiable etiology* or distinct medical cause. Only 5% of pediatric obesity appears to have an underlying cause such as neurologic injury, endocrine dysfunction, or a hereditary disease or syndrome. *Hereditary or other genetic disorders* account for about 1% of cases (Prader-Willi, Cushing's, Frohlich's, and Laurence-Moon-Biedl syndromes as well as other inborn errors of metabolism, glycogen storage diseases, and isolated gene defects including leptin receptor mutations and melanocortin 4 gene mutations) (5).

Caloric excess appears to be the primary contributor to child and adolescent obesity. Fundamentally, overweight and obesity may result from high caloric intake and low energy output. Inactivity is the most important determinant of increased obesity in children (TV watching, computer usage, video gaming) (6).

Neonatal factors may also contribute to the development of childhood obesity. Breast-fed babies appear less likely to be obese in later childhood (7). Formula-fed babies demonstrate higher plasma insulin levels with greater fat deposition and early adipocyte development (8,9). Breast milk contains factors which inhibit adipocyte formation in vitro (10). Breast-fed infants generally have a lower overall protein intake than formula-fed infants. High neonatal protein intake also has been shown to increase the risk of developing childhood obesity (11). Small for gestational age infants who have rapid post-partum weight gain have been shown to be more likely to develop obesity (12).

Hormonal factors. Twin studies suggest that genetic factors may play an important role as well (13). Dysregulation or imbalance of any of a number of known and hitherto unknown hormonal pathways may contribute to the development of pediatric obesity.

Restricted sleep time. A recent 32-year prospective birth cohort study suggested that sleep restriction in childhood increases the long-term risk for obesity (14).

Shorter childhood sleep times were significantly associated with higher adult BMI values, and remained so after adjustment for adult sleep time and the potential confounding effects of early childhood BMI, childhood socioeconomic status, parental BMIs, child and adult television viewing, adult physical activity, and adult smoking. Notably, evidence suggests that children on average may be going to bed as much as two hours later today than they did 20 years ago (15).

PATHOPHYSIOLOGY
In general, most obese children will not have significant non-psychiatric complications related to obesity for decades. Very few of the medical complications seen in adult obesity and overweight are seen in children. Nevertheless, some children may experience significant morbidity and are predisposed to more significant obesity-related complications in adulthood (16).

Respiratory
Pulmonary function and the respiratory mechanics of overweight and obese children are influenced by the amount and distribution of adipose tissue.

Restrictive disease. Overweight and obese children demonstrate altered pulmonary dynamics with reductions in FVC and FRC typical of a restrictive pattern. Chest wall compliance is reduced and anterior chest wall excursion is limited. Reductions in forced *expiratory reserve volumes* and flows (e.g., FEV_1 and FEF_{25-75}) are common (17). Impairment of the *diffusing capacity* for lung CO_2 has also been noted (18).

Obstructive disease.   Pediatric obesity may produce elements of obstructive disease as well, with overweight and obese children having a higher incidence of asthma (especially exercise-induced asthma) than other children (19).

Atelectasis.   At rest, obese pediatric patients have significantly more atelectasis than non-obese children (20). When tidal volumes approximate closing capacity in such patients, they are more prone to shunting and hypoxia. This effect is enhanced in the supine position as the abdominal wall and intraabdominal contents both exert diaphragmatic pressure and limit diaphragmatic excursion (21).

Obstructive sleep apnea is seen in 7% to 17% of obese children with a BMI greater than the 150th percentile (22). Obesity hypoventilation syndrome, defined as extreme obesity and alveolar hypoventilation in wakefulness, has also been recognized in children. Such hypoventilation in the absence of frank airway obstruction is more common during sleep (and less easily identified without a sleep study), likely due to the restrictive ventilatory pattern of obesity (23).

Asthma.   Overweight and obese children demonstrate a greater frequency and degree of bronchospasm compared to other children (24). Overweight children have been shown to have more severe asthma symptoms than age-matched children below the 85th percentile for BMI (25).

Infections.   Overweight infants have more frequent and severe respiratory infections than other infants, a trend that persists into childhood (26).

Airway narrowing and other anatomic abnormalities secondary to both the amount of adipose tissue and the location of its deposition have been described (27).

Cardiovascular
Both obesity and overweight have long been associated with the development of cardiovascular risk factors such as hypertension, left ventricular hypertrophy, pulmonary hypertension, dyslipidemia, and both insulin resistance and Type 2 diabetes. Despite the increasing prevalence of pediatric overweight and obesity, there is little evidence to date of increased cardiac morbidity in childhood, though almost certainly these risks are perpetuated into adulthood.

Hypertension.   Obesity during childhood is associated with hypertension in childhood, with persistence into adulthood (28). Suggested mechanisms for obesity related hypertension include sympathetic nervous system hyperactivity, insulin resistance, and vascular abnormalities (29). Higher resting heart rates, as well as greater variability of heart rate and blood pressure, have been identified in obese adolescents, thought to be due to sympathetic nervous system overactivity (30).

Blood volume.   Pediatric obesity is associated with increased blood volume (likely due to increased renal sodium retention related to hyperinsulinism as well as the added vascularization of adipose tissue), increased stroke volume, increased cardiac output, and increased left ventricular mass (31). Increases of oxygen consumption and carbon dioxide production are proportional to increasing weight, aggravating the workload of the heart (32). Severely obese adolescents may demonstrate significant cardiac deconditioning, with many unable to achieve the anaerobic threshold during stress testing (27).

Atherosclerosis.   There is no evidence of cardiac disease or atherosclerosis in the otherwise normal obese pediatric population, though there may be significant obesity-related mortality seen in adulthood (33). As is the case with obese adults, an android fat pattern in pediatric obesity may be associated with less favorable plasma lipid profiles.

Hepatic and Gastrointestinal

Hepatic steatosis, or fatty liver, is commonly seen in obese children. Non-alcoholic steatohepatitis may also be seen, with resultant fibrosis, cirrhosis, and liver failure if not identified and appropriately managed (34). Cholelithiasis, while rarely symptomatic in the pediatric population, may cause abnormal elevations of liver enzymes (35).

Gastroesophageal reflux disease, thought to be secondary to increased intraabdominal pressure, is seen in a minority of obese children. However, no significant difference in gastric emptying time has been observed between obese, overweight, and normal-weight children (36).

Endocrine

Insulin dependent diabetes, often seen in obese adults, is increasingly being diagnosed amongst the growing population of overweight and obese adolescents (37). *Non-insulin dependent diabetes mellitus* is increasingly seen in the overweight and obese pediatric population, especially in those children with a family history of diabetes (38). This is commonly associated with other elements of the metabolic syndrome, including hyperlipidemia and hypertension.

Accelerated growth. Overweight and obesity in children and adolescents have been associated with accelerated linear growth and bone age (39).

Sexual maturation. Overweight has been associated with an earlier onset of sexual maturation in girls and, conversely, a delay in sexual maturation in boys (40). Overweight and obese adolescent females are at increased risk of hyperandrogenism, early onset of the polycystic ovary syndrome and its associated gynecological abnormalities (e.g., amenorrhea, dysfunctional uterine bleeding) (41).

Hematological

Obesity is well recognized in adults to be a risk factor for venous thromboembolic disease (42). While the same association has not yet been shown in children (43), it is reasonable to believe that obesity may pose an increased risk for the development of deep venous thrombosis and subsequent pulmonary embolism in children as well.

Abnormal endothelial function. Obesity has also been shown to be associated with abnormal endothelial function and structure, with an increased intimal-medial thickness in otherwise healthy young children (44). Intimal-medial thickness is a noninvasive marker for early atherosclerotic changes in pediatric patients and is related to the cardiovascular risk factors of obesity, especially hypertension, chronic inflammation, and impaired glucose metabolism (45).

Thromboembolism. These vascular changes and associated cardiovascular risk factors have been linked to venous thromboembolism and pulmonary embolism in surgical patients (46), suggesting that obesity may place children and adolescents at risk for thromboembolic complications.

Musculoskeletal

Secondary to excess weight load upon an immature skeletal, muscular, and synovial system, orthopedic comorbidities are common in the overweight and obese pediatric population. In general, such children with *orthopedic comorbidities* are at increased risk for fractures, musculoskeletal pain (particularly of the back, lower extremities, and lower extremity joints), lower extremity misalignment, and impaired mobility (47). *Slipped capital femoral epiphysis* (or SCFE) is common amongst overweight and obese adolescents, characterized by displacement of the capital femoral epiphysis from the femoral neck through to the growth plate (48). Surgical management is generally required. *Tibia vara (or Blount disease)* results from inhibited growth of the medial proximal tibial growth plate resulting from excessive abnormal weight bearing (49). Clinically this is seen as progressive bowed legs and tibial torsion.

Neurological
Neurological complications of overweight and obesity in children appear to be limited to an increased prevalence of idiopathic intracranial hypertension (or pseudotumor cerebri).

Idiopathic intracranial hypertension. As many as 50% of children who present with idiopathic intracranial hypertension are obese, though it appears that onset of symptoms does not correlate with weight gain (50). Typical presentation includes headache, nausea, vomiting, retroocular pain, transient visual changes, diplopia, and visual loss. In severe cases, idiopathic intracranial hypertension may lead to significant visual impairment or visual loss, necessitating aggressive weight management.

Psychiatric and Psychosocial
Psychiatric and psychosocial consequences of pediatric overweight and obesity are common: alienation, distorted peer relationships, poor self-esteem, distorted body image, anxiety, and depression. Such morbidities appear to increase with increasing age and disproportionately affect females (51).

Quality of life. Overweight children and adolescents report a decreased health-related quality of life compared to non-obese peers, a decrease similar to that typical of children and adolescents with cancer (52). *Developed negative self-image* appears to persist into adulthood, particularly amongst females, and has been associated with fewer years of completed advanced education, lower marriage rates, and higher rates of poverty compared to non-obese peers (53).

Pharmacology
As is the case with much pediatric pharmacology, inference frequently must be made from adult studies owing to the paucity of study data in children. Pharmacologic implications of pediatric overweight and obesity are even less studied, again requiring inferences from both adult and other pediatric literatures. What data there are regarding the pharmacokinetic and pharmacodynamics of common drugs in obese children are often conflicting or inconsistent. Dosages in the obese and overweight pediatric population may be difficult to estimate. While pediatric anesthesiologists are accustomed to adjusting dose by weight, adjusting for body composition adds a challenging dimension to such calculations. General considerations for drug dosing in obese patients may be found in chapter 9, "Anesthetic Drug Administration." Specific recommendations for pediatric patients may be found below in Section IV, subsections F, G, and H.

SURGICAL AND ANESTHETIC MORBIDITY AND MORTALITY
There is limited and frequently conflicting data regarding perioperative outcomes in the overweight and obese pediatric population.

Adverse Events
In a single center analysis of more than 100,000 patients, 9.56% of obese pediatric patients were found to have had an adverse perioperative event, compared to 5.89% of adult obese patients (54).

Airway Events
More recent studies have identified overweight and obese children as being at increased risk for significant airway events, such as difficult mask ventilation, airway obstruction (in both the OR and PACU), and major desaturation (>10% of baseline) (55). *Contributory risk factors* for such events have been shown to include procedures involving the airway, obesity (versus overweight), age younger than 10 years, and OSA. Significant differences in critical airway events related to *inhalation induction* or *intravenous induction* have not been demonstrated in the pediatric obese and overweight population (56).

Studies have variably shown no difference or a small difference (1.3%) in the rate of *difficult intubation* for pediatric overweight and obese children, significantly less than published rates for adults (57).

Postanesthesia Care Unit (PACU) Stays
Overweight and obese children are at increased risk for extended PACU stays (>3 hours) and unplanned hospital admission, though data is limited and conflicting. PACU delays appear to be due largely to post-operative airway obstruction (56).

Postoperative nausea and vomiting (PONV) has not conclusively been shown to be a cause of extended PACU stay or unplanned hospital admission (55,57).

Other Anesthetic and Procedural Morbidities
These morbidities have not been shown to be different. Rates of grade 1 pressures sores (assessed in the PACU), surgical site problems and return to activity were not shown to be significantly different between all groups of obese, overweight, and lean children in one large prospective trial (55).

Hospital Charges
Hospital charges and the overall burden on the healthcare system may be greater in overweight and obese children. In a study of pediatric adenotonsillectomy, obese and overweight children were more likely to be admitted than their peers, and among those admitted, length of stay correlated with BMI. Total hospital charges, as well as anesthesia, PACU, pharmacy and laboratory charges, were significantly higher for obese versus normal weight children (58).

ANESTHETIC MANAGEMENT
There is relatively little published data regarding anesthetizing overweight and obese pediatric patients. Again, guidance must be sought from the adult obesity literature, with careful attention to the specific pathophysiologic and pharmacologic considerations for pediatric overweight and obesity outlined above.

Preoperative
A thorough history and physical exam should be performed with particular attention to the specific morbidities and predictors of adverse outcomes in this

population. Poor self-esteem mandates that tact should be used during the preoperative assessment. *Respiratory symptoms* such as OSA, asthma, and recurrent infections should be identified. A *complete airway exam* should be performed and a gastroesophageal reflux history should be elicited as a part of the routine review of systems. *Physical examination* should include evaluation of potential venous access, arterial access (depending upon the procedure to be performed), and appropriateness for regional and neuraxial blocks should such be indicated.

For severely obese children, or those for whom many comorbidities exist, an *arterial blood gas* (to exclude hypoxemia and hypercapnia) as well as a *chest X-ray* and *electrocardiogram* (to evaluate for right ventricular strain and increased pulmonary pressures) may be indicated. Evaluation of the proper postoperative disposition of the patient should be made, paying particular attention to the known perioperative risks of the overweight and obese pediatric patient in relation to the planned procedure.

Premedication
Heavy sedation may cause respiratory depression, especially in the severely obese, and must be undertaken with caution. These risks must be balanced against the need for anxiolysis in many children. Often discussion and distraction (TV, hand-held video games, etc.) alone may alleviate the patient's anxiety (59). Small doses of *midazolam* or, in some cases, *ketamine* or *clonidine* may be used for patient relaxation (60). Intramuscular approaches should be avoided when possible due to the variable absorption of drugs following intra-adipose deposition. In the absence of intravenous access, oral midazolam and/or oral ketamine may serve as a premedication, being aware in the latter case of increased oral secretions for which glycopyrrolate may be added as an adjunct. The application of topical anesthetic creams (or other transdermal preparations) should be considered if a pre-induction IV is planned.

Reflux Precautions
Recent work has challenged the assumption of elevated reflux and aspiration risk in overweight and obese children. Recent studies in adults have shown a lower incidence of high gastric volume and low gastric pH in obese compared to non-obese adults (61). A review of over 50,000 patients demonstrated no incidences of aspiration (62). Other reviews of perioperative complications have similarly demonstrated no increased incidence of aspiration in obese children during general anesthesia. Overweight and obese children should be managed by the same perioperative NPO guidelines as other patients.

Monitoring
The use of standard ASA monitoring is generally sufficient, unless the procedure indicates invasive monitoring. Low voltages secondary to excess subcutaneous tissue can complicate *ECG monitoring* (63). Soft tissue excess can also limit the reliability of *pulse oximetry*, a critical monitor in this population especially given their lower tissue oxygen tensions relative to arterial values. Alternative sites, such as the ear, lip, or smallest fingers may be tried to improve accuracy (64).

Non-invasive blood pressure measurement may be inaccurate or unreliable in obese children given the lack of appropriate sizes and the conical shape of overweight and obese patients' upper arms, necessitating placement of an arterial catheter. Alternatively, forearm pressure measurement appears reproducible, though this technique may overestimate arterial pressure (65).

Monitoring of *neuromuscular blockade* may also prove difficult in the obese patient, necessitating use of percutaneous needle electrodes—a practice widely described though rarely reported. *End-tidal CO_2 monitoring* may also be complicated by factors such as decreases in FRC, VQ mismatch, and the dead-space to tidal volume ratio changes seen with obesity (66). Transcutaneous CO_2 monitoring has been described, but has yet to be validated in children.

Positioning

Positioning is critically important for procedures involving both overweight and obese children in order to protect the patient from iatrogenic injury and to optimize pulmonary and hemodynamic mechanics. Especially with older and larger overweight and obese children, it is important to handle them with great care so as to prevent falls and other injuries related to patient transfer and operative positioning. Induction on the OR table, rather than the patient bed is recommended (unless the patient is expected to be in the prone position).

Positioning has significant cardiopulmonary ramifications. The *supine* and *head-down positions* are tolerated relatively poorly compared to the prone and head-up positions, as cardiopulmonary changes worsen with increasing BMI. Supine position is associated with increased venous return, pulmonary blood flow, cardiac output, and arterial pressure increases secondary to vascular redistribution (67). Although changes of these indices are usually well-tolerated in non-obese patients, they may lead to cardiovascular collapse in obese individuals, though this is rarely described in the pediatric literature. Abdominal contents decrease diaphragmatic travel and lung volumes in the supine position, an effect enhanced by anesthetics and muscle relaxants. This is amplified dramatically by head-down positioning. A mildly head-up position or patient ramping if possible is recommended.

The *prone position* is generally well-tolerated so long as the abdomen is free, therefore unloading the diaphragm and augmenting FRC. Cardiovascular function is generally preserved. Great care must be taken in flipping the patient and ensuring airway patency.

Induction

Difficult intravenous (IV) access and airway difficulties associated with overweight and obese children present a challenge to the pediatric anesthetist. The chief consideration is whether to pursue an intravenous or inhalational induction. Given the potential for airway management difficulties, concerns about potential reflux, and numerous recommendations to perform rapid sequence inductions, many practitioners will attempt IV placement and an intravenous induction. With a cooperative (or suitably premedicated) child, *transillumination* may be used to facilitate IV placement. Even with premedication this may be extraordinarily difficult in young overweight or obese children.

Inhalation inductions in overweight and obese children have been shown to have similar rates of adverse airway-related events (e.g., airway obstruction, significant desaturation, aspiration) compared to normal children, leading to greater frequency of mask induction in this population (56). Randomized trials of inhalational versus intravenous inductions have yet to be performed and retrospective comparative data is lacking. Inhalation inductions and mask ventilation may be compromised by high inspiratory pressures, leading to gaseous distention of the stomach, further compromise of FRC, and rapid desaturation. Great care must be taken to avoid excess inspiratory force.

Inhalational inductions (and efficient rise of alveolar concentrations of inhaled anesthetic) may be hampered by intermittent airway obstruction (68). This is generally remedied by placement of an appropriately sized oral airway after sufficient anesthetic depth has been reached. Children have a lower FRC and higher metabolic oxygen requirement than adults; therefore, they tend to desaturate rapidly when apneic. Obesity further impairs FRC in the pediatric patient, amplifying this effect. As a general rule, a variety of airway management tools should be readily available to assist with intubation, should difficulty be encountered. *Awake intubation*, while technically possible, is rarely feasible in the overweight and obese pediatric population given the difficulty of gaining IV access and the distinct lack of patient cooperation.

Maintenance
The literature regarding anesthetic technique for overweight and obese pediatric patients is quite limited, requiring significant derivation of technique from the more established adult literature. The applicability of this data is open to debate.

Pulmonary effects. Anesthesia generally promotes degrees of hypoventilation with an increased A-a gradient and reduced FRC when patients are allowed to breathe spontaneously (69). This effect is particularly pronounced in obese infants and children, generally mandating some form of controlled mechanical ventilation via an endotracheal tube. *Tidal volumes* of approximately 8 to 10 ml/kg of ideal body weight are generally sufficient. Any intraabdominal procedure, or any procedure that involves increasing intraabdominal pressure (e.g., laparoscopy, retraction), will further limit FRC and pulmonary compliance.

Application of PEEP may be utilized to enhance oxygenation when arterial hypoxemia is present in the setting of a high FiO_2 (70). PEEP limits small airway closure, atelectasis, and desaturation. High levels of PEEP may impair venous return and otherwise depress cardiac output and should be managed carefully (71).

Hepatic steatosis and related hepatic dysfunction may predispose overweight and obese children to inhalational anesthetic-related hepatitis.

Obese adults have been shown to have higher plasma concentrations of metabolites related to volatile anesthetic exposure than non-obese patients, suggesting increased risk for hepatotoxicity; however, with the progressive discontinuation of halothane use, such events are increasingly rare. *Sevoflurane* is believed to have enhanced biotransformation in obese adults and hence greater plasma fluoride concentrations (72). No such studies have been performed in children (73). *Isoflurane* appears to have a lesser degree of metabolism in nor mal-weight patients and may therefore be a reasonable choice for use in the overweight and obese pediatric population, (74) though its strong odor and slower onset make it a poor choice for inhalational induction. *Desflurane*, while having a very low solubility in blood and fat and as such appearing to be an ideal agent, is very irritating to the pediatric airway and should be used with caution (75).

Total intravenous anesthesia (TIVA) is also an option for the overweight or obese child, with or without and inhalational induction. *Propofol*, while not licensed for children under three years of age and also having been implicated in cases of refractory metabolic acidosis in pediatric patients, has been widely used for anesthesia induction and maintenance, even in the under three age group (76). Induction doses of propofol should be based on ideal body weight, generally 2.5 to 4.0 mg/kg (77). Maintenance (or infusion) dosing should be based on total body weight. Special attention should be paid to the possibility of prolonged emergence following such anesthetics. *Remifentanil*, which demonstrates a reduced volume of distribution in obese children, should be dosed by ideal body weight initially and adjusted as necessary (78).

Analgesia
As is the case with adult patients, short acting analgesics and regional techniques are preferred when possible, though there is little current literature to support these recommendations. *Short-acting opioids* (e.g., fentanyl) are preferred for surgical analgesia, limiting the possibility of respiratory depression in overweight and obese pediatric patients, particularly those with obstructive sleep apnea who may demonstrate greater sensitivity to the respiratory depressant side-effects of narcotics. *Remifentanil* has been used in children for adenotonsillectomy with a profile similar to that seen in adults (79).

In non-obese infants undergoing major abdominal surgery, a shorter recovery time and time to extubation has been demonstrated when using remifentanil in conjunction with combined regional and general anesthetics (80). *Ketorolac*, or other non-narcotic analgesics, should be used when possible. *Regional techniques*, while technically more challenging in this population, should be considered. For most pediatric patients, regional anesthetics must be initiated following induction of a general anesthetic, with regional-only anesthetics being quite rare. Regional and neuraxial anesthetics generally reduce opioid requirements, reduce or eliminate the need to neuromuscular blockade (and its reversal), allow for earlier extubation, and provide excellent post-operative analgesia (81). Adult studies have shown reduced incidence of respiratory complications in such patients as compared to those receiving opioids only, though there is little confirmatory data in children.

While there is little data presently available on the effect of obesity upon the spread of neuraxial blockade in children, the experience from the adult literature should be considered. In adults, the height of neural blockade in both spinal and epidural anesthetics appears to be related to the degree of obesity (82,83). The decreased CSF volume thought to result from increased intraabdominal pressure in obese adults may produce more extensive blockade via reduced dilution of the injected local anesthetic.

Post-Operative Care
Post-Operative Care for overweight and obese children follows similar principles and patterns as seen with overweight and obese adults. *Post operative mechanical ventilation* is infrequently required except in cases of significant volume resuscitation or ongoing pressor requirement, prolonged prone position with associated facial edema, or major airway surgery. *Post-operative hypoxemia* is common and mandates extubation of overweight and obese children only when fully awake and without evidence of persistent neuromuscular blockade. Patients should be extubated in a *semi recumbent position* to decrease abdominal pressure upon the diaphragm and optimize the ratio of FRC to closing capacity (84).

Children with a history of obstructive sleep apnea are at increased risk for post-operative respiratory complications and should be monitored closely during the immediate post-operative period (85). This is particularly true for patients following major abdominal or airway surgery.

Nasal continuous positive airway pressure (N-CPAP) or bilevel positive airway pressure (Bi-PAP) may be used for patients with OSA or other post-operative hypoventilation syndromes (86). Caution must be exercised when using these modalities in patients with nasogastric tubes as gastric distention may result.

Thromboembolism, a major cause of postoperative morbidity in obese adult post-operative patients, may be mitigated by the judicious use of anticoagulants and pneumatic compression devices (87). While thromboembolic risk has not been well-documented on the overweight and obese pediatric populations, such therapies may be warranted.

Chest physical therapy, coughing, incentive spirometry, and early ambulation are to be encouraged, mandating appropriate post-operative analgesia.

ADOLESCENT BARIATRIC SURGERY
In adults, weight loss surgeries have demonstrated significant and sustained reductions in BMI, diabetes, and dyslipidemia as well as reduced mortality. Bariatric surgeries (i.e., gastric bypass and gastric banding) have been performed in a limited number of adolescents as early as the 1970s, however by 2003 there were greater than 700 such surgeries performed on adolescents in the United States (88). Adolescents currently comprise less than 1% of the bariatric surgery population, though 42% of bariatric surgeons have reported plans to develop multidisciplinary weight loss surgery programs (89).

Risk for Comorbidities
Overweight and obese children and adolescents with severe obesity (generally speaking the 99th percentile of BMI for age and gender) are at risk for numerous comorbidities such as OSA, diabetes, hypertension, left ventricular hypertrophy, nonalcoholic steatohepatitis, and depression. Early intervention may treat or prevent these problems and improve long-term health outcomes. As surgical weight loss entails risk, the American Academy of Pediatrics currently recommends a stepwise approach to weight management that promotes non-invasive, multidisciplinary behavioral approaches for treatment of obesity (90). Limited available data suggest that dietary and behavioral interventions generally have poor success rates for adolescents with severe obesity. Weight loss is generally less than 3% following program initiation, with little sustained weight loss (91).

Outcomes studies following adolescent bariatric surgery are also limited, but as a group appear to demonstrate that such procedures performed in adolescents lead to clinically significant and sustained reductions in BMI. Overall reductions in BMI at one year average 37% in the largest study to date, with significant decrease in body fat (51% to 30%) and preservation of lean body mass (92). Obesity-related diseases generally resolve or improve following adolescent bariatric surgery; most notably improvements in insulin resistance, triglyceride levels, OSA, depression, and quality of life scores (93,94). Improvements in cardiac abnormalities have also been found approximately 1 year post-procedure, specifically in LVH and diastolic function (95).

Maintenance. It is not yet clear the extent to which such surgical weight loss will be maintained. Two studies with 4 to 10 years follow up suggest that 10% to 15% of gastric bypass patients will regain significant weight while those patients with gastric banding procedures may see a significant regression (from 52% to 42% excess weight loss) at three years (96). There is not yet enough data to directly compare gastric bypass and banding-type procedures.

Inclusion criteria.   Given significant mounting evidence of adverse long term consequences of childhood and adolescent obesity along with the limited, though favorable, outcome data of bariatric surgery trials, many practitioners are endorsing more aggressive patient selection criteria (97). Such criteria include:

1. BMI > 35 and a severe comorbidity (OSA, type 2 diabetes, pseudotumor cerebri or clinically significant steatohepatitis) or BMI > 40 with only minor comorbidities. Most centers use a flat BMI threshold (rather than an age and gender based BMI percentile) which has the benefit of being more conservative at younger ages. However, this approach may underestimate the severity of obesity in younger adolescents
2. Physical maturity (i.e., 95% of predicted adult stature) or Tanner IV staging
3. Failure of sustained efforts to lose weight through diet and exercise programs. While participation in such programs may not improve patient selection for surgical intervention per se, consistent attendance may be a useful indicator of the patient's willingness to pursue appropriate post-operative follow up

Appropriate criteria for exclusion include:

1. Known medically correctable causes for obesity
2. Ongoing (or within one year) substance abuse problems
3. Any condition (medical, psychiatric, or other) that might prevent appropriate postoperative dietary and medical management as well as adherence to appropriate follow up
4. Current or planned pregnancy within 18 months of planned procedure. Severe obesity can lead to irregular menstruation, anovulation, and infertility while surgically induced weight loss may lead to resumption of ovulation and fertility leading to higher-than-expected rates of pregnancy (12.8%) in female adolescents who have undergone weight reduction surgery (98)
5. Inability to appropriately comprehend and consent to the risks and benefits of the surgical procedure

Multidisciplinary approach.   These criteria by themselves are not sufficient for operative patient selection. This task must be undertaken by an appropriate multidisciplinary team that can evaluate a patient's and family's readiness for such a procedure, their ability to comply with post-operative management including the specific nutritional requirements of gastric bypass patients, and maturity of decision-making ability.

Weight loss surgery has yet to be extensively studied in syndromic and otherwise genetic causes for pediatric obesity (e.g., Prader Willi syndrome, leptin gene mutations). It is unclear whether there is added benefit and/or risk to such procedures in the pediatric or adolescent populations.

REFERENCES

1. Deurenberg P, Weststrate JA, Seidell JC. Body mass index as a measure of body fatness: age- and sex-specific prediction formulas. Br J Nutr 1991; 65: 105.
2. Baker S, Barlow SS, Cochran W, et al. Overweight children and adolescents: a clinical report of the North American Society for Pediatric Gastroenterology, Hepatology and Nutrition. J Pediatr Gastroenterol Nutr 2005; 40: 533.

3.   Ogden CL, Carroll MD, Flegal KM. High body mass index for age among US children and adolescents, 2003–2006. JAMA 2008; 299: 2401.
4.   Ogden CL, Flegal KM, Carroll MD, et al. Prevalence and trends in overweight among US children and adolescents, 1999–2000. JAMA 2002; 288: 1728.
5.   Clement K. Leptin and the genetics of obesity. Acta Paediatr Suppl 1999; 428: 51–7.
6.   Dietz WH, Gortmaker SL. Do we fatten our children at the TV set? Television viewing and obesity in children and adolescents. Pediatrics 1985; 75: 807–12.
7.   von Kries R, Koletzko B, Sauerwald T, et al. Breast feeding and obesity: cross sectional study. Br Med J 1999; 319: 147–50.
8.   Lucas A, Sarson DL, Blackburn AM, et al. Breast vs bottle: endocrine responses are different with formula feeding. Lancet 1980; 1: 1267–9.
9.   Lucas A, Boyes S, Bloom SR, et al. Metabolic and endocrine responses to a milk feed in six-day-old term infants: differences between breast and cow's milk formula feeding. Acta Paediatr Scand 1981; 70: 195–200.
10. Petruschke T, Rohrig K, Hauner H. Transforming growth factor beta (TGF-beta) inhibits the differentiation of human adipocyte precursor cells in primary culture. Int J Obes Relat Metab Disord 1994; 18: 532–6.
11. Owen CG, Martin RM, Whincup PH, et al. Effect of infant feeding on the risk of obesity across the life course: a quantitative review of published evidence. Pediatrics 2005; 115: 1367.
12. Yeung MY. Postnatal growth, neurodevelopment and altered adiposity after preterm birth—from a clinical nutrition perspective. Acta Paediatr 2006; 95: 909.
13. Feldman W, Beagen BL. Screening for childhood obesity. In: Canadian Task Force on the Periodic Health Examination Canadian Guide to the Clinical Preventive Health Care. Ottawa: Health Canada, 1994: 334–44.
14. Landhuis CE, Poulton R, Welch D, et al. Childhood sleep time and long-term risk for obesity: a 32-year prospective birth cohort study. Pediatrics 2008; 122: 955–60.
15. Kohyama J, Shiiki T, Ohinata-Sugimoto J, et al. Potentially harmful sleep habits of 3-year-old children in Japan. J Dev Behav Pediatr 2002; 23: 67–70.
16. Must A, Jacques PF, Dallal GE, et al. Long-term morbidity and mortality of overweight adolescents. A follow-up of the Harvard Growth Study of 1922 to 1935. N Engl J Med 1992; 327: 1350.
17. Lazarus R, Colditz G, Berkey CS, et al. Effects of body fat on ventilatory function in children and adolescents: cross-sectional findings from a random population sample of school children. Pediatr Pulmonol 1997; 24: 187–94.
18. Inselman LS, Milanese A, Deurloo A. Effect of obesity on pulmonary function in children. Pediatr Pulmonol 1993; 16: 130–7.
19. Kaplan TA, Montana E. Exercise-induced bronchospasm in non-asthmatic obese children. Clin Pediatr 1993; 32: 220–5.
20. Eichenberger AS, Proietti S, Wicky S, et al. Morbid obesity and postoperative pulmonary atelectasis: an underestimated problem. Anesth Analg 2002; 95: 1788–92.
21. Buckley FP. Anesthesia and obesity and gastrointestinal disorders. In: Barash PG, Cullen BF, Stoelting RK, eds. Clinical Anesthesia. Philadelphia: Lippincott, 1989: 1117–31.
22. Slyper AH. Childhood obesity, adipose tissue distribution, and the pediatric practitioner. Pediatrics 1998; 102: e4.
23. Wing YK, Hui SH, Pak WM, et al. A controlled study of sleep-related disordered breathing in obese children. Arch Dis Child 2003; 88: 1043–7.
24. Unger R, Kreeger L, Christoffel KK. Childhood obesity: medical and familial correlates and age of onset. Clin Pediatr 1990; 29: 368–73.
25. Luder E, Melnik TA, DiMaio M. Association of being overweight with greater asthma symptoms in inner city black and Hispanic children. J Pediatr 1998; 132: 699–703.
26. Tracey VVNC, Harper JR. Obesity and respiratory infection in infants and young children. Br Med J 1971; 1: 16–18.

27. Smith HL, Meldrum DJ, Brennan LJ. Childhood obesity: a challenge for the anaesthetist? Paediatric Anaesthesia 2002; 12: 750–61.
28. Gortmaker SL, Dietz WH, Sobol AM, et al. Increasing pediatric obesity in the United States. Am J Dis Child 1987; 141: 535–40.
29. Sorof J, Daniels S. Obesity hypertension in children: a problem of epidemic proportions. Hypertension 2002; 40: 441–7.
30. Martini G, Riva P, Rabbia F, et al. Heart rate variability in childhood obesity. Clin Auton Res 2001; 11: 87–91.
31. Daniels SR, Kimball TR, Morrison JA, et al. Effect of lean body mass, fat mass, blood pressure, and sexual maturation on left ventricular mass in children and adolescents. Statistical, biological, and clinical significance. Circulation 1995; 92: 3249–54.
32. Gidding SS, Nehgme R, Heise C, et al. Severe obesity associated with cardiovascular deconditioning, high prevalence of cardiovascular risk factors, diabetes mellitus/hyperinsulinemia, and respiratory compromise. J Pediatr 2004; 144: 766–9.
33. Berenson GS, Srinivasan SR, Nicklas TA. Atherosclerosis: a nutritional disease of childhood. Am J Cardiol 1998; 82: 22T–29T.
34. Lavine JE, Schwimmer JB. Nonalcoholic fatty liver disease in the pediatric population. Clin Liver Dis 2004; 8: 549.
35. World Health Organisation. Obesity: Preventing and Managing the Global Epidemic. Geneva: WHO/NUT/NCD/98.1, 1998.
36. Chiloiro M, Caroli M, Guerra V, et al. Gastric emptying in normal weight and obese children—an ultrasound study. Int J Obesity 1999; 23: 1303–6.
37. Sinha R, Fisch G, Teague B, et al. Prevalence of impaired glucose tolerance among children and adolescents with marked obesity. N Engl J Med 2002; 346: 802.
38. Williams DE, Cadwell BL, Cheng YJ, et al. Prevalence of impaired fasting glucose and its relationship with cardiovascular disease risk factors in US adolescents, 1999–2000. Pediatrics 2005; 116: 1122.
39. Garn SM, Clark DC. Nutrition, growth, development, and maturation: findings from the ten-state nutrition survey of 1968–1970. Pediatrics 1975; 56: 306.
40. Wang Y. Is obesity associated with early sexual maturation? A comparison of the association in American boys versus girls. Pediatrics 2002; 110: 903.
41. Leibel NI, Baumann EE, Kocherginsky M, et al. Relationship of adolescent polycystic ovary syndrome to parental metabolic syndrome. J Clin Endocrinol Metab 2006; 91: 1275.
42. Stein PD, Beemath A, Olson RE. Obesity as a risk factor in venous thromboembolism. Am J Med 2005; 118: 978–80.
43. Parasuraman S, Goldhaber SZ. Venous thromboembolism in children. Circulation 2006 Jan 17; 113: e12–e16.
44. Woo KS, Chook P, Yu CW, et al. Overweight in children is associated with arterial endothelial dysfunction and intima–media thickening. Int J Obes Relat Metab Disord 2004; 28: 852–7.
45. Reinehr T, Kiess W, de Sousa G, et al. Intima media thickness in childhood obesity: relations to inflammatory marker, glucose metabolism, and blood pressure. Metabolism 2006; 55: 113–18.
46. Edmonds MJ, Crichton TJ, Runciman WB, et al. Evidence-based risk factors for postoperative deep vein thrombosis. Aust N Z J Surg 2004; 74: 1082–97.
47. Taylor ED, Theim KR, Mirch MC, et al. Orthopedic complications of overweight in children and adolescents. Pediatrics 2006; 117: 2167.
48. Krebs NF, Himes JH, Jacobson D, et al. Assessment of child and adolescent overweight and obesity. Pediatrics 2007; 120(Suppl 4): S193.
49. Henderson RC. Tibia vara: a complication of adolescent obesity. J Pediatr 1992; 121: 482.

50. Weisberg LA, Chutorian AM. Pseudotumor cerebri of childhood. Am J Dis Child 1977; 131: 1243.
51. Reilly JJ, Methven E, McDowell ZC, et al. Health consequences of obesity. Arch Dis Child 2003; 88: 748.
52. Schwimmer JB, Burwinkle TM, Varni JW. Health-related quality of life of severely obese children and adolescents. JAMA 2003; 289: 1813.
53. Gortmaker SL, Must A, Perrin JM, et al. Social and economic consequences of overweight in adolescence and young adulthood. N Engl J Med 1993; 329: 1008.
54. Smith HL, Meldrum DJ, Brennan LJ. Childhood obesity: a challenge for the anaesthetist? Paediatr Anaesth 2002; 12: 750–61.
55. Tait AR, Voepel-Lewis T, Burke C, et al. Incidence and risk factors for perioperative adverse respiratory events in children who are obese. Anesthesiology 2008; 108: 375–80.
56. Setzer N, Saade E. Childhood obesity and anesthetic morbidity. Perdiatr Anesth 2006; 17: 321–6.
57. Nafiu OO, Reynolds PI, Bamgbade OA, et al. Childhood body mass index and perioperative complications. Pediatr Anesth 2007; 17: 426–30.
58. Nafiu OO, Chimbira WT, Woolford SJ, et al. Does high BMI influence hospital charges in children undergoing adenotonsillectomy? Obesity 2008; 16: 1667–71.
59. Bellieni CV, Cordelli DM, Raffaelli M, et al. Analgesic effect of watching TV during venipuncture. Arch Dis Child 2006; 91: 1015–17; Epub 2006 Aug 18.
60. Schmidt AP, Valinetti EA, Bandeira D, et al. Effects of preanesthetic administration of midazolam, clonidine, or dexmedetomidine on postoperative pain and anxiety in children. Pediatr Anesth 2007; 17: 667–74.
61. Harter RL, Kelly WB, Kramer MG, et al. A comparison of the volume and pH of gastric contents of obese and lean surgical patients. Anesth Analg 1998; 86: 147–52.
62. Borland LM, Sereika SM, Woelfel SK, et al. Pulmonary aspiration in pediatric patients during general anesthesia: incidence and outcome. J Clin Anesth 1998; 10: 95–102.
63. Alpert MA, Terry BE, Cohen MV, et al. The electrocardiogram in morbid obesity. Am J Cardiol 2000; 85: 908–10.
64. Grant P, Newcombe M. Emergency management of the morbidly obese. Emerg Med Australas 2004; 16: 309–17.
65. Emrick DR. An evaluation of non-invasive blood pressure (NIBP) monitoring on the wrist: comparison with upper arm NIBP measurement. Anaesth Intens Care 2002; 30: 43–7.
66. Griffin J, Terry BE, Burton RK, et al. Comparison of end-tidal and transcutaneous measures of carbon dioxide during general anaesthesia in severely obese adults. Br J Anaesth 2003; 91: 498–501.
67. Brodsky JB. Positioning the morbidly obese patient for anesthesia. Obes Surg 2002; 12: 751–8.
68. Fisher A, Waterhouse TD, Adams AP. Obesity: its relation to anaesthesia. Anaesthesia 1975; 30: 633–47.
69. Hedenstierna G, Santesson J. Breathing mechanics, dead space and gas exchange in the extremely obese, breathing spontaneously and during anaesthesia with intermittent positive pressure ventilation. Acta Anaesth Scand 1976; 20: 248–54.
70. Oberg B, Poulsen TD. Obesity: an anaesthetic challenge. Acta Anaesthesiol Scand 1996; 40: 191–200.
71. Santesson J. Oxygen transport and venous admixture in the extremely obese. Influence of anaesthesia and artificial ventilation with and without positive end-expiratory pressure. Acta Anaesth Scand 1976; 20: 387–94.
72. Higuchi H, Satoh T, Arimura S, et al. Serum inorganic fluoride levels in the mildly obese patients during and after sevoflurane anesthesia. Anesth Analg 1993; 77: 1018–21.

73. Frink EJ Jr, Malan P Jr, Brown EA, et al. Plasma inorganic fluoride levels with sevoflurane anesthesia in morbidly obese and nonobese patients. Anesth Analg 1993; 76: 1333–7.
74. Strube PJ, Hulands GH, Halsey MJ. Serum fluoride levels in morbidly obese patients: enflurane compared with isoflurane anaesthesia. Anaesthesia 1987; 42: 685–9.
75. Zwass MS, Fisher DM, Welborn LG, et al. Induction and maintenance characteristics of anesthesia with desflurane and nitrous oxide in infants and children. Anesthesiology 1992; 76: 373–8.
76. Reinhold P, Kraus G, Schluter E. Propofol for anesthesia and short-term sedation. The final word on use in children under three years. Anaesthesist 1998; 47: 229–37.
77. Saint-Maurice C, Cockshott ID, White M, et al. Pharmacokinetics of propofol in young children after a single dose. Br J Anaesth 1989; 63: 667–70.
78. Davis PJ, Ross AK, Stiller RL, et al. Pharmacokinetics of remifentanil in anesthetized children 2–12 yrs of age. Anesth Analg 1995; 80: S93.
79. Davis PJ, Finkel JC, Orr RJ, et al. A randomized, double-blind syudy of remifentanil versus fentanyl for tonsillectomy and adenoidectomy surgery in pediatric ambulatory surgical patients. Anesth Analg 2000; 90: 863–71.
80. Wee LH, Moriarty A, Cranston A, et al. Remifentanil infusion for major abdominal surgery in small infants. Paed Anaesth 1999; 9: 415–18.
81. Shenkman Z, Shir Y, Brodsky JB. Perioperative management of the obese patient. Br J Anaesth 1993; 70: 349–59.
82. Taivainen T, Tuominen M, Rosenberg PH. Influence of obesity on the spread of spinal analgesia after injection of plain 0.5% bupivacaine at the L3–4 or L4–5 interspace. Br J Anaesth 1990; 64: 542–6.
83. Hodgkinson R, Husain FJ. Obesity and the cephalad spread of analgesia following epidural administration of bupivacaine for Cesarean section. Anesth Analg 1980; 59: 89–92.
84. Vaughan RW, Bauer S, Wise L. Effect of position (semirecumbent versus supine) on postoperative oxygenation in markedly obese subjects. Anesth Analg 1976; 55: 37–41.
85. Dearlove OR, Dobson A, Super M. Anaesthesia and Prader–Willi syndrome. Paed Anaesth 1998; 8: 267–71.
86. Rennotte MT, Baele P, Aubert G, et al. Nasal continuous positive airway pressure in the perioperative management of patients with obstructive sleep apnea submitted to surgery. Chest 1995; 107: 367–74.
87. Kalfarentzos F, Stavropoulou F, Yarmenitis S, et al. Prophylaxis of venous thromboembolism using two different doses of low-molecular-weight heparin (nadroparin) in bariatric surgery: a prospective randomized trial. Obes Surg 2001; 11: 670–6.
88. Tsai WS, Inge TH, Burd RS. Bariatric surgery in adolescents: recent national trends in use and in-hospital outcome. Arch Pediatr Adolesc Med 2007; 161: 217.
89. Allen SR, Lawson L, Garcia V, Inge TH. Attitudes of bariatric surgeons concerning adolescent bariatric surgery (ABS). Obes Surg 2005; 15: 1192.
90. Barlow SE. Expert committee recommendations regarding the prevention, assessment, and treatment of child and adolescent overweight and obesity: summary report. Pediatrics 2007; 120(Suppl 4): S164.
91. Berkowitz RI, Fujioka K, Daniels SR, et al. Effects of sibutramine treatment in obese adolescents: a randomized trial. Ann Intern Med 2006; 145: 81.
92. Lawson ML, Kirk S, Mitchell T, et al. One-year outcomes of Roux-en-Y gastric bypass for morbidly obese adolescents: a multicenter study from the Pediatric Bariatric Study Group. J PediatrSurg 2006; 41: 137.
93. Kalra M, Inge T, Garcia V, et al. Obstructive sleep apnea in extremely overweight adolescents undergoing bariatric surgery. Obes Res 2005; 13: 1175.
94. Fielding GA, Duncombe JE. Laparoscopic adjustable gastric banding in severely obese adolescents. Surg Obes Relat Dis 2005; 1: 399.

95. Ippisch HM, Inge TH, Daniels SR, et al. Reversibility of cardiac abnormalities in morbidly obese adolescents. J Am Coll Cardiol 2008; 51: 1342.
96. Nadler EP, Youn HA, Ren CJ, et al. An update on 73 US obese pediatric patients treated with laparoscopic adjustable gastric banding: comorbidity resolution and compliance data. J Pediatr Surg 2008; 43: 141.
97. Pratt JSA, Lenders CM, Dionne ED, et al. Best practice updates for pediatric/adolescent weight loss surgery. Obes Res 2008, in press.
98. Roehrig HR, Xanthakos SA, Sweeney J, et al. Pregnancy after gastric bypass surgery in adolescents. Obes Surg 2007; 17: 873.

20 | The Obese Trauma Patient

Heena P. Santry[1] and Marc de Moya[2]

[1]Fellow and Assistant in Surgery [2]Assistant Professor of Surgery, Division of Trauma, Emergency Surgery, and Surgical Critical Care, Massachusetts General Hospital, Boston, Massachusetts, U.S.A.

INTRODUCTION

Trauma was the fifth overall leading cause of death in the United States from 2001 to 2005 (1). From 1985 to 2004, the rate of trauma related deaths was stable with trauma accounting for 167,184 deaths (7% of all deaths) in 2004 (2). In 2004, trauma also accounted for 31 million initial emergency department (ED) visits (32% of all ED visits) and 1.9 million hospital discharges (6% of all discharges) (2). Since the late 1980s, emergency care providers have had increasing numbers of obese trauma victims as the prevalence of overweight [body mass index (BMI) > 25–30 kg/m²], obese (BMI > 30–40 kg/m²), and morbidly obese (BMI > 40 kg/m²) people has increased (3). The obese trauma patient poses significant diagnostic and therapeutic challenges.

EPIDEMIOLOGY
Variable Estimates of Obesity Among Trauma Victims

The proportion of obese subjects in studies of critically ill trauma patients has ranged from 5% to 26% (4–6). Estimates vary according to the type of mechanism and/or data source as detailed below:

1. In a study of blunt trauma patients, 24% of patients were obese (7).
2. The proportion of obese subjects in studies of all-cause trauma patients has ranged from 12% to 21% (8,9).
3. The proportion of obese subjects in motor vehicle crash databases has ranged from 24% to 27% (10,11).

Female Predominance

Trauma patients overall are disproportionately male with men accounting for approximately 70% to 75% of all trauma patients. However, there is a higher prevalence of obesity among female trauma victims. Evidence of higher prevalence of obesity among female trauma patients includes the following studies:

1. Bochicchio's study of 1167 all-cause adult trauma patients admitted to a Level I trauma center over a two-year period found that 48% of obese patients were female compared to only 24% of non-obese patients (p < 0.001) (4)
2. Byrnes' study of 1179 all-cause adult trauma patients evaluated at a Level I trauma center over a one-year period found that 43.4% of obese patients were female compared to only 33% of non-obese patients (p = 0.03) (8)
3. Newell's study of 1543 consecutive adult blunt trauma patients with an injury severity score (ISS, see below) >15 admitted to a Level I trauma center over a 4.5-year period found that 47% of obese patients were female compared to only 25% of normal weight patients (p < 0.0001) (7)

Paucity of Height and Weight Data

Height and weight are often not recorded in the trauma population which suggests that the prevalence quoted above may be underestimated. There is evidence of poor BMI data collection:

1. Only 83% of Newell's original study population of 2108 patients had BMI data available (7).
2. 63% of Byrnes's original study population of 1877 patients had BMI data available (8).
3. Only 83.8% of the 10,656 patients in the National Automotive Sampling System Crashworthiness Data System for 2003 (NASS-CDS) had BMI data available (12).
4. Only 11.6% of 7030 patients evaluated at a Level I trauma center by Duane et al. had BMI data available (13).

PATHOPHYSIOLOGY
Obesity and the Response to Acute Injury

Excess adiposity is associated with pro-inflammatory cytokines that also play a role in response to trauma (14). Evidence of pro-inflammatory effects of adiposity (9,15) include insulin resistance, endothelial cell dysfunction, and atherogenesis. The hypothesized impacts of pro-inflammatory state on trauma (9) are unbridled post-injury inflammation and decreased resistance to infection. Insensitivity to immunomodulator leptin among obese patients is theorized as a cause of differences in inflammatory response among obese trauma patients (5).

PATTERNS OF INJURY
Mechanism of Injury Similar Across BMI Groups (5,8,16)

None of the epidemiological studies of trauma and obesity have shown differences in mechanism of injury. Obese and normal weight trauma victims are equally as likely to be injured by blunt (inclusive of auto collisions, falls, and assaults) and penetrating (inclusive of gunshot wounds, shotgun wounds, and stab wounds) mechanisms. There is no evidence of differences in risk taking behaviors between obese and normal weight subjects in the general population.

Injury Severity Score

ISS is a validated metric applied to polytrauma patients based on unweighted scoring of anatomic regions of injury at the time of presentation (17). In ISS, six regions [head, face, chest, abdomen, extremity (includes pelvis), and external] are assigned an abbreviated injury score (AIS). By convention, researchers have used $ISS \geq 15$ and/or $ISS \geq 20$ to identify critically injured patients. There is evidence of obesity's impact on ISS.

1. Newell's study of critically injured blunt trauma patients found increasing ISS with increasing BMI (24 ± 8 for BMI 18.5–24.9 kg/m^2, 25 ± 10 for BMI 25–29.9 kg/m^2, 26 ± 10 for BMI 30–39.9 kg/m^2, 27 ± 10 for BMI ≥ 40 kg/m^2; $p < 0.001$) (7).
2. Byrnes' study of all-cause trauma patients found increasing likelihood of $ISS \geq 16$ with increasing BMI ($p = 0.021$ calculated from data presented in text) (8).

Distribution of Body Mass Among Obese Trauma Victims Associated with Patterns of Injury

Detailed studies of injury patterns have revealed predictable patterns related to overweight and obesity. As exemplified in the studies below, obese trauma victims have lower incidences of head injury (18,19) and abdominal injury (10,18,19). Causality is unknown for most injuries but hypothesized as a "cushion effect" for decreased incidence of head and abdominal injuries (10).

1. Neville's study of 242 adult blunt trauma patients admitted to a Level I trauma center intensive care unit (ICU) over a one-year period found fewer basilar skull fractures among obese patients compared to normal weight patients (2% vs. 13%, respectively, p = 0.01) (5).
2. The Crash Injury Research and Engineering Network (CIREN) database of 1615 patients older than 15 years injured between 1996 and 2005 found that the rate of head injury among obese patients was 20% compared to 29% among normal weight patients (<0.05) (11).
3. The University of Michigan Program of Injury Research and Education (UMPIRE) database of motor vehicle collisions (MVC) study of 189 patients older than 12 years found a significant decrease of 0.7 in abdominal AIS in obese patients compared to normal weight patients (p = 0.008) (10).

Meanwhile, obese trauma victims have higher incidence of chest injury (rib fractures, pulmonary contusions) (18) and lower extremity fractures (5,18). Unlike with head and abdominal trauma, the higher incidence of long bone fractures is hypothesized as due to increased loading on the injured extremity by patient weight (20).

1. Brown's study of 690 brain injured adult patients admitted to a Level I trauma center ICU over a five-year period found that the rate of chest injury was 46% among obese patients versus 35% among normal weight patients (p = 0.03) (16).
2. The CIREN study found that the rate of lower extremity fractures was 54% among obese patients versus 44% for normal weight patients (p < 0.05) (11).
3. The UMPIRE study found that the average extremity AIS was higher among obese patients whose mean was 2.5 compared to normal weight patients whose mean was 1.9 (p < 0.05) (10).
4. Brown's study of brain injured patients found that the rate of severe long bone fractures was 29% among obese patients versus 20% among normal weight patients (p = 0.03) (16).
5. Neville's study of blunt trauma patients found that obese patients had a 22% rate of femur fractures compared to 10% among normal weight patients (p = 0.01) (5).

Obesity and the Role of Motor Vehicle Restraints

MVCs accounted for 37.1% of accidental deaths in the United States from 2001 to 2005 (1). When it comes to motor vehicle restraints and injury, restraints are estimated to prevent up to 200,000 injuries annually in the United States. Based on 2006 data, proper use of lap/shoulder belts could reduce front-seat passenger fatalities by 45% and reduce the risk of moderate to critical injury of front seat passengers by 50% (21). However, motor vehicle restraints have been developed and safety tested based on an idealized 1.8 m, 77 kg male body (BMI = 24kg/m^2; the 50th percentile male Hybrid Crash Dummy) and the utility of restraints in obese subjects has been questioned (20).

Older data showed that obese individuals were less likely to use or to properly use motor vehicle restraint systems (22–24). More recently, the CIREN study showed decreased usage of restraints among obese patients (54% vs. 61%, p = 0.032) (11). Poor seat belt compliance among the obese may be attributable to the discomfort or lack of ease of use associated with seatbelts originally designed for smaller patients. Belted obese patients were more likely than non-belted obese patients to suffer abdominal wall injuries in a large cohort of 7459 patients weighted to represent 3.4 million occupants involved in MVCs in the United States in 2003 (12).

CHALLENGES IN PRE-HOSPITAL CARE OF THE OBESE TRAUMA PATIENT (25)
Ambulance Transfer
1. Patients too heavy to be lifted by a single EMS team
   Strategy: Additional first responder(s) assistance in lifting patient
2. Patients too heavy/wide for standard transport gurney
   Strategy: Lay the patient on floor of ambulance

Immobilization
1. Patients do not fit across standard board
   Strategy: Use several boards placed on wide axis under patient
2. Patients do not fit into standard adult sized C-collars
   Strategy: Stabilize neck between rolls of towels

RESUSCITATION CHALLENGES IN THE OBESE TRAUMA PATIENT (25)
Assessment of the acutely injured patient occurs in two phases known as primary and secondary surveys. The primary survey consists of rapid evaluation and initial resuscitation of the patient with the goals of identifying and treating immediate life threats (tension pneumothorax, cardiac tamponade, obvious source of massive hemorrhage, etc.) while quickly addressing the ABCDEs (A = airway, B = breathing, C = circulation, D = disability, E = exposure). The mnemonic ABCDE outlines the order of priorities for trauma resuscitation and does not vary between obese and normal weight patients.

Airway
The various physiologic and physical challenges in management of the obese patient's airway have been detailed at length in chapter 10. However, trauma patients pose two additional challenges:

1. Inability to manipulate the neck in the presence of c-collar or other mode of immobilization
   Strategy: Always use in-line stabilization of C-spine for trauma patients regardless of BMI
2. Higher risk of aspiration as trauma victims often have a full stomach on presentation. In the obese patient, this is exacerbated by baseline increased likelihood of reflux or gastric outlet obstruction
   Strategy: Early gastric decompression with nasogastric tube (or orogastric tube if midface fractures are present)

Breathing (25)

The altered respiratory mechanics of non-injured obese persons is discussed in detail in chapter 2. However, certain aspects of these baseline findings will impact the resuscitation of the obese trauma patient:

1. CO_2 retention results in baseline respiratory acidosis with metabolic compensation
    Strategy: Careful analysis of serum bicarbonate levels should be supplemented by ABG analysis and lactate levels to monitor degree of shock and response to resuscitation
2. Inability to sit upright or in semi-recumbant position to maximize pre-oxygenation because patient must be supine until TLS spine cleared
    Strategy: Reverse Trendelenburg position, which may assist recruitment of airways
    Strategy: Additional PEEP while supine to maintain oxygenation

Circulation

The obese patient's altered circulatory system and its monitoring are discussed in chapters 6, 7, and 11. However, a history of trauma suggests that these patients are more likely to present with hypovolemic shock than their non-injured counterparts. Thus, assessing and addressing the circulatory status of obese patients is perhaps of greater importance in the setting of trauma.

1. Standard blood pressure cuffs are often unreliable in detecting hypovolemia
    Strategy: BP cuff should be 2:5 cuff width to arm circumference ratio and bladder length should be 80% arm circumference
    Strategy: Low threshold for arterial line
    Strategy: CVP monitoring to guide adverse effects of resuscitation
2. Difficult venous access—worsened by emergent nature (two large bore PIVs still preferred but lower threshold for CVL)
    Strategy: U.S. guidance for PIV or CVL placement
    Strategy: Interosseus line at tibia (even obese patients have easily palpable tibial prominence)

Disability

The Glasgow Coma Score can be universally applied to all trauma victims irrespective of the presence or absence of obesity.

Exposure

1. The traditional teaching of removing all clothing is not adequate in obese patients
    Strategy: Explore all pannus areas including axillary folds, gluteal folds, and abdominal folds that may harbor otherwise hidden injury

DIAGNOSTIC CHALLENGES IN THE OBESE TRAUMA PATIENT (25)

The secondary survey follows the primary survey and consists of a thorough head to toe evaluation looking for non-life threatening injuries. A diagnostic work-up is directed towards areas clinically suspicious for injury or occult injury as suspected by mechanism. If the patient's condition deteriorates at any time during the secondary survey, the ABCDEs are immediately reassessed and treated. Obesity poses diagnostic challenges during the secondary survey.

Plain Radiographs
1. Generally are under-penetrated due to overlying fat
2. Difficult to get entire area of interest in a standard sized radiographic plate
   Strategy: Double flat plates (e.g., CXR would mean an x-ray of the right and left lung fields separately)
   Strategy: Tape away overlying fat out of the field (e.g., breasts) for flat plates

CT/MRI
1. Equipment has weight limits that may exclude use
   Strategy: Practitioners should always know the weight limitations and gantry size limitations (for machines where girth rather than weight is the limiting factor) of hospital equipment

Ultrasound
1. Decreased visualization of fat/organ/fluid planes
   Strategy: Use 2-MHz transducer to maximize power and gain of ultrasound machines

DPL
1. Standard needle lengths not long enough
   Strategy: Use modified Seldinger technique (expose down to fascia with as long an incision as needed then insert needle directly into fascia) and longer needles

THE IMPACT OF OBESITY ON POST-INJURY OUTCOMES
Increased Mortality
There is evidence for increased mortality in all-cause trauma (4–6,8,19).

1. Choban's early study of 184 blunt trauma patients found higher death rates among all obese blunt trauma patients (42% vs. 5% for the normal weight group, $p < 0.001$) (19).
2. Neville's study of critically injured blunt trauma patients found higher death rates among the obese group (32% vs. 16% for the normal weight group, $p = 0.008$) with the odds of death 5.7 (95% CI 1.9–19.6, $p = 0.003$) times higher in obese patients compared to normal weight patients (5).
3. Byrnes found the greatest rise in mortality to begin at a BMI of 35 kg/m^2. Patients in that BMI group were 2.8 times more likely to die after trauma than patients with a BMI < 35 kg/m^2 ($p = 0.003$) (8).

In addition, there is evidence for higher death rates among obese MVC patients (10,11,26).

1. In the CIREN study, the death rate was 20.5% for the obese group versus 9.4% for the normal weight group ($p < 0.001$) (11). The odds ratio for death was 1.013 (95% CI 1.007–1.018) for each kilogram increase in body weight (26).
2. In the UMPIRE study, the odds ratio for death was 4.2 (95% CI 1.1–16.2, $p = 0.04$) times higher for obese patients compared to normal weight patients (10).

Differences in injury patterns and injury severity cannot explain the independent effect of obesity on mortality after trauma found in the majority of studies.

Differences in mortality are possibly attributable to the known higher prevalence of co-morbidities such as hypertension and diabetes among obese patients discussed elsewhere in this text.

Increased Risk of Systemic Complications

Evidence for increased multisystem organ failure (MOF) among obese trauma patients is found in several sources.

1. Ciesla's study of 716 all-cause adult trauma victims with ISS > 15 treated at a Level I trauma center over 6.5 years found that MOF is 1.81 (95% CI 1.21– 2.71, $p = 0.004$) times more likely to develop in obese injured patients compared to normal weight injured patients, even after controlling for age, injury severity, and transfusion requirement (all factors also shown to independently increase the odds of MOF) (9).
2. Neville's study of critically ill blunt trauma patients found a 13% rate of MOF in obese patients compared to a 3% rate in normal weight patients ($p = 0.02$) (5).
3. Brown's study of brain injured patients found that the rate of MOF in the obese group was 19% compared to 10% for the normal weight group ($p < 0.01$) (16).
4. Newell's study of blunt trauma patients found that the odds of developing MOF was 2.64 (95% CI 1.09–6.42, $p = 0.032$) times higher for morbidly obese patients compared to normal weight patients (7).

There is also evidence for increased pulmonary complications/respiratory failure/ARDS among obese trauma patients.

1. Newell's study of blunt trauma patients found that the odds of developing pneumonia were 1.72 (95% CI 1.21–2.45, $p < 0.001$) times higher for obese patients and 2.49 (95% CI 1.48–4.30, $p < 0.001$) times higher for morbidly obese patients compared to normal weight patients. The odds of developing respiratory failure were 1.76 (95% CI 1.27–2.45, $p < 0.001$) times higher for obese patients and 2.79 (95% CI 1.63–4.78, $p < 0.001$) times higher for morbidly obese patients compared to normal weight patients. The odds of developing ARDS were 3.68 (95% CI 1.23–10.9, $p = 0.026$) times higher for morbidly obese patients compared to normal weight patients (7).
2. Byrnes' study of all-cause trauma patients found that pulmonary complications (pneumonia, ARDS, need for mechanical ventilation) occurred in 18% of morbidly obese patients compared to only 11.3% of patients who were not morbidly obese ($p = 0.04$) (8).
3. Brown's study of brain injured patients found that the rate of respiratory failure was 12% among obese patients compared to 6% among normal weight patients ($p < 0.01$) (16).
4. A study of 1565 all-cause trauma patients requiring emergent intubation in the field or the resuscitation unit over a 3.5-year period found that the odds of early respiratory complications in emergently intubated obese patients were 1.04 (95% CI 1.01–1.06, $p = 0.004$) times higher than for emergently intubated normal weight patients (27).

There is also evidence for increased renal failure among obese trauma patients.

1. Newell's study of critically ill blunt trauma patients found that the odds of developing acute renal failure was 13.5 (95% CI 2.39–76.4, $p = 0.008$)

times higher for morbidly obese patients compared to normal weight patients (7).

2. Byrnes' study of all-cause trauma patients found that renal complications (not further defined) occurred in 6.6% of morbidly obese patients versus only 1% of patients who were not morbidly obese (p < 0.001) (8).

Evidence for increased thromboembolic complications among obese trauma patients is provided in the trauma literature as well.

1. Brown's study of brain injured patients found an increased rate of DVT (5%) among the obese group compared to the lean group (1%) (p < 0.01) (16).
2. Newell's study of critically ill blunt trauma patients found that the odds of DVT was significantly increased (OR 4.11, 95% CI 1.25–13.50, p < 0.014) among morbidly obese patients compared to normal weight patients (7).

Increased Risk of Infectious Complications

Obese trauma patients also suffer from higher rates of infectious complications. Bochicchio's study of critically ill all-cause trauma patients found that the rate of infections (bacteremia, pneumonia, and UTI) among obese patients was 61% compared to 34% for normal weight patients (p < 0.001) (4). Other studies have individually addressed infectious complications including urinary tract infections (UTI) (4,7,19) and pneumonia (4,7,19) as detailed below.

1. Newell's study of critically ill blunt trauma patients found that the odds of developing UTI was 1.82 (95% CI 1.16–2.86, p = 0.013) times higher for obese patients and 2.33 (95% CI 1.23–4.43, p = 0.013) times higher for morbidly obese patients compared to normal weight patients (7).
2. Newell's study also addressed pneumonia separately in its analysis of pulmonary complications and found an increased risk among both obese and morbidly obese patients (see data above) (7).

Increased Interventions

Obese trauma patients are also more likely to require instrumentation and have been found to have increased usage and duration of mechanical ventilation (28), increased foley catheter days, and increased CVL days.

1. A study limited to 3649 patients with blunt and penetrating thoracic injury (thoracic AIS ≥ +2) found that the odds of requiring mechanical ventilation was 1.53 (95% CI 1.17–1.99, p = 0.0019) times higher in the obese group compared to the normal weight group (28).
2. Byrnes' study of all-cause trauma patients found that the proportion of patients requiring mechanical ventilation was higher among the morbidly obese group with 17.2% requiring ventilators compared to the group that was not morbidly obese in whom only 9.9% required ventilators (p = 0.02) (8).
3. Newell's study of critically ill blunt trauma patients found that the number of ventilator days increased with increasing BMI (4.5 days for BMI 18.5–24.9 kg/m^2, 4.3 days for BMI 25–29.9 kg/m^2, 7.4 days for BMI 30–39.9 kg/m^2, 9.2 days for BMI ≥ 40 kg/m^2; p < 0.001) (7).

4. Bochicchio's study of critically ill all-cause trauma patients found that obese patients averaged 8.2 (95% CI 5.5–11.0, p < 0.0001) ventilator days more than normal weight patients (4).
5. Bochicchio's study also found that foley catheter use averaged 10.9 (95% CI 8.14–13.5, p < 0.0001) days more for obese patients (4).
6. Bochicchio's study also found that central venous line (CVL) use averaged 11.1 (95% CI 9.2–13.9, p < 0.0001) days more for obese patients (4), providing evidence for increased CVL days.

Longer ICU Length of Stay (LOS)

Obese injured patients have longer lengths of stay both in the ICU and overall as reported in a number of studies.

1. Byrnes' study of all-cause trauma patients found that ICU LOS increased slightly among morbidly obese patient who averaged 8.7 days compared to patients who are not morbidly obese who averaged 6.1 days (p = 0.045) (8).
2. Newell's study of critically ill blunt trauma patients found that ICU LOS increased with increasing BMI (4.8 days for BMI 18.5–24.9 kg/m², 4.9 days for BMI 25–29.9 kg/m², 7.5 days for BMI 30–39.9 kg/m², 10.4 days for BMI ≥ 40 kg/m²; p < 0.001) (7).
3. Bochicchio's study of critically ill all-cause trauma patients found that ICU LOS averaged 7.7 (95% CI 5.1–10.4, p < 0.0001) days longer for obese patients compared to normal weight patients (4).
4. Ciesla's study of critically ill all-cause trauma patients found that ICU LOS was 21.3 ± 1.4 days for obese patients compared to 16.1 ± 0.6 for normal weight patients (p > 0.0001) (9).
5. Byrnes' study also found that hospital LOS averaged 10 days for morbidly obese patients compared to 4.7 days for patients who were not morbidly obese (p = 0.001) (8).
6. Newell's study also found that hospital LOS increased with increasing BMI (11.7 days for BMI 18.5–24.9 kg/m², 12.6 days for BMI 25–29.9 kg/m², 16.6 days for BMI 30–39.9 kg/m², 22 days for BMI ≥ 40 kg/m²; p < 0.001) (7).
7. Bochicchio's study found that hospital LOS averaged 10.1 (95% CI 6.8–13.4, p < 0.0001) days longer for obese patients compared to normal weight patients (4).
8. Ciesla's study found that hospital LOS was 25.2 ± 1.4 days for obese patients compared to 20.1 ± 1.6 for normal weight patients (p = 0.02) (9).

Longer Hospital Length of Stay

Evidence of increased hospital LOS can be found in Byrnes's study which found that hospital LOS averaged 10 days for morbidly obese patients compared to 4.7 days for patients who were not morbidly obese (p = 0.001) (8). Newell's study found that hospital LOS increased with increasing BMI (11.7 days for BMI 18.5–24.9 kg/m², 12.6 days for BMI 25–29.9 kg/m², 16.6 days for BMI 30–39.9 kg/m², 22 days for BMI ≥ 40 kg/m²; p < 0.001) (7). Bochicchio's study found that hospital LOS averaged 10.1 days longer (95% CI 6.8–13.4, p < 0.0001) for obese patients compared to normal weight patients (4).

Ciesla's study found that hospital LOS was 25.2 ± 1.4 days for obese patients compared to 20.1 ± 1.6 for normal weight patients (p = 0.02) (9).

CONCLUSIONS

The rising prevalence of obesity among the U.S. population translates to larger numbers of obese trauma patients. Obesity poses challenges to the primary and secondary surveys of the trauma victim. Timely and accurate diagnosis may be aided by improvements in imaging technology. Obesity influences injury patterns. Awareness of such patterns may heighten clinical suspicion during the secondary survey.

Obesity adversely affects a number of trauma outcomes. Adverse outcomes may be reduced by reducing the overall societal burden of obesity or designing motor vehicle restraint systems to better protect riders of large body mass. Research concerning obesity and trauma may be greatly improved by more accurate and standardized recording of height and weight for all trauma patients.

REFERENCES

1. WISQARS Leading causes of death reports, 1999–2005. National Center for Injury Prevention and Control, Centers for Disease Control, 2008. [Accessed August 25, 2008, at http://www.cdc.gov/ncipc/wisqars/].
2. Bergen GC, Chen LH, Warner M, Fingerhut LA. Injuries in the United States: 2007 Chart Book. Hyattsville, MD: The National Center for Health Statistics, Centers for Disease Control, 2008.
3. US Obesity Trends, 1997–2005. Division of Nutrition, Physical Activity and Obesity, National Center for Chronic Disease Prevention and Health Promotion, Centers for Disease Control 2008. [Accessed August 25, 2008, at http://www.cdc.gov/nccdphp/dnpa/obesity/trend/maps/index.htm].
4. Bochicchio GV, Joshi M, Bochicchio K, et al. Impact of obesity in the critically ill trauma patient: a prospective study. J Am Coll Surg 2006; 203: 533–8.
5. Neville AL, Brown CV, Weng J, et al. Obesity is an independent risk factor of mortality in severely injured blunt trauma patients. Arch Surg 2004; 139: 983–7.
6. Brown CV, Neville AL, Rhee P, et al. The impact of obesity on the outcomes of 1,153 critically injured blunt trauma patients. J Trauma 2005; 59: 1048–51; discussion 51.
7. Newell MA, Bard MR, Goettler CE, et al. Body mass index and outcomes in critically injured blunt trauma patients: weighing the impact. J Am Coll Surg 2007; 204: 1056–61; discussion 62–4.
8. Byrnes MC, McDaniel MD, Moore MB, et al. The effect of obesity on outcomes among injured patients. J Trauma 2005; 58: 232–7.
9. Ciesla DJ, Moore EE, Johnson JL, et al. Obesity increases risk of organ failure after severe trauma. J Am Coll Surg 2006; 203: 539–45.
10. Arbabi S, Wahl WL, Hemmila MR, et al. The cushion effect. J Trauma 2003; 54: 1090–3.
11. Ryb GE, Dischinger PC. Injury severity and outcome of overweight and obese patients after vehicular trauma: a crash injury research and engineering network (CIREN) study. J Trauma 2008; 64: 406–11.
12. Zarzaur BL, Marshall SW. Motor vehicle crashes obesity and seat belt use: a deadly combination? J Trauma 2008; 64: 412–19; discussion 9.
13. Duane TM, Dechert T, Aboutanos MB, et al. Obesity and outcomes after blunt trauma. J Trauma 2006; 61: 1218–21.
14. Coppack SW. Pro-inflammatory cytokines and adipose tissue. Proc Nutr Soc 2001; 60: 349–56.
15. Bastard JP, Maachi M, Lagathu C, et al. Recent advances in the relationship between obesity, inflammation, and insulin resistance. Eur Cytokine Netw 2006; 17: 4–12.
16. Brown CV, Rhee P, Neville AL, et al. Obesity and traumatic brain injury. J Trauma 2006; 61: 572–6.

17. Baker SP, O'Neill B, Haddon W Jr, et al. The injury severity score: a method for describing patients with multiple injuries and evaluating emergency care. J Trauma 1974; 14: 187–96.
18. Boulanger BR, Milzman D, Mitchell K, et al. Body habitus as a predictor of injury pattern after blunt trauma. J Trauma 1992; 33: 228–32.
19. Choban PS, Weireter LJ Jr, Maynes C. Obesity and increased mortality in blunt trauma. J Trauma 1991; 31: 1253–7.
20. Moran SG, McGwin G Jr, Metzger JS, et al. Injury rates among restrained drivers in motor vehicle collisions: the role of body habitus. J Trauma 2002; 52: 1116–20.
21. Traffic Safety Facts: Occupant Protection. Washington, DC: National Center for Statistics and Analysis, National Highway Traffic Safety Administration, 2007.
22. Cooper WE, Salzberg P. Safety restraint usage in fatal motor vehicle crashes. Accid Anal Prev 1993; 25: 67–75.
23. Hunt DK, Lowenstein SR, Badgett RG, et al. Safety belt nonuse by internal medicine patients: a missed opportunity in clinical preventive medicine. Am J Med 1995; 98: 343–8.
24. Campbell BJ, Stewart JR, Reinfurt DW. Change in injuries associated with safety belt laws. Accid Anal Prev 1991; 23: 87–93.
25. Brunette DD. Resuscitation of the morbidly obese patient. Am J Emerg Med 2004; 22: 40–7.
26. Mock CN, Grossman DC, Kaufman RP, et al. The relationship between body weight and risk of death and serious injury in motor vehicle crashes. Accid Anal Prev 2002; 34: 221–8.
27. Sifri ZC, Kim H, Lavery R, et al. The impact of obesity on the outcome of emergency intubation in trauma patients. J Trauma 2008; 65: 396–400.
28. Reiff DA, Hipp G, McGwin G Jr, et al. Body mass index affects the need for and the duration of mechanical ventilation after thoracic trauma. J Trauma 2007; 62: 1432–5.

Index

Printed in the United States
by Baker & Taylor Publisher Services